Effective Leadership & Management in Nursing

SIXTH EDITION

Effective Leadership & Management in Nursing

SIXTH EDITION

Eleanor J. Sullivan, PhD, RN, FAAN
School of Nursing
University of Kansas
Kansas City, KS

Phillip J. Decker, PhD
School of Business and Public Administration
University of Houston—Clear Lake
Houston, TX

PEARSON

Prentice
Hall

Upper Saddle River, New Jersey 07458

Library of Congress Cataloging-in-Publication Data

Sullivan, Eleanor J. (date)
    Effective leadership & management in nursing / Eleanor J. Sullivan, Phillip J. Decker.—6th ed.
      p .; cm.
    Includes bibliographical references and index.
    ISBN 0-13-178094-8 (pbk.)
    1. Nursing services—Administration. 2. Leadership. I. Decker, Phillip J. II. Title.
    [DNLM: 1. Nurse Administrators. 2. Leadership. 3. Nursing Care—organization & administration.
      WY 105 S949ea 2004]
  RT89.S85 2004
  362.17′3′068—dc22

                                                      2004041537

Notice: Care has been taken to confirm the accuracy of information presented in this book. The authors, editors, and the publisher, however, cannot accept any responsibility for errors or omissions or for consequences from application of the information in this book and make no warranty, express or implied, with respect to its contents.

    The authors and publisher have exerted every effort to ensure that drug selections and dosages set forth in this text are in accord with current recommendations and practice at time of publication. However, in view of ongoing research, changes in government regulations, and the constant flow of information relating to drug therapy and drug reactions, the reader is urged to check the package inserts of all drugs for any change in indications of dosage and for added warnings and precautions. This is particularly important when the recommended agent is a new and/or infrequently employed drug.

Publisher: Julie Levin Alexander
Publisher's Assistant: Regina Bruno
Editor-in-Chief: Maura Connor
Editorial Assistant: Malgorzata Jaros-White
Director of Manufacturing and Production:
  Bruce Johnson
Managing Production Editor: Patrick Walsh
Production Liaison: Cathy O'Connell
Production Editor: Trish Finley,
  Carlisle Communications
Manufacturing Manager: Ilene Sanford
Manufacturing Buyer: Pat Brown
Design Director: Cheryl Asherman

Cover Designer: Wanda España
Senior Design Coordinator: Maria Guglielmo Walsh
Director of Marketing: Karen Allman
Executive Marketing Manager: Nicole Benson
Channel Marketing Manager: Rachele Strober
Marketing Coordinator: Janet Ryerson
Assistant Editor: Sladjana Repic
Media Editor: John Jordan
Media Production Manager: Amy Peltier
Media Project Manager: Stephen Hartner
Composition: Carlisle Communications
Printer/Binder: Courier/Westford
Cover Printer: Phoenix Color

Pearson Prentice Hall™ is a trademark of Pearson Education, Inc.
Pearson® is a registered trademark of Pearson plc
Prentice Hall® is a registered trademark of Pearson Education, Inc.

Pearson Education Ltd.
Pearson Education Singapore, Pte. Ltd.
Pearson Education Canada, Ltd.
Pearson Education—Japan

Pearson Education Australia PTY, Limited
Pearson Education North Asia Ltd.
Pearson Educación de Mexico, S.A. de C.V.
Pearson Education Malaysia, Pte. Ltd.
Pearson Education, Upper Saddle River, New Jersey

10 9 8 7 6 5 4 3 2 1
ISBN: 0-13-178094-8

This book is dedicated to my family for their continuing love and support.

Eleanor J. Sullivan

Contents

PART 2

KEY SKILLS IN NURSING MANAGEMENT   99

Preface

Leading and managing are essential skills for all nurses in today's rapidly changing health care arena. New graduates find themselves managing unlicensed assistive personnel, and experienced nurses are managing groups of health care providers from a variety of disciplines and educational levels. Declining revenues and increasing costs mandate that every organization use its resources efficiently. Thus, nurses are challenged to manage effectively with fewer resources. Never has the information presented in this textbook been needed more. *Effective Leadership & Management in Nursing*, Sixth Edition, can help both student nurses and those with practice experience acquire the skills needed to ensure success in today's dynamic health care environment.

FEATURES OF THE SIXTH EDITION

Effective Leadership & Management in Nursing has made a significant and lasting contribution to the education of nurses and nurse managers in its five previous editions. Used worldwide, this award-winning textbook is now offered in an updated and revised edition to reflect changes in the current health care system and in response to suggestions from the book's users. The Sixth Edition builds upon the work of previous contributors to provide the most up-to-date and comprehensive learning package for today's busy students and professionals.

Student-Friendly Learning Tools

Designed with the adult learner in mind, the book focuses on the application of the content presented with specific guidelines for implementing the skills included. To further illustrate and emphasize key points, each chapter in this edition includes these features:

- Chapter outline and preview
- New *MediaLink* boxes in each chapter introduce readers to resources and activities on the Companion Website at www.prenhall.com/sullivan-decker. *MediaLink* tabs in the chapter margins encourage students to use the website activities.

- Key terms defined on the pages where they first appear
- *What You Know Now* lists at end of each chapter
- A list of "tools," or key behaviors, for using the skills presented in the chapter
- *Case Studies* with *Manager's Checklist* to demonstrate application of content
- *Questions to Challenge You* to help students relate concepts to their experience
- Up-to-date references

RESOURCES FOR LEARNING AND TEACHING

Companion Website

Students and instructors can use the updated and greatly enhanced Companion Website at www.prenhall.com/sullivan-decker to apply textbook concepts to real practice scenarios experienced in a variety of healthcare settings. This *free* on-line Study Guide is designed to help students apply the concepts presented in the book. Each chapter-specific module features Objectives, NCLEX Review with rationales, Chapter Outlines for lecture notes, Critical Thinking Activities, Current Event Activities, MediaLinks, Glossary, and more. Additionally, each chapter in the Companion Website features *Nursing Leadership & Management in Action* activities, such as "Managing Staff Resources," "Identifying Variance," and "Personal Motivation." These activities serve as an excellent tool designed to enhance the understanding of leadership and management principles and to apply the theoretical concepts of leadership and management in a safe environment.

Syllabus Manager

Faculty adopting this textbook have *free* access to the online **Syllabus Manager** feature of the Companion Website, www.prenhall.com/sullivan-decker. Syllabus Manager offers a host of features that facilitates the students' use of the Companion Website and allows faculty to post syllabi and course information online for their students. For more information or a demonstration of Syllabus Manager, please contact your Prentice Hall Sales Representative.

Online Course Management

Online companions are available for schools using course management systems. The online course management solutions feature all instructor and student online course materials for this book, such as interactive assessment modules, electronic test bank, PowerPoint slides, online grade books, communication between students and instructors, and much more. For more information about adopting an online course management system to accompany *Effective Leadership & Management in Nursing*, Sixth Edition, please contact your Prentice Hall Sales Representative or go to the appropriate website below:

 http://cms.prenhall.com/webct/index.html

 http://cms.prenhall.com/blackboard/index.html

 www.prenhall.com/onekey

Instructor's Resource CD-ROM

To assist instructors in using this book, the Instructor's Resource CD-ROM provides an electronic test bank, PowerPoint slides, and a complete Instructor's Resource Manual in Word with chapter outlines, discussion questions, and guidelines for using the Companion Website and online course management (i.e., Blackboard, WebCt, or OneKey) in the course. The Instructor's Resource Manual is also available through secure download only to instructors at www.prenhall.com/nursing. Please contact your Prentice Hall Sales Representative for more information.

HALLMARK FEATURE: MULTIDISCIPLINARY AUTHORS

This book has been a success for many reasons. It combines practicality with conceptual understanding; is responsive to the needs of faculty, nurse managers, and students; and taps the expertise of contributors from a variety of disciplines, especially management professionals whose work has been adapted by nurses for current nursing practice. The expertise of management professors in schools of business and practicing nurse managers is seldom incorporated into nursing textbooks. This unique approach provides students with invaluable knowledge and skills and sets the book apart from others.

ORGANIZATION

The text is organized into three sections that address the essential information and key skills that nurses must learn to succeed in today's volatile health care environment.

Part 1. Understanding Nursing Management and Organizations. Part 1 introduces the concepts of organizations and organizational theory and design with an emphasis on health care system mergers, integrated care networks, and managed care. Leadership is presented within a theoretical framework, and management functions are explained. Also included in Part 1 is information about legal challenges, ethical dilemmas, power, and politics, all necessary for nurses to succeed and prosper.

Part 2. Key Skills in Nursing Management. Essential skills for today's managers comprise Part 2. These include thinking critically, making decisions, solving problems, communicating with a variety of individuals and groups, resolving conflicts, delegating, working in teams, creating and managing resources, promoting quality management, using health care technology, managing time and stress, and effecting change.

Part 3. Human Resource Management. Human resources are the health care system's most valuable asset, so nurses must be adept at handling staffing and scheduling, recruiting and selecting staff, motivating and developing staff, evaluating staff performance, coaching, disciplining and terminating staff, reducing turnover and retaining staff, managing absenteeism and handling the inevitable personnel problems. In addition, collective bargaining—a key issue today in many organizations—is included in Part 3.

Acknowledgments

The success of previous editions of this book has been due to the expertise of many contributors. Nursing administrators, management professors, and faculty in schools of nursing all made significant contributions to earlier editions. I am enormously grateful to them for sharing their knowledge and experience to help nurses learn leadership and management skills. Without them, this book would not exist.

At Prentice Hall Health, Editor-in-Chief Maura Connor and former nursing editor Nancy Anselment guided this revision throughout. Editorial Assistant Gosia Jaros-White was especially attentive to details in this revision. The production staff, including Cathy O'Connell and Patrick Walsh, helped bring this book to publication.

Because health care continues to change, reviewers who are using the book in their management practice and in their classes provided invaluable comments and suggestions (see list on page xx). Susan Fry, a leading nurse executive, offered valuable insights on what really matters in today's fast-paced health care environment. Tona Leiker provided library and research assistance.

I am especially grateful to experienced nurse manager Elaine Level, who created case scenarios to exemplify the real-life experience of nurses in management roles. In addition, she assisted throughout with ideas and suggestions.

To everyone who has contributed to this fine book over the years, I thank you.

Eleanor J. Sullivan, PhD, RN, FAAN
www.EleanorSullivan.com

About the Author

Eleanor J. Sullivan, PhD, RN, FAAN, is the former dean of the University of Kansas School of Nursing and past president of Sigma Theta Tau International. She has served on the board of directors of the American Association of Colleges of Nursing and on the advisory council of the National Institute on Alcohol Abuse and Alcoholism at the National Institutes of Health, among other professional positions.

Dr. Sullivan is known for her publications in nursing, including this award-winning textbook, *Effective Leadership & Management in Nursing*, and most recently, *Becoming Influential: A Guide for Nurses* from Prentice Hall. Other publications include *Creating Nursing's Future: Issues, Opportunities and Challenges* and *Nursing Care for Clients with Substance Abuse*. From 1997 to 2002, she served as editor of the *Journal of Professional Nursing*, the official journal of the American Association of Colleges of Nursing.

Today Dr. Sullivan is a professional speaker and mystery author. Her first mystery, *Twice Dead*, features nurse sleuth Monika Everhardt. By showing nursing realistically, she hopes that readers will understand the complexity of nursing care and the skills and knowledge involved in being a nurse. *Deadly Diversion*, the second book in the series, was recently released by Hilliard & Harris.

Learn more at www.EleanorSullivan.com

MEDIA SUPPLEMENTS CONTRIBUTORS

Maureen Cluskey, DNSc, RN
Associate Chairperson
Bradley University
Department of Nursing
Peoria, Illinois
Instructor's Resource CD-ROM

Peggy Craik, MBA, MS, RN
Associate Professor
University of Mary-Hardin Baylor
Belton, Texas
Instructor's Resource CD-ROM

Cynthia A. Hornberger, PhD, RN, MBA
Associate Professor and Dean
Washburn University
School of Nursing
Topeka, Kansas
Instructor's Resource CD-ROM

Elaine Blake, PhD, RN, MSN
Nursing Professor
Belmont University
School of Nursing
Nashville, Tennessee
Companion Website

Rebecca Gesler, RN, MSN
Lecturer
Bellarmine University
Louisville, Kentucky
Companion Website

Mary A. Helms, PhD, RN, MSN
Nursing Professor
Tennessee State University
Department of Nursing
Nashville, Tennessee
Companion Website

Virginia Rogers, RN, MSN, ANP/CNP, HNC
Associate Professor
Oakton Community College
Department of Nursing
Des Plaines, Illinois
Companion Website

Susan Parnell Scholtz, RN, DNSc
Associate Professor of Nursing
St Luke's School of Nursing at Moravian College
Bethlehem, Pennsylvania
Instructor's Resource CD-ROM

REVIEWERS

Rebecca Gesler, RN, MSN
Lecturer
Bellarmine University
Louisville, Kentucky

Gladys L. Husted, RN, PhD
Distinguished Professor
Duquesne University School
of Nursing
Pittsburgh, Pennsylvania

Bonnie Kirkpatrick, RN, MS, CNS
Clinical Instructor
Ohio State University College
of Nursing
Columbus, Ohio

Shirley McIntosh, RN, C, MSN, LNC
Instructor
Kent State University College
of Nursing
Kent, Ohio

Donna M. Nickitas, PhD, RN, CNAA
Associate Professor
Hunter College School of Nursing
New York, New York

PART 1

Understanding Nursing Management and Organizations

Introduction to Nursing Management

Looking Ahead

Rapid changes in today's health care industry are continuing to reshape the nurse's role. The emergence of integrated health care systems and the shift from a service orientation to a business orientation directly affect where and how nursing care is delivered, as well as those who deliver the care. If we as nurses are to succeed in this new health care environment, we must learn how to manage ourselves and others effectively within the context of these changes and decreasing resources. This opening chapter introduces those challenges and the management education essential to all nurses.

Objectives

In this chapter, you will learn

- How efforts to contain costs have changed today's health care industry.
- How changes in the health care system affect nursing.
- What the future of health care might be.
- Why cultural diversity is essential to health care managers.
- How patient care and communications technology are changing the way care is delivered.
- What role nurse managers play in the success of health care organizations.

MediaLink 🌐 **www.prenhall.com/ sullivan-decker**

Additional resources for this chapter can be found on the Companion Website at www.prenhall.com/ sullivan-decker. Click on "Chapter 1" to select the activities for this chapter.

- NCLEX Review
- Critical Thinking Activities
- Current Events

- MediaLinks
- *Nursing Leadership & Management in Action*: Planning for Your Future: Transition to Professional Practice; Health Care Change: Impact on Nurses

Today, all nurses are managers. Whether you work on a medical floor in an acute care hospital, in a critical care unit, in an ambulatory care clinic, or in home care, you must deal with staff, including other nurses and unlicensed assistive personnel, who work with you and for you, and you must use resources wisely. To manage well, you must understand the health care system and the organizations where you work. You need to recognize what external forces affect your work and how to influence those forces. You need to know what motivates people and how you can help create an environment that inspires and sustains the individuals who work in it. You must be able to collaborate with others, both as a leader and as a team member, in order to become confident in your ability to be a leader and a manager.

This book is designed to provide new graduates or novice managers with the information they need to become effective managers and leaders in health care. More than ever before, today's rapidly changing health care environment demands highly refined management skills and superb leadership.

The Changing Health Care System

Today's health care system is continuing to undergo significant changes. Costly lifesaving medicines, tele-health, and innovations in imaging technologies, noninvasive treatments, and surgical procedures have combined to produce the most sophisticated and effective health care ever—and the most expensive. Skyrocketing costs and inaccessibility to health care are ongoing concerns for employers, health care providers, state legislatures, the U. S. Congress, and the public at large.

The Cost of Health Care

Health care spending continues to rise. Health care consumed 14.8 percent of the gross domestic product (the measure of output of goods and services) in the United States in 2002 (Congressional Budget Office [CBO], 2003). New medical technology, expanding insurance coverage, increased spending for prescription drugs, and the aging of the population account for the greatest increases in spending in recent years.

KEY TERMS

Diagnosis-related group   A system of prospective payment used by Medicare that pays a provider a set amount for a specific condition.

Although the United States spends more money on health care than any other country, millions of Americans have no access to basic health care. For some, this is a temporary situation, such as changing jobs, but many others continue to go without health care because they work only part-time without benefits or because they have a preexisting health condition that makes them ineligible for coverage. When the uninsured receive care, it is provided at great expense in emergency rooms, often after the condition has progressed and requires more complex and long-term care. Some of the costs of this unnecessarily expensive care are borne by the health care organization, and some costs are passed on to other payers, such as Medicare and private insurance companies, who pass on their costs to their constituents: taxpayers and customers.

Medicare is the government's largest health care financing program, paying out more than $277 million in 2003 to 40 million elderly and disabled people (CBO, 2003). The federal government has made several attempts to contain Medicare costs. In the mid-1980s, a system of prospective, rather than retrospective, payment for health care was introduced for all Medicare recipients. Other third-party payers soon followed suit. This system, based on **diagnosis-related groups** (DRGs), pays a provider (individual or organization) a set amount for a specific condition, stipulated ahead of time, instead of paying the bill after care is rendered. Health care providers have responded to these restrictions by instituting cost-cutting measures, by drastically reducing hospital stays, and by limiting time spent with patients in all settings, including hospitals, offices, and clinics. Despite these changes, health care costs have continued to rise.

In 1997 the Balanced Budget Act was passed by Congress in an attempt to control Medicare expenditures by reducing payments to providers. Deemed too radical, 1999 Balanced Budget Reform Act and the Budget Improvement and Protection Act in 2000 restored some of these cuts. Providing care to the uninsured, however, remains an unresolved problem.

Cost containment has had an especially deleterious effect on rural communities. A smaller population, a larger proportion of whom are elderly, makes it difficult to maintain cost efficiency in isolated rural areas.

MEDIALINK   Health Care Change

The rapid growth in nurse practitioner education, especially programs targeted to rural areas, is one attempt to meet rural residents' needs for primary care. Another is telehealth, discussed later in the chapter.

Integrated Systems of Care

Besides government action, marketplace changes radically altered the way health care organizations operate. Competition forced hospitals, physicians, and home care agencies into mergers, networks, and integrated systems of care. **Integrated health care networks** emerged as organizations have struggled to find ways to survive in today's cost-conscious environment, and the major driver for forming networks was savings on payroll, including nurses' salaries (McConnell, 2000). Integrated systems encompass a variety of model organizational structures, but certain characteristics are common. Network systems

- Deliver a whole continuum of care;
- Provide geographic coverage for the buyers of health care services; and
- Accept the risk inherent in taking a fixed payment in return for providing health care for all persons in the selected group, such as all employees of one company.

To provide such services, networks of providers have emerged to encompass hospitals and physician practices. Most importantly, the focal point for care is primary care rather than the hospital. The goal is to keep patients healthy by treating them in the setting that incurs the lowest cost and thereby reducing expensive hospital treatments. The former goal—to keep hospital beds filled—has been replaced with a new goal: to keep patients out of them!

A variety of other arrangements have emerged, varying from loose affiliations between hospitals to complete mergers of hospitals, clinics, and physician practices. These arrangements continue to move and shift as alliances fail and new affiliations are established but, regardless, providing care through systems and networks is expected to continue throughout the 21st century.

Health care is now a competitive, market-based enterprise. This change has transformed health care from an industry with a service orientation to one with a business orientation. Scrutinizing costs is a way of life in health care today. Every expenditure, including supplies, equipment, and—most important—staff time, is closely examined.

KEY TERMS

Integrated health care networks   Organizational health care structures that deliver a continuum of care, provide coverage for a group of individuals, and accept fixed payments for that group.

Quality management   A preventive approach designed to address problems efficiently and quickly.

Benchmarking   A method of comparing performance using identified quality indicators across institutions or disciplines.

Quality in Health Care

Medical Errors

When the Institute of Medicine (IOM, 1999) reported that 98,000 deaths occurred each year from preventable medical mistakes in hospitals, health care organizations and the public alike were astounded. More recently, medical injuries have been found to increase length of stay and patients' costs in addition to an increased risk of mortality (Zhan & Miller, 2003). Health care organizations have been scrambling to design and develop systems to prevent such errors. Computerized systems for pharmacy that alert staff to possible drug interactions or adverse reactions based on the patient's condition or other medications is an example.

Consumers, employers, and third-party payers are also demanding that organizations demonstrate accountability in preventing errors. The Leapfrog Group is a coalition of public and private employers organized to bring attention to consumers about quality indicators in health care and mobilize employers to reward health care organizations that demonstrate quality outcome measures (Leapfrog Group, 2003). The Leapfrog Group is focusing on computer physician order entry systems, evidence-based hospital referrals, and ICU physician staffing, the three practices that have demonstrated the most significant impact on preventing medical errors.

Quality Management

Quality management is a preventive approach designed to address problems before they become crises. The quality movement began in post–World War II Japan, when Japanese industries adopted a system that W. Edwards Deming designed to improve the quality of manufactured products. Its philosophy is that the consumers' needs should be the focus and that employees should be empowered to evaluate and improve quality. Besides businesses in the United States and elsewhere, the health care industry also has adopted total quality management or variations on it.

Built into the system is a mechanism for continuous improvement of products and services through constant evaluation of how well the consumers' needs are met and devising plans to perfect the process. Patient satisfaction surveys exemplify how health care organizations evaluate their customers' needs.

Benchmarking

More recently performance initiatives by the government and professional organizations have been instituted. Known as **benchmarking**, outcome indicators are identified that can be used to compare performance across disciplines or organizations. In contrast to quality management that compares internal measures across comparable units, benchmarking compares an organization's data with similar organizations (Tran, 2003). Once the results are known, health care organizations can address areas of weakness and enhance areas of strength.

Nursing Care and Outcomes

Recently research has confirmed what nurses intuitively knew: that fewer nurses translates into poorer care for patients. Two studies have shown that the number of nurses available to provide care has a direct effect on patient care outcomes. In the first study, researchers found that nurse staffing levels had a direct, negative effect on outcomes of surgical patients in the United States (Kovner & Gergen, 1998). Later, Aiken and colleagues discovered that patient mortality was directly related to hospital nurse staffing (Aiken, Clarke, Sloane, Sochalski, & Silber, 2002).

What Is the Future of Health Care?

Nursing Shortage

Today's nursing shortage is predicted to worsen in the coming years, climbing as high as 20 percent fewer nurses than those needed by the year 2020

(Buerhaus, Staiger, & Auerback, 2000). Contributing factors include a shortage of nursing faculty that limits enrollment in schools of nursing (American Association of Colleges of Nursing [AACN], 2003), the rising average age of the current nursing workforce (Buerhaus, Staiger, & Auerback, 2000), and the aging of the population.

Efforts are being made to address the shortage. The Nurse Reinvestment Act passed by Congress in 2002 includes scholarships to students and future faculty members, among other initiatives. The American Hospital Association (2002) has addressed workforce shortages in a report titled "In Our Hands: How Hospital Leaders Can Build a Thriving Workforce." Its recommendations include developing new work designs, improving workplace partnerships, and aggressively recruiting diverse populations to health care.

Two national media campaigns are addressing the public image of nursing. In 2002 Johnson & Johnson launched a television ad campaign called "Be a Nurse," and a coalition of health care organizations are addressing recruitment of middle and high school students with print ads and public service announcements, called "Nurses for a Healthier Tomorrow." Regardless, the nursing shortage will not abate anytime soon, and it threatens the quality of health care as well as the quality of life for nurses.

Cultural Diversity

According to the U.S. Census Bureau, the current population of the United States is 75.0 percent Caucasian, 12.5 percent Hispanic/Latino, 12.3 percent African American, 3.6 percent Asian, and less than 1.0 percent Native American, Eskimo, or Native Hawaiian. In addition, more than 11 percent are foreign-born residents, with Latin America and Asia accounting for 78 percent of this population (U.S. Census Bureau, 2000).

One obvious barrier to health care delivery to people of foreign-born cultures is language. The U.S. Census Bureau (2000) estimates that for 47 million people, English is a second language. To meet the needs of these individuals, health care providers need to be fluent in the language of their patients or be able to identify interpreters who can translate for them.

Another barrier is socioeconomic status, a concern for both native- and foreign-born minorities. If you can pay for health care, access is not an issue; but for those who can't, health care may not be accessible.

MEDIALINK Benchmarking

MEDIALINK Nursing Shortage Fact Sheet

The challenge for health care policymakers and the public is to find ways to provide universal access regardless of race, ethnic origin, or socioeconomic status.

In addition, prejudice toward a particular group of people hinders the health care they receive. Prejudice, a strongly held opinion about a group of people that often leads to discrimination and differential treatment, is not limited to people from other countries or minorities. Some maintain negative attitudes toward the elderly, others toward women, and still others toward lesbians and gay men. Religious intolerance is an additional concern.

Diversity also is uneven, varying in different geographical areas. For example, in California only 48 percent of the population is Caucasian, whereas in Maine 97 percent are Caucasian (Orndoff, 2003). Some areas have attracted large numbers of immigrants from specific war-torn countries. Bosnians, for example, have immigrated in large numbers to St. Louis (Moore, 2003).

The influx of immigrants means that health care must assume a transcultural focus. Those who decide health care policies and those who offer clinical services must consider the values, beliefs, and lifestyles of a number of diverse cultures. This is no small challenge. Becoming aware of the differences and similarities among cultures, being sensitive to different perspectives, and providing care within the cultural belief system of the patient requires commitment, respect, and persistence. Leininger (2001) suggests that culturally congruent care is provided by (a) accepting and complying with an individual's beliefs; (b) planning, negotiating, and accommodating culturally specific practices; and (c) restructuring care based on knowledge about the culture.

The cultural diversity seen in the general population is also reflected in nursing. The Health Resources and Services Administration (HRSA, 2000) reports that about 12 percent of nurses identify themselves as from one or more racial minority groups, up from 7 percent in 1980. African American and Hispanic backgrounds are the most frequently reported minorities.

The gender mix of people who are nurses differs from other professions. Only about 5 percent of nurses are men although the number has grown from approximately 2 percent in 1980 (HRSA, 2000).

Nurse managers must develop sensitivity to cultural differences among their staff as well as their patients and be responsive to these differences within the context of the work environment.

KEY TERMS

Telehealth   Using telecommunications technology to provide medical and nursing services from afar.

Telehealth

Called by various names—telehealth, telemedicine, telenursing—**telehealth** uses sophisticated patient care technology and evolving communications connections to provide medical and nursing services from distant geographic locations. Both home and office sites are used. Cost, convenience, and conservation of resources are driving factors in the development and expansion of telehealth technologies.

Providers can view X-ray films, observe and interview patients, take vital signs, study lab results, suggest procedures and treatments, and even do surgery, all from a distance far from their patients. Technologies also include devices that alert patients to take medications, in-home monitoring medical devices, telephone systems that track patients' vital signs at specified times, and even televideo systems to manage patients' care in their homes (Salvatore, 2002). Both the technology to provide care and that which connects distant sites are predicted to grow exponentially in the coming decades, allowing greater flexibility in accessing services, more options for consultation, and a reduction in costs.

More Change

Health care exists because society deems it worthy of support. Beliefs about what support and to whom it should be given depend on societal decisions in the form of public and private policies. Today health care is in flux. Government agencies and private citizens alike share concern about the future ability to pay for care. Thus, cost will continue to drive policy decisions.

Other challenges continue. An aging population and the increasing incidence of life-threatening diseases, such as HIV/AIDS and hepatitis, intensify the demand for care. Informed consumers insist on participating in decisions regarding their care. Accountability for performance and cost requires providers to justify their actions and expenses. Adding to the demands of an already overburdened system is the need to prepare for bioterrorism, violence, and disasters.

Additionally, rapidly advancing technology in genomics, nanotechnology, and virtual care, among others, promise emerging treatments, and citizens will most certainly demand access to them. All these innovations require financing, adding to an already overburdened system.

Health care will continue to move beyond hospital walls into less-expensive settings. Health care employers, as other businesses, are finding innovative ways to staff. Outsourcing is one of those trends. Using contract employees from temporary staffing agencies began as a stopgap measure for hospitals. Such outsourcing for services has become a major method of staffing for many industries. Services include public relations, office support, informational technology staffing, Web hosting, housekeeping, and maintenance, among others. Businesses, including health care organizations, avoid the expense of salaries and benefits for specialty staff especially if the work demands are not steady or consistent.

Information technology will become increasingly integrated into systems of care (Kerfoot & Simpson, 2002). Evidence-based practice, integrated clinical and financial systems, point-of-care technology, and distance interventions will define care in the future. Preparing nurses to function successfully in this environment will challenge nursing educational systems to provide compatible learning environments (Connors, Weaver, Warren, & Miller, 2002).

The system of health care in the United States continues to shift, change, and adjust to market forces, political pressures, and consumer demands. The radical changes in health care systems are still evolving. No one knows yet exactly how the system of the future will look. What seems certain is that the system will continue to evolve and be decidedly different from today. The way that nursing services are delivered will also continue to change in response to the delivery system, but regardless of how the health care system evolves, nurses and nurse managers are key to its success.

Nursing's Role in Today's Health Care System

Cost containment has significantly affected the manner in which care is being delivered. As a result of restructuring health care delivery systems into integrated networks, the numbers of registered nurses in acute care have diminished to 59 percent in 2000, down from 66 percent in 1980 (HRSA, 2000). The largest gains in areas of employment for nurses are in public and community health and ambulatory care.

Because there are fewer registered nurses (RNs) in relation to assistive personnel, all nurses today are managers. They manage the care of a defined group of patients, doing some of the care themselves, directing others to provide care, and collaborating with still others. Nurses participate in teams of care providers and lead teams of professionals and nonprofessionals. Nurses therefore need new skills, especially management skills. Nurses must know how to delegate, supervise, evaluate, motivate, and communicate with practitioners of other disciplines, other nurses, and unlicensed personnel. They must be skilled in negotiation, conflict resolution, and collaboration, and they must be able to participate in, as well as lead, teams.

Preparation for management must be an integral part of nursing education, and specific training in management skills is needed in nursing school as well as in the work setting. Most important, however, is that nurses be able to transfer their newly acquired skills to the job itself. Thus, nurse managers must be experienced in management themselves and be able to assist their staff in developing adequate management skills. Management training for nurses at all levels is essential for any organization to be efficient and effective in today's cost-conscious and competitive environment.

Challenges for Nurse Managers

The challenge for nurse managers and administrators is how to manage in a constantly changing system. Working with teams of administrators and providers to deliver quality health care in the most cost-effective manner offers opportunity as well. Nurses' unique skills in communication, negotiation, and collaboration position them well for the system of today and for the future.

The one constant of today's health care system is that tomorrow it will change. Tim Porter-O'Grady (2003) challenges nursing leaders to help staff "close the door" on allegiance to past practices and turn toward emerging practice opportunities. Leaders themselves must learn new skills as well as convey enthusiasm and commitment for change. Everyone in health care must learn to live with ambiguity and be flexible enough to adapt to the changes it brings.

Nurse managers today are challenged to manage with decreasing resources, to help design new systems of care, to supervise teams of professionals and nonprofessionals from a variety of cultures, and, finally, to teach personnel how to function well in the new system. This is no small task. It requires that nurses and

MEDIALINK   U.S. Department of Labor Bureau of Labor Statistics

their managers be committed, involved, enthusiastic, flexible, and innovative; above all else, it requires that they have good mental and physical health. Because the nurse manager of today is responsible for others' work, the nurse manager must also be a coach, a teacher, and a facilitator. The manager works through others to meet the goals of individuals, of the unit, and of the organization. Most of all, the manager must be a leader who can motivate and inspire.

Nurse managers must address the interests of both administrators and employees. Both want the same result—quality care. Administrators, however, must focus on cost and efficiency in order for the organization to compete and survive. Employees want to be supported in their work with adequate staffing, supplies, equipment, and, most of all, time. Therein lies the conflict. Between the two is the nurse manager, who must balance the needs of both. Being a nurse manager today is the most challenging opportunity in health care. This book is designed to prepare you to meet these challenges.

What You Know Now

- Health care is radically changing today and is expected to continue to change in the foreseeable future.
- Health care structures have become integrated networks of care designed to reduce costs and maximize the organization's competitive advantage.
- To survive in a competitive environment, health care has adopted a market-based approach that includes a focus on customers, attention to cost, and quality improvement.
- The tension between providing adequate nursing care and paying for that care will continue.
- Patient care technologies and distance connections are expected to expand in the coming decade.
- Cultural diversity will continue to demand nurses' attention and to shape nursing's workforce.
- The nurse manager is an active participant and plays a key role in the success of health care organizations.

Questions to Challenge You

1. What would you suggest that would reduce the cost of health care without compromising patients' health and safety? Name three changes. Consider how you could help make these changes.

2. Because health care today is being provided by networks, how could nurses gain power to enhance their ability to provide care in these systems? (See Chapter 6 for help.)

3. What mechanisms could you suggest to improve and ensure the quality of care? (Don't just suggest adding nursing staff!)

4. What are some ways that nurses could take advantage of emerging technologies in health care and information systems? Think big.

5. What steps do you plan to take to transfer the knowledge and skills you learn in this book into your work setting?

Explore 🌐 MediaLink

NCLEX review questions, essay activities, group activities, and other interactive resources for this chapter can be found on the Web site at http://www.prenhall.com/sullivan-decker. Click on "Chapter 1" to select activities for this chapter.

References

Aiken, L. H., Clarke, S. P., Sloane, D. M., Sochalski, J., & Silber, J. H. (2002). Hospital nurse staffing and patient mortality, nurse burnout, and job dissatisfaction. *Journal of the American Medical Association, 288*(16), 1987–1993.

American Association of Colleges of Nursing. (2003). *Nursing shortage fact sheet.* Retrieved July 2003 from www.aacn.nche.edu

American Hospital Association. (2002). *In our hands: How hospital leaders can build a thriving workforce.* Chicago, IL: Author.

Buerhaus, P. I., Staiger, D. O., & Auerback, D. I. (2000). Implications of an aging registered nurse workforce. *Journal of the American Medical Association, 283*(22), 2948–2954.

Congressional Budget Office. (March 20, 2003). Testimony to the Senate Special Committee on Aging.

Connors, H. R., Weaver, C., Warren, J., & Miller, K. L. (2002). An academic-business partnership for advancing clinical informatics. *Nursing Education Perspectives, 23*(5), 228–233.

Health Resources & Services Administration [HRSA]. (2000). *National sample survey of registered nurses 2000.* Retrieved September 30, 2003, from http://bhpr.hrsa.gov

Institute of Medicine. (1999). *To err is human: Building a safer health system.* Washington, DC: National Academy Press.

Kerfoot, K., & Simpson, R. (2002). Knowledge-driven care: Powerful medicine. *Reflections on Nursing Leadership, 28*(3), 22–24, 44.

Kovner, C., & Gergen, P. J. (1998). Nurse staffing levels and adverse events following surgery in U.S. hospitals. *Image: Journal of Nursing Scholarship, 30*(4), 315–321.

Leapfrog Group. (2003). *The Leapfrog Group for patient safety: Rewarding higher standards.* Retrieved July 2003 from http://www.leapfroggroup.org

Leininger, M. M. (2001). *Culture care diversity and universality: A theory of nursing.* Sudbury, MA: Jones & Bartlett.

McConnell, C. R. (2000). The manager and the merger: Adaptation and survival in the blended organization. *Health Care Manager, 19*(1), 1–11.

Moore, D. (2003, July 13). Dreaming big. *St. Louis Post-Dispatch*, p. C1.

Orndoff, K. (2003). Assessing American diversity. *The Futurist, 37*(1), 22–26.

Porter-O'Grady, T. (2003). A different age for leadership, Part 2: New rules, new roles. *Journal of Nursing Administration, 33*(3), 173–178.

Salvatore, T. (2002). A telehealthcare primer for managers. *Home Healthcare Nurse, 20*(2), 127–130.

Tran, M. N. (2003). Take benchmarking to the next level. *Nursing Management, 34*(6), 19–23.

U.S. Census Bureau. (2000). *2000 census of population.* Washington, DC: Government Printing Office. Retrieved September 30, 2003, from http://www.census.gov

Zhan, C., & Miller, M. R. (2003). Excess length of stay, charges, and mortality attributable to medical injuries during hospitalization. *Journal of the American Medical Association, 290*(14), 1868–1874.

CHAPTER 2

How Organizations Are Designed

Organizational Theories

Classical Theory
Neoclassical Theory
Systems Theory
Contingency Theory
Chaos Theory

Health Care Organizations

Types of Health Care
    Organizations
Interorganizational Relationships
Diversification

Traditional Organizational Structures

Functional Structure
Service-Line Structure
Hybrid Structure
Matrix Structure
Parallel Structure

Relationship-Oriented Structures

Shared Governance
Heterarchy Structure
Self-Organizing Structures

Redesigning, Restructuring, and Reengineering

Barriers to Job Redesign
Restructuring and Reengineering

Strategic Planning

Values
Vision
Mission
Philosophy
Goals

Organizational Environment and Culture

Magnet Hospital Designation
Generational Differences

Looking Ahead

Understanding the health care environment, a crucial element of management, begins with understanding organizational theory. These theories lay the foundation for the types of health care organizations in existence today. Hospitals, home care agencies, clinics, and other health care organizations are designed by integrating goals, size, technology, and environment, and a variety of structures are used in health care organizations. This chapter outlines broad-based theories and discusses specific challenges nurses face in designing and implementing organizational structures.

Objectives

In this chapter, you will learn

- How organizational theories evolved.
- What different types of health care organizations exist.
- How health care organizations are structured.
- How structures are changing.
- How strategic planning shapes the future.
- How organizational culture affects success.

MediaLink www.prenhall.com/
sullivan-decker

Additional resources for this chapter can be found on the Companion Website at www.prenhall.com/sullivan-decker. Click on "Chapter 2" to select the activities for this chapter.

- NCLEX Review
- Critical Thinking Activities
- Current Events
- MediaLinks
- *Nursing Leadership & Management in Action*: Recognizing the Impact of Organizational Culture; Defining Organizational Structures; Developing strategic plan

Within our society are numerous organizations— schools, churches, businesses, and so on. An **organization** is a collection of people working together under a defined structure to achieve predetermined outcomes using financial, human, and material resources. The justification for developing organizations is both rational and economic. Coordinated efforts capture more information and knowledge, purchase more technology, and produce more goods, services, opportunities, and securities than individual efforts. This chapter discusses organizational theory, structures, and functions.

Organizational Theories

The earliest recorded example of organizational thinking comes from the ancient Sumerian civilization, around 5000 B.C. The early Egyptians, Babylonians, Greeks, and Romans also gave thought to how groups were organized. Later, Machiavelli in the 1500s and Adam Smith in 1776 established the management prin-

ciples we know as specialization and division of labor (Cannon, 1925). Nevertheless, organizational theory remained largely unexplored until the Industrial Revolution. During the late 1800s and early 1900s, a number of approaches to the structure and management of organizations developed. These approaches, or schools of thought, are traditionally labeled classical theory, neoclassical theory, systems theory, contingency theory, and chaos theory.

Classical Theory

The classical approach to organizations focuses almost exclusively on the structure of the formal organization. The main premise is efficiency through design. People are seen as operating most productively within a rational and well-defined task or organizational design. Therefore, one designs an organization by subdividing work, specifying tasks to be done, and only then fitting people into the plan. Theorists who significantly contributed to this school of thought include Frederick Taylor, the founder of scientific management; Frank and Lillian Gilbreth; Henri Fayol; and Max Weber, the founder of organizational theory. Classical theory is built around four elements: division and specialization of labor, chain of command, organizational structure, and span of control.

Division and Specialization of Labor Dividing the work reduces the number of tasks that each employee must carry out, thereby increasing efficiency and improving the organization's product. This concept lends itself to proficiency and specialization. Therefore, division of work and specialization are seen as economically beneficial. In addition, managers can standardize the work to be done, which in turn provides greater control.

Chain of Command The **chain of command** is the hierarchy of authority and responsibility within the organization. *Authority* is the right or power to direct

MediaLink ● Organizational Theory: Determinants of Structure

activity, whereas *responsibility* is the obligation to attain objectives or perform certain functions. Both are derived from one's position within the organization and define accountability. The line of authority is such that higher levels of management delegate work to those below them in the organization.

There are two types of authority. Command or **line authority** is the linear hierarchy through which activity is directed. **Staff authority** is an advisory relationship; recommendations and advice are offered, but responsibility for the work is assigned to others. In Figure 2-1, the relationships among the chief nurse executive, nurse manager, and staff nurse are examples of line authority. The relationship between the clinical nurse specialist and the nurse manager illustrates staff authority. Neither the clinical nurse specialist nor the nurse manager is responsible for the work of the other; instead, they collaborate to improve the efficiency and productivity of the unit for which the nurse manager is responsible.

Organizational Structure Organizational structure describes the arrangement of the work group. It is a rational approach for designing an effective organization. Classical theorists developed the concept of departmentation as a means to maintain command, reinforce authority, and provide a formal system for communication. The design of the organization is intended to foster the organization's survival and success.

Characteristically, the structure takes shape as a set of differentiated but interrelated functions. Max Weber (1958) proposed the term **bureaucracy** to define the ideal, intentionally rational, most efficient form of organization. Today this word has a negative connotation, suggesting long waits, inefficiency, and red tape.

Span of Control Span of control is a concept related to organizational structure that addresses the pragmatic concern of how many employees a manager can

---

KEY TERMS

Line authority The linear hierarchy of supervisory responsibility and authority.

Staff authority The advisory relationship in which responsibility for actual work is assigned to others.

Bureaucracy A term proposed by Max Weber to define the ideal, intentionally rational, most efficient form of organization.

Span of control The number of employees that can be effectively supervised by a single manager.

Hawthorne effect The tendency for people to perform as expected because of special attention.

---

effectively supervise. Complex organizations usually have numerous departments that are highly specialized and differentiated; authority is centralized, resulting in a *tall* organizational structure with many small work groups. Less complex organizations have *flat* structures; authority is decentralized, with several managers supervising large work groups. Figure 2-2 depicts the differences.

Using a classical perspective, Mintzberg (1989) described five organizational designs: simple structure, machine bureaucracy, professional bureaucracy, divisionalized form, and adhocracy. The designs differ in their executive-level management (strategic apex); the individuals responsible for doing the organizational work (operating core); the managers; the individuals who help standardize and improve the work, such as accountants, in-service educators, and nurse recruiters (technostructure); and the support staff, individuals supporting others who provide the basic work, such as housekeepers and unit secretaries.

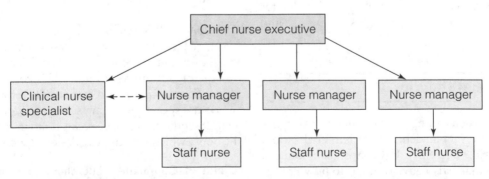

Figure 2-1   Chain of authority.

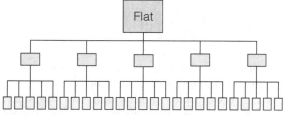

Figure 2-2 **Contrasting spans of control.**
From *Managing Health Services Organizations and Systems*, 4th ed. (p. 124), by B. B. Longest, J. S. Rakich, and K. Darr, 2000, Baltimore: Health Professions Press. Reprinted by permission.

An organization with a *simple structure* design consists of only a strategic apex and an operating core. The private physician's office, in which the physician is the strategic apex and the staff are the operating core, is an example of a simple structure design.

The *machine bureaucracy* is representative of the bureaucracy described by Weber (1958). A tall structure with centralized decision making and departmentalization is characteristic. Government-owned hospitals frequently are machine bureaucracies.

In the *professional bureaucracy*, the operating core of professionals is the dominant feature. Decision making is usually decentralized, and the technostructure is underdeveloped. The support staff, however, is well developed. Most hospitals are professional bureaucracies.

The *divisionalized form* is characterized by a number of independent divisions that are joined by a mutual administration. Decision making is decentralized; both technostructure and support staffs are minimal. A multiorganizational health system is an example of the divisionalized design.

Adhocracy represents a fluid structure in which management, staff, and experts work together on teams. Power, coordination, and control are constantly shifting. Relationship-oriented structures (discussed later in this chapter) are particularly prone to change, and as relationships among and between health care providers shift and evolve so do power, coordination, and control.

Neoclassical Theory

Criticism of classical theory led to the development of neoclassical or humanistic theory, an approach identified with the human relations movement of the 1930s. The neoclassical theorists had a common desire to humanize classical theory without totally rejecting the structural view. All recognized the need to design a rational organizational structure, but the neoclassicists proposed that it be done through cooperation and participation, tapping the motivation of the individual.

A major assumption of this theory is that people desire social relationships, respond to group pressures, and search for personal fulfillment. This theory was developed as the result of a series of studies conducted by the Western Electric Company at their Hawthorne plant in Chicago. The first study was conducted to examine the effect of illumination on productivity. However, this study failed to find any relationship between the two. In most groups, productivity varied at random, and in one study productivity actually rose as illumination levels declined. The researchers concluded that unforeseen "psychological factors" were responsible for the findings. Further studies of working conditions, such as rest breaks and the length of the workweek, still failed to reveal a relationship to productivity. The researchers concluded that the social setting created by the research itself—that is, the special attention given workers as part of the research—enhanced productivity. This tendency for people to perform as expected because of special attention became known as the **Hawthorne effect.**

Although the findings are controversial, they led organizational theorists to focus on the social aspects of work and organizational design. (See Chapter 19 for a description of motivational theories.) One important assertion of this school of thought was that individuals cannot be coerced or bribed to do things they consider unreasonable; formal authority does not work without willing participants (Barnard, 1938).

Systems Theory

Organizational theorists who maintain a systems perspective view productivity as a function of the interplay among structure, people, technology, and environment. Like nursing theories based on systems theory (such as those of Roy and Neuman), organizational theory defines *system* as a set of interrelated parts arranged in a unified whole (Robbins, 1983). Systems can be closed or open. Closed systems are self-contained and usually can be found only in the physical sciences. An open system, in contrast, interacts both internally and with its environment.

In organizational systems theory, an organization is defined as a complex, sociotechnical, open system. This theory provides a framework by which the interrelated parts of the system and their functions can be studied. According to Katz and Kahn (1978), resources, or **input,** such as employees, patients, materials, money, and equipment, are imported from the environment. Within the organization, energy and resources are utilized and transformed; work, a process called **throughput,** is performed to produce a product. The product, or **output,** is then exported to the environment. An organization, then, is a recurrent cycle of input, throughput, and output. Each health care organization—whether a hospital, outpatient clinic, home health care agency, and so on—requires human, financial, and material resources. Each also provides a variety of services to treat illness, restore function, provide rehabilitation, and protect or promote wellness.

In this model, the manager is the catalyst for the input–throughput–output process. The manager is also the interface with the environment. Managers are responsible for integrating information and other stimuli from the environment, such as legislation or changes in health care delivery, to coordinate and facilitate the work of the organization. Figure 2-3 depicts a systems model of a health care organization.

Other systems theorists include March and Simon (1958), who view an organization as an information-processing network with many decision points for both individual members and the organization. Galbraith (1977) views the organization as a large communication system. He proposed a number of strategies for increasing capacity and decreasing uncertainty within the system. Examples of such systems are the matrix structure and the heterarchy structures discussed later in this chapter.

Systems theorists have provided great insight into important organizational and human variables. However,

---

KEY TERMS

Input   Resources such as employees, patients, materials, money, and equipment.

Throughput   The work process to produce a product.

Output   The product of a work process.

---

systems theory does not recognize the vast complexity of organizations or the interactive effects of many variables.

Contingency Theory

Contingency theorists believe organizational performance can be enhanced by matching an organization's structure to its environment. The environment is defined as the people, objects, and ideas outside the organization that influence the organization. The environment of a health care organization includes patients and potential patients; third-party payers, including Medicare and managed-care companies; regulators; competitors; and suppliers of physical facilities, personnel (such as schools of nursing and medicine), equipment, and pharmaceuticals.

Health care organizations are unique with respect to the kinds of products and services they offer. However, like all other organizations, health care organizations are shaped by external and internal forces. These forces stem from the economic and social environment, the technologies used in patient care, organizational size, and the abilities and limitations of the personnel involved in the delivery of health care, including nurses, physicians, technicians, administrators, and, of course, patients.

Given the variety of health care services and patients served today, it should come as no surprise that organizations differ with respect to the environments they face, the levels of training and skills of their caregivers, and the emotional and physical needs of patients. It is naive to think that the form of organization best for one type of patient in one type of environment is appropriate for another type of patient in a completely different environment. We would not expect to see the same staffing, rules and procedures, or chain of command in an inner-city substance abuse center as in a suburban women's health center. Thus, the optimal form of the organization is contingent on the circumstances faced by that organization.

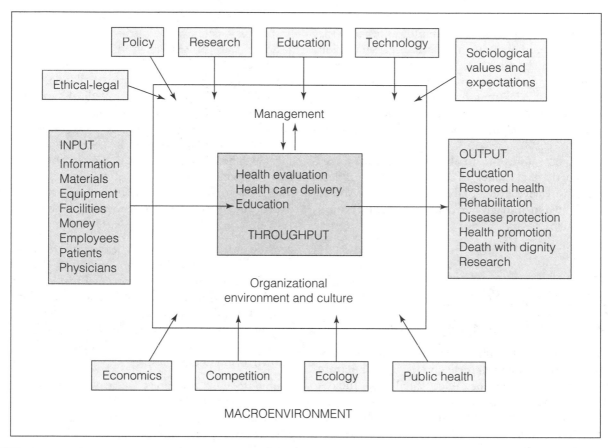

Figure 2-3   **The health care organization as an open system.**

Chaos Theory

The work of industrial theorists focused on linear cause-and-effect relationships. But as the proponents of chaos theory maintain, the universe is not an orderly place; instead, it is filled with chaos, unpredictability, and uncertainty (Kellert, 1994). This theory, which was inspired by the finding of quantum mechanics, challenges us to look at organizations and the nature of relationships and work from new perspectives.

Chaos theory proposes that nature's work does not follow a straight line. The elements of nature often move in a circular, ebbing fashion; a stream destined for the ocean, for example, never takes a straight path. In fact, very little in life operates as a straight line; people's relationships to each other and to their work certainly do not. This notion challenges traditional thinking regarding the design of organizations. According to chaos theory, "organizations are made up of intertwined links and diversified choices that generate unanticipated consequences" (Tetenbaum, 1998, p. 1).

Organizations are living, self-organizing systems that are complex and self-adaptive.

The life cycle of an organization is fully dependent on its adaptability and response to changes in its environment. The tendency is for the organization to grow. When it becomes a large entity, it tends to stabilize and develop more formal standards. From that point, however, the organization tends to lose its adaptability and responsiveness to its environment. Its new challenge is to avoid centralization, remain flexible, and redesign the structure to support the culture that provides the context for its purpose. The set of rules that guided the industrial notions of organizational function and integrity must be discarded, and newer principles that ensure flexibility, fluidity, speed of adaptability, and cultural sensitivity must emerge. Thus, the new definition of a system is a set of cyclic processes that are only temporarily manifested in stable structures that move between order and chaos as the demand on the system requires.

Chaos theory suggests that the drive to create permanent organizational structures is doomed to fail. The assumptions on which the work of the organization is built do not remain relevant. The role of leadership in these changing organizations is to build resilience in the midst of change, to maintain a balance between tension and order, which promotes creativity and prevents instability. Managers also are responsible for creating and maintaining a learning organization, one that tolerates conflict and supports experimentation, risk taking, and trial-and-error modes of problem solving (Tetenbaum, 1998).

This theory requires us to abandon our attachment to any particular model of design and to reflect instead on creative and flexible formats that can be quickly adjusted and changed as the organization's realities shift.

Health Care Organizations

Types of Health Care Organizations

The types of health care organizations in existence today vary from acute care hospitals to ambulatory care facilities to long-term–care facilities. Today's health care organizations differ in ownership, role, activity, and size. Ownership can be either private or government, voluntary (not for profit) or investor-owned (for profit), and sectarian or nonsectarian (Figure 2-4). Private organizations are usually owned by corporations or religious entities, whereas government organizations are operated by city, county, state, or federal entities, such as the Indian Health Service. Voluntary organizations are usually not for profit, meaning that surplus monies are reinvested into the community. Investor-owned, or for-profit corporations, distribute surplus monies back to the investors, who expect a profit. Sectarian agencies have religious affiliations.

Hospitals Hospitals are frequently classified by length of stay and type of service. Most hospitals are acute (short-term or episodic) care facilities. The American Hospital Association (1995) defines an acute care hospital as a facility in which the average length of stay is less than 30 days; chronic or long-term hospitals are designed to care for patients whose average length of stay is longer than 30 days. In addition, hospitals may be classified as general or special care facilities, such as pediatric, rehabilitative, and psychiatric facilities. Many hospitals also serve as teaching institutions for nurses, physicians, and other health care professionals.

The term *teaching hospital* commonly designates a hospital associated with a medical school that maintains a house staff of residents on call 24 hours a day. Nonteaching hospitals, in contrast, have only private physicians on staff. Because private physicians are less accessible than house staff, the medical supervision of patient care differs, as may the role of the nurse. This designation is changing dramatically as new forms of physician groups and allied practices emerge in partnerships with hospitals and medical schools. Some hospitals have adopted "hospitalists," physicians who provide care only to hospital inpatients; those who care for patients in intensive care are known as "intensivists."

Long-Term–Care Facilities Long-term–care facilities provide professional nursing care and rehabilitative services, or the facility may not include skilled nursing care. Facilities that provide professional nursing care may be freestanding or part of a hospital, and length of stay is limited. Residential care facilities are sheltered environments in which no skilled care is provided. The final years of life are often spent in these facilities, also known as nursing homes.

Ambulatory Care Centers A growing proportion of health care is delivered in ambulatory settings. Physician's offices, health maintenance organizations, emergency rooms, surgical centers, birthing centers, diagnostic imaging centers, and family planning clinics are just a few examples of the variety of ambulatory services available. Many hospitals offer both on- and off-campus outpatient sites to compete in this growing area of health care.

Home Health Care Agencies Another growth area is in home health care. Home health care is the intermittent, temporary delivery of health care in the home by skilled or unskilled providers. With shortened lengths of hospital stay, more acutely ill patients are discharged to recuperate at home. Furthermore, more people are surviving life-threatening illnesses or trauma and require extended care. The primary service provided by home care agencies is nursing care; however, larger home care agencies also offer other professional services, such as physical or occupational therapy, and durable medical equipment, such as ventilators, hospital beds, home oxygen equipment, and other medical supplies.

Temporary Service Agencies An outgrowth of the home health care industry is the temporary service agency. These agencies provide nurses and other health care workers to hospitals that are temporarily short-staffed; they also provide private duty nurses to individual patients.

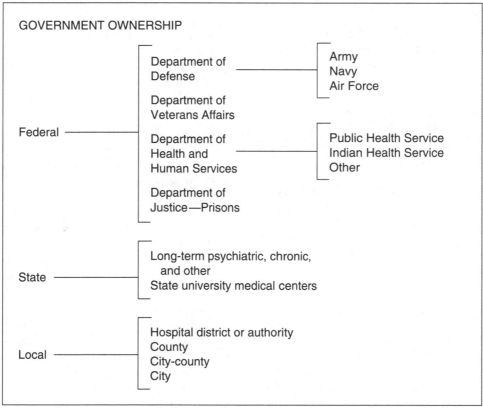

Figure 2-4   **Types of ownership in health care organizations. From *Managing Health Services Organizations and Systems*, 4th ed. (p. 173), by B. B. Longest, J. S. Rakich, and K. Darr, 2000, Baltimore: Health Professions Press. Reprinted by permission.**

Managed Health Care Organizations The managed health care organization is the newest form of health care delivery. In this system, a group of providers is responsible for delivering services (that is, managing health care) through an organized arrangement with a group of individuals (for example, all employees of one company, all Medicaid patients in the state). Different types of managed-care organizations exist: health maintenance organizations (HMOs), preferred provider organizations (PPOs), and point-of-service plans (POS).

The HMO is a geographically organized system that provides an agreed-on package of health maintenance and treatment services. There are four different types of HMOs:

1. *Staff Model.* Physicians are HMO employees paid a salary.
2. *Independent Practice Association (IPA).* Physicians maintain individual or group practices, but contract with an HMO to serve enrollees for a negotiated fee.
3. *Group Model.* The HMO contracts with a multi-specialty group to provide enrollees' services for a negotiated fee.
4. *Network Model.* The HMO contracts with two or more IPAs (independent or group practices) to provide enrollee services at a fixed monthly fee per enrollee, called **capitation.**

In a PPO, the managed-care organization contracts with independent practitioners to provide enrollees with established discounted rates. If an enrollee obtains services from a nonparticipating provider, significant copayments are usually required.

The POS is considered to be an HMO–PPO hybrid. In a POS, enrollees may use the network of managed-care providers to go outside the network as they wish. However, use of a provider outside the network usually results in additional costs in copayments, deductibles, or premiums.

Interorganizational Relationships

With increased competition for resources and public and governmental pressures for better efficiency and effectiveness, organizations have been forced to establish relationships with one another for their continued survival. Multihospital systems and multi-organizational arrangements, both formal and informal, are mechanisms by which these relationships have formed.

Arrangements between or among organizations that provide the same or similar services are examples of

---

KEY TERMS

Capitation A fixed monthly fee for providing services to enrollees.

Horizontal integration Arrangements between or among organizations that provide the same or similar services.

Vertical integration An arrangement between or among dissimilar but related organizations to provide a continuum of services.

Diversification The expansion of an organization into new arenas of service.

Joint venture A partnership in which each partner contributes different areas of expertise, resources, or service to create a new product or service.

---

horizontal integration. For instance, all hospitals in the network provide comparable services, as shown in Figure 2-5.

Vertical integration, in contrast, is an arrangement between or among dissimilar but related organizations to provide a continuum of services. An affiliation of a health maintenance organization with a hospital, pharmacy, and nursing facility represents vertical integration (see Figure 2-6).

Besides enhancing survival, vertical integration is thought to improve coordination of services, quality, cost effectiveness, efficiency, and bargaining power; promote continuity of care and improve community service; expand services, which enhances competition; strengthen education and research opportunities; and use human resources more efficiently (Newhouse & Mills, 1999).

Numerous arrangements using horizontal and vertical integration can be found, and these models likely will become the common structure for delivery of health care. Examples of such arrangements include affiliations, consortia, alliances, mergers, and consolidations. An assortment of health care agencies under the umbrella of a corporate network is shown in the example in Figure 2-7.

Diversification

Diversification provides another strategy for survival in today's economy. Diversification is the expansion of an organization into new arenas. Two types of diversification are common: concentric and conglomerate.

Figure 2-5   Horizontal integration.

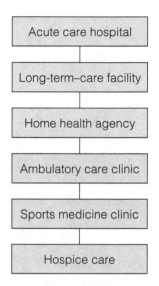

Figure 2-6   Vertical integration.

Concentric diversification occurs when an organization complements its existing services by expanding into new markets or broadening the types of services it currently has available. For example, a children's hospital might open a day-care center for developmentally delayed children or offer drop-in facilities for sick child care.

Conglomerate diversification is the expansion into areas that differ from the original product or service. The purpose of conglomerate diversification is to obtain a source of income that will support the organization's product or service. For example, a long-term–care facility might develop real estate or purchase a company that produces durable medical equipment.

Another type of diversification common to health care is the **joint venture**. A joint venture is a partnership in which each partner contributes different areas of expertise, resources, or services to create a new product or service. In one type of joint venture, one partner (general partner) finances and manages the venture, whereas the other partner (limited partner) provides a needed service. Joint ventures between health care organizations and physicians are becoming increasingly common. Integrated health care organizations, hospitals, and clinics seek physician and/or practitioner groups they can bond (capture) in order to obtain more referrals. The health care organization as financier and manager is the *general partner,* and physicians are *limited partners.*

A joint venture also might involve two organizations with different areas of expertise who join together to create a new product or service. An alliance between the Cerner Corporation who supplies hospital information systems and the University of Kansas School of Nursing to develop a clinical system for teaching students evidence-based practice is an example of combining resources of both organizations to develop an innovative new product (Connors, Weaver, Warren, & Miller, 2002).

Traditional Organizational Structures

The optimal organizational structure integrates organizational goals, size, technology, and environment. When structure is not aligned with organizational needs, the organization's response to environmental change diminishes; decisions are delayed, overlooked, or poor; conflict results; and performance deteriorates (Porter-O'Grady, 1994). Organizational structure is an important tool through which managers can increase

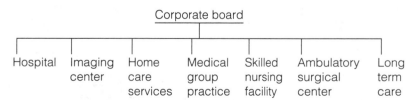

Figure 2-7   Corporate health care network.

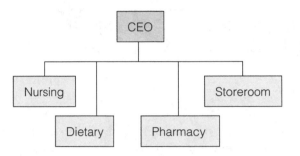

Figure 2-8   Functional structure.

organizational efficiency. Reorganization occurs in response to changes in organizational goals, size, technology, or environment.

Functional Structure

In *functional structures,* employees are grouped in departments by specialty, with similar tasks being performed by the same group, similar groups operating out of the same department, and similar departments reporting to the same manager (Figure 2-8). In a functional structure, all nursing tasks fall under nursing service; the same is true of other functional areas. Functional structures tend to centralize decision making because the functions converge at the top of the organization.

Functional structures have several weaknesses. Coordination across functions is poor. Decision-making responsibilities can pile up at the top and overload senior managers, who may be uninformed regarding day-to-day operations. Responses to the external environment that require coordination across functions are slow. General management training is limited because most employees move up the organization within functional departments. Many health care organizations have a function-like structure.

Service-Line Structure

Service-line structures also are called product-line or service-integrated structures. In a service-line structure, all functions needed to produce a product or service are grouped together in self-contained units (Figure 2-9). A large health care institution that acquires a smaller clinic may operate it as a self-contained unit. The service-integrated structure is decentralized; units are based on product, service, geographical location, or type of customer.

Integrated structures are preferred in large and complex organizations because the same activity (for example, hiring) is assigned to several self-contained units, which can respond rapidly to the unit's immediate needs. This is extremely appropriate when environmental uncertainty is high and the organization requires frequent adaptation and innovation.

Figure 2-9   Service-line structure.

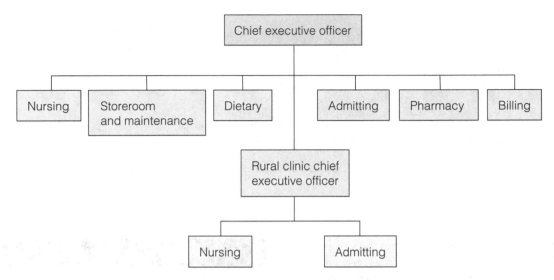

Figure 2-10 Hybrid structure.

One of the strengths of the service-line structure is its potential for rapid change in an unstable environment. Because each division is specialized and its outputs can be tailored to the situation, client satisfaction is high. Coordination across function (nursing, dietary, pharmacy, and so on) occurs easily; work partners identify with their own service and can compromise or collaborate with other service functions to meet service goals and reduce conflict. Service goals receive priority under this organizational structure because employees see the service outcomes as the primary purpose of their organization.

The major weaknesses of service-integrated structures include possible duplication of resources (such as ads for new positions) and lack of in-depth technical training and specialization. Coordination across service categories (oncology, cardiology, and the burn unit, for example) is difficult; services operate independently and often compete. Each service category, which is independent and autonomous, has separate and often duplicate staff and competes with other service areas for resources.

With a service-line structure, a department of nursing may not be shown on the organizational chart. This presents a challenge to nursing administrators and managers to maintain nursing standards across service lines (Fitzpatrick, McElroy, & DeWoody, 2001).

Hybrid Structure

When an organization grows, it typically organizes both self-contained units and functional units; the result is a hybrid organization (Figure 2-10). The strengths of the hybrid structure are that it (a) provides simultaneous coordination within product divisions while maintaining the quality of each function, (b) improves the alignment between corporate and service or product goals, and (c) fosters better adaptation to the environment while still maintaining efficiency.

The weakness of hybrid structures is conflict between top administration and managers. Managers often resent administrators' intrusions into what they see as their own area of responsibility. Over time, organizations tend to accumulate large corporate staffs to oversee divisions in an attempt to provide functional coordination across service or product structures.

Matrix Structure

The matrix structure is unique and complex (Figure 2-11); it integrates both product and functional structures into one overlapping structure. In a matrix structure, different managers are responsible for function and product. For example, the nurse manager for the oncology clinic may report to the vice president for nursing as well as the vice president for outpatient services.

Matrices tend to develop where there are strong outside pressures for a dual organizational focus on product and function. The matrix is appropriate in a highly uncertain environment that changes frequently but also requires organizational expertise.

A major weakness of the matrix structure is its dual authority, which can be frustrating and confusing for departmental managers and employees. Excellent interpersonal skills are required from the

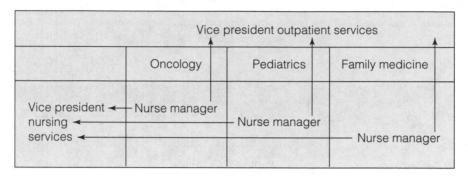

Figure 2-11　**Matrix structure.**

managers involved. A matrix organization is time consuming, because frequent meetings are required to resolve problems and conflicts; the structure will not work unless participants can see beyond their own functional area to the big organizational picture. Finally, if one side of the matrix is more closely aligned with organizational objectives, that side may become dominant.

Parallel Structure

Parallel structure is a structure unique to health care. It is the result of complex relationships that exist between the formal authority of the health care organization and the authority of its medical staff. In a parallel structure, the medical staff is separate and autonomous from the organization. The result is an organizational dilemma: two lines of authority. One line extends from the governing body to the chief executive officer and then to the managerial structure; the other line extends from the governing body to the medical staff. These two intersect in departments such as nursing, in which decision making involves both managerial and clinical elements.

Parallel structures are found in health care institutions with a functional structure and separate medical governance structure (Figure 2-12). Parallel structures are becoming less successful as health care organizations integrate into newer models that incorporate physician practice under the organizational umbrella.

Relationship-Oriented Structures

Shared Governance

A recent phenomenon in the structuring of nursing departments has evolved from the desire to build accountable decision making in hospitals, especially

KEY TERMS

Shared governance　An organizational paradigm based on the values of interdependence and accountability that allows nurses to make decisions in a decentralized environment.

among the nursing staff. These innovations may simply take the form of participative decision making or more substantive systems known as **shared governance.** Shared governance presents the values of interdependence and accountability as a basis for constructing a new organizational paradigm. Shared governance is based on a philosophy that nursing practice is best determined by nurses. It is a network of making nursing practice decisions in a decentralized environment. As a result, nurses gain significant control over their practice, efficiency and accountability are improved, and feelings of powerlessness are mitigated.

Shared governance is by design and concept an invitational process. Because of its dynamic nature, it cannot be contained or owned in any exclusive framework and cannot be limited to any specific work group. If it is, it simply fails to maintain itself and eventually dissipates into parochialism, paternalism, and organizational isolation (Porter-O'Grady & Tornebini, 1993).

Shared governance allows staff nurses significant control over major decisions about nursing practice. These systems usually are built on a foundation of primary nursing, peer review, and some provision for clinical advancement. Most shared governance systems are similar to and reflect the principles often found in academic or medical governance models. For example, nurses may elect a council to represent the nursing staff collectively. Other councils may exist, such as a human resources council in charge of staffing levels, recruitment, and

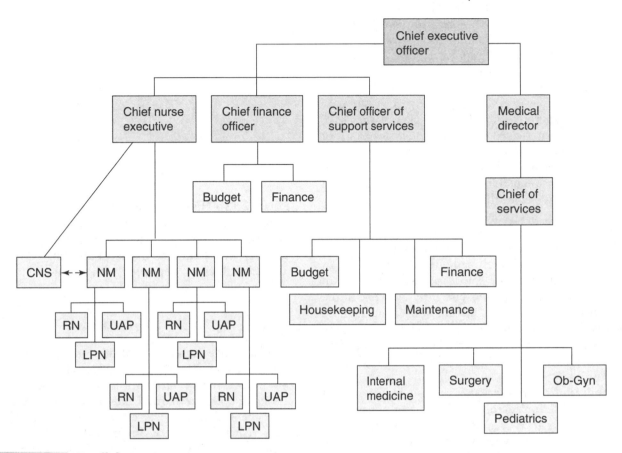

Figure 2-12   Parallel structure.

retention; a nursing council in charge of care standards, audit criteria, research, and staff education; and individual unit councils.

Some shared governance systems incorporate elected advisory boards for each service or clinical department. From these boards is elected a senate or congress that meets several times a year to decide larger policy issues.

The ultimate outcome of shared governance is that nurses participate in an accountable forum to control their own practice within the health care organization. The assumption is that nursing staffs, like medical staffs, will predetermine the clinical skills of staff nurses and monitor the work of each through peer review while deciding on other practice issues through accountable forums or councils.

Increasingly, shared governance principles integrate disciplines within newer service settings. As the continuum of care and the linkage of services become more important components of organizational design, shared governance provides a process and structure that supports decision making, quality imperatives, and collaboration among disciplines. Departmental

and divisional structures are disappearing, and soon discipline-specific structures may give way to service configurations that address the continuum of care in a large health plan. Shared governance principles are increasingly being used as a framework for the models of structure that will integrate the organization's functions and structures.

The shared governance movement began purposefully with nursing. Major organizational transformation rarely succeeds if it exists only at the top of an organization or system. Such change generally succeeds at the place closest to where the work gets done. In a service organization, that means that major change begins in the settings closest to the patient. Indeed, if the major purveyors of the organization's service, in this case nurses, are not fully invested in the change process, it doesn't matter where else it works. Because of the large number of players and their varying proximity to the patient, it is reasonable to begin structural redesign with nurses and to create a milieu that supports the movement of such change to other parts of the patient care system. If successful, such movement is inevitable and essential. The literature is replete with information regarding its implementation and effectiveness as a process for empowering nurses (DeBaca, Jones, & Tornebini, 1993).

Partners in care include all the professional and technical workers that operate within the patient care continuum. This group includes physicians, who have historically been viewed as working independently of the functional relationship of institutional providers. Because partnership is the driving theme of shared leadership and decision making, bringing the physician into the partnership creates the essential relationship necessary to initiate effective service arrangements, evaluate care, and build effective supporting structures.

Integrative care models and multidisciplinary team approaches to care further facilitate the demand for an organizational structure more supportive of team members than that which is currently available in the more traditional hospital hierarchies. Creating more collateral structures that reflect the relationship of the players to each other acts more clearly in concert with interdisciplinary work than do more traditional structures.

Implications for altering service, operations, and governance are considerable. The fact that principles of shared governance reflecting partnership, equity, accountability, and ownership form the basis for these newer approaches indicates the strong foundations that shared governance has established in successfully structuring an empowered nursing organization. It is natural to assume that these processes would expand as the health system moves to point-of-service design and constructs the empowerment processes necessary to make these more integrated systems function effectively.

The continuum of care and the structures that support it will have a major impact on nurses and the design of patient service organizations of the future. The configuration of these systems will be radically different from those found in the past. New foundations for building knowledge and conducting research will emerge as newer organizational forms take shape.

Heterarchy Structure

One such innovative structure has been suggested by organizational consultant, nurse Tim Porter-O'Grady (Porter-O'Grady & Malloch, 2002). **Heterarchy** is a relational design based on the concept of connections (see Figure 2-13). In contrast to organizational structures based on industrial models, heterarchy acknowledges the linkages among people and their relationships.

Figure 2-13 **Heterarchy structure. From *Quantum Leadership: A Textbook of New Leadership* (p. 5), by T. Porter-O'Grady and K. Malloch, 2002, Sudbury, MA: Jones and Bartlett Publishers (www.jbpub.com). Reprinted with permission.**

Self-Organizing Structures

A new adaptive organizational structure evolves from organizational tasks (Wheatly, 1992). This self-organizing (self-renewing) structure is flexible and able to respond to both internal and external change. The only requirement of this structure is self-reference; that is, future structures are consistent with the previously established identity and its past. Rigid, permanent structures are avoided; the organizational structure changes when the need arises. Roles and structures are created out of need and interest; relationships, exchanges, and connections among employees are nurtured as the primary source of organizational creativity and success.

Redesigning, Restructuring, and Reengineering

To reduce the cost of delivering health care and maintain market positions, jobs have been redesigned, organizations restructured, and systems reengineered. In **redesign**, the distribution of activities, role overlap, excess specialization, and waste are examined. The goal is to design each job according to appropriate tasks and necessary qualifications and to have all jobs fit together so that the organization's work gets done in the most efficient and effective manner. Redesign usually focuses on the individual jobs in one clinical specialty area, although each area may be undergoing job redesign simultaneously or consecutively (see job analysis in Chapter 18).

Barriers to Job Redesign

The nurse manager should be aware of some common problems in the redesign of jobs. For example, the nurse manager's role may change from leader and director of unit staff to that of coordinator of staff activities. Somehow, the notion of coordinator seems inconsistent with our cultural stereotypes of leadership. We usually think of a leader as the person in charge, or the boss. That stereotype of leadership tends to include the unilateral and unquestioned use of power with objectives, strategies, and evaluation defined strictly from the leader's perspective.

A number of factors other than the power afforded by virtue of job title and reporting relationships are involved in effective leadership. Effective leadership is accepted leadership, and there are many ways to foster acceptance of the nurse manager's legitimate organizational power (see Chapter 6). If effectiveness means being a coordinator as opposed to being the boss, then the strategies and techniques involved in carrying out that role are what the nurse manager should use.

Another barrier to job redesign is that the values implicit in job redesign may be at odds with those of the organization's administration. The notion of providing autonomy, feedback, greater responsibility, and self-direction in the performance of jobs may not be in tune with the philosophy and history of the organizational hierarchy—matters that are not under the nurse manager's immediate discretion or control. However, different management areas afford different degrees of responsibility, and there may be a good deal of flexibility within the limits of the organization's rules, especially with the flux in today's environment. Job redesign is just another tool to use within the limits of the situation at hand.

In some cases, staff members are reluctant to engage in job redesign or other motivational efforts because they fear that increased productivity may have implications for their job security. They are concerned that if productivity increases sufficiently, some people may lose their jobs because they are no longer needed to accomplish the work. Increased productivity, however, not only eases the workload but also, if properly managed (for example, rewarded), is likely to result in greater satisfaction and organizational commitment as well as less absenteeism and turnover. Also, fears regarding job security usually focus solely on the quantity of work and ignore the quality of work as a separate, but equally important, dimension. Effective motivation of staff members involves both of these dimensions, but job enrichment most consistently increases job satisfaction and work quality rather than the quantity of work produced.

> ### KEY TERMS
>
> *Heterarchy* A relational design based on the concept of connections.
>
> *Redesign* A technique that examines the tasks within each job with the goal of combining appropriate tasks to improve efficiency.
>
> *Restructuring* An examination of a health care organization's structure to improve the organization's productivity.
>
> *Reengineering* A complex and often radical approach to the organization of patient care in which new relationships and expectations are adopted.
>
> *Downsizing* Cutting the number of positions in an organization.

The fourth major barrier to job redesign is that not everyone desires change or growth in his or her job. Some people prefer to have their work clearly prescribed, unvarying in its content or procedure, and highly predictable from day to day. Job redesign is appropriate only for staff members whose jobs are too highly structured to suit their needs.

Still another major barrier to job redesign is the lack of exact specifications of what is to be accomplished by redesigning an individual's job. For that reason, organizations may restructure and reengineer systems.

Restructuring and Reengineering

Job redesign focuses on individual jobs; **restructuring** and **reengineering** examine the entire health organization's structure with a goal of improving the organization's functioning and productivity. Restructure means to change the structure of the organization. The administrative structure changes, as do reporting relationships and communication channels. Restructuring naturally follows organizational affiliations, mergers, and the establishment of integrated health care systems as efforts to reduce duplication among the network's various entities ensue. In restructuring, coordination of work effort is stressed and interdependence valued. Organizationally based models, such as case management, total quality management, and product-line management, are used in system reorganization.

Another type of restructuring is downsizing. **Downsizing** or *right-sizing* simply means cutting the number of staff positions. The workload may or may not be the same as it was before the cuts; most often the degree of downsizing depends on the number of patients in the system, the care they need, and the mix of staff skills.

Downsizing without job redesign encourages self-promotion, reduces trust, destroys morale, and consumes inordinate amounts of the time and energy of the staff and management. Mortality and malpractice exposure may increase. The organization operates in a continuous crisis mode, with those most affected assuming a bunker mentality in an attempt to protect their own turf. Although cost containment is the impetus for downsizing, the acuity of today's hospitalized patients makes downsizing imprudent. Similarly, reducing the number and qualifications of staff in outpatient settings may contribute to increased complications and concomitant higher costs due to repeat hospitalizations.

Reengineering involves examining and improving the process by which health care is delivered. Reengineering is collaborative, data driven, and patient focused. Reengineering usually involves the entire organization and results in major change to both the organization and its members.

Reengineering is very complex and often radical. A new approach to the organization of patient care is adopted. Nurses, physicians, and other health care professionals develop different teams and the use of patient outcomes are integral parts of restructuring and reengineering. Working in collaborative teams and using a multidisciplinary approach requires open communication, the ability to accept and give criticism, clarity about responsibilities, and accountability by all. Adopting these behaviors is challenging and stressful, and some individuals resist it. The challenge for nurse managers is to help staff members understand the ultimate goal, participate in the process, and use their professional expertise to contribute to the well-being of the organization's patients, both now and in the future.

Restructuring and reengineering also may be used in system redesign. Common themes in system redesign are integration/coordination across department lines; critical path/protocol development; management restructuring; multiskilled worker development; implementation of patient-focused care and case management (Gellinas & Manthey, 1997).

Nurse managers are key players in the redesign efforts. They are expected not only to initiate change while reducing costs, maintaining or improving quality of care, coaching and mentoring, and team building, but also to do so in an ever-changing environment full of ambiguities while their own responsibilities are expanded.

Strategic Planning

Successful organizations, both for profit and not for profit, have learned that they must focus their resources on a limited number of activities. **Strategic planning** involves projecting the organization's goals and activities into the future, usually 2 to 5 years ahead. Based on the values, philosophy, and mission of the organization and the vision of its leaders, strategic planning guides the direction the organization is to take.

Values

Values are the beliefs or attitudes one has about people, ideas, objects, or actions that form a basis for behavior. Organizations use value statements to identify those beliefs or attitudes esteemed by the organizational leaders.

Vision

A **vision statement** describes the goal to which the organization aspires. The vision statement is designed to inspire and motivate employees to achieve a desired state of affairs. "Our vision is to be a regional integrated healthcare delivery system providing premier healthcare services, professional and community education, and healthcare research," is an example of a vision statement for a health care system.

Mission

The **mission** of an organization is a broad, general statement of the organization's reason for existence. Developing the mission is the necessary first step to designing a strategic plan. "Our mission is to improve the health of the people and communities we serve," is an example of a mission statement that guides decision making for the organization. If, for example, a proposed activity does not promote the organization's stated mission, it probably would not be pursued. Purchasing a medical equipment company, for example, might not be considered an activity that helps meet the mission of improving the community's health.

Philosophy

The **philosophy** is a written statement that reflects the organizational values, vision, and mission.

Goals

Goals are specific statements of what is to be achieved. They follow the mission and vision of the organization. Goals are measurable and precise. "Every patient will

KEY TERMS

Strategic planning   A process of long-range and ongoing planning for the future.

Values   The beliefs or attitudes one has about people, ideas, objects, or actions that form a basis for behavior.

Vision statement   A description of the goal to which an organization aspires.

Mission   A general statement of the purpose of an organization.

Philosophy   The mission, values, and vision of an organization.

Goals   Specific statements of achievement that provide direction.

Objectives   Statements of achievement specific to abilities within the organization.

Strategies   Actions by which objectives are to be achieved.

Organizational climate   The perceived characteristics of an organization.

Organizational culture   The norms and traditions within an organization.

be satisfied with his or her care" is an example of a goal. Goals apply to the entire organization, whereas **objectives** are specific to an individual unit. A nursing objective to meet the above goal might be "Provide appropriate information and education to patients from preadmission to discharge." **Strategies** follow objectives and specify what actions will be taken. "Implement patient education classes for prenatal patients" is an example of a strategy to meet the patient satisfaction objective.

Other categories in a strategic plan include the personnel responsible for each activity, the projected cost, criteria to establish that the goal has been met, expected date of completion, and the current status.

The process of doing strategic planning involves gathering a planning committee composed of (at least)

- Top-level administrators,
- Representatives of those closest to the work,
- Staff to collect data and distribute information, and
- Willingness by all involved to contribute.

It is best to use those people who are enthusiastic, experienced, and committed to the organization. Naysayers can be included once some parts of the plan are formulated. It is essential to involve everyone in the organization, however, albeit peripherally. "Buy-in" is critical to the plan's success.

The planning group assesses the environment and the organization's assets and areas of weakness and balances those with the organization's values and goals. This is a time-consuming and demanding process and should not be undertaken hurriedly. Put in use, however, a well-thought-out strategic plan guides the organization toward its goals, helps all the staff stay directed, and prevents the organization from responding to inappropriate requests.

Strategic planning is an ongoing process, not an end in itself. It requires a continual focus on the goal and meticulous attention to progress; the organization's mission and vision must always guide activities.

Organizational Environment and Culture

The environment within an organization can be defined in terms of its climate and culture. **Organizational climate** is the perceived characteristics of the organization—its physical attributes, organizational structure, lines of communication, policies and procedures. For example, some aspects of an organization's climate are its benefits offered, staffing ratios, the location of employee parking, and the layout of the nursing unit.

Organizational culture, on the other hand, consists of the norms and traditions maintained. Organizational culture affects the practices and procedures of the organization. For example, are uniforms or scrubs worn? When is report given? To whom? Is tardiness tolerated? How late is acceptable?

Like climate, organizational culture varies from one institution to the next and subcultures and even countercultures, groups whose values and goals differ significantly from those of the dominant organization, may exist. A subculture is a group that has shared experiences or like interests and values. Nurses form a subculture within health care environments. They share a common language, rules, rituals, and dress. Individual units also can become subcultures.

Besides organizational cultures differing between institutions, culture may differ between the organization and its subculture. If the subculture's norms and traditions are in agreement with the organization's, then consonance occurs; if not, dissonance occurs.

MEDIALINK   The Center of Organizational Design

Cooke and Lafferty (1989) have identified three types of culture:

- Constructive or positive, where the focus is on self-actualization, humanism, affiliation, and achievement
- Passive or defensive, where the focus is on approval, dependence, convention, and avoidance
- Aggressive or defensive, where the focus is on competition, perfectionism, power, and opposition

The presence of a constructive culture promotes employee retention and decreases patient mortality (McDaniel & Stumpf, 1993). Similarly, Shortell and colleagues (1991) found a correlation between a constructive or positive work culture in the intensive care unit and a decrease in mortality for acutely ill patients. More recent studies as well indicate that a positive culture affects patient outcomes (Kovner & Gergen, 1998; Aiken et al., 2002).

Evaluating an organization's culture is essential when a merger is being considered. Ignoring issues of organizational culture can result in one culture becoming dominant (McConnell, 2000). Unintended consequences may result, including poor morale and, ultimately, loss of employees. More than one merger, established for financial reasons without consideration of people issues, has failed.

One way to assess the organizational environment or culture is to evaluate the hiring preferences for key positions in the organization. An organization in which nursing leaders are innovative, creative, and energetic will tend to operate in a fast-moving, goal-oriented fashion. If humanistic, interpersonal skills are sought in candidates for leadership positions, the organization will focus on human resources, employees, and patient advocacy (Hersey, Blanchard, & Johnson, 2001).

Magnet Hospital Designation

Developed in 1994 by the American Nurses Credentialing Center (ANCC), the magnet recognition program designates health care organizations that "demonstrate sustained excellence in nursing care" (ANCC, 2003). The program is based on the magnet hospital program begun in the early 1980s. To qualify for recognition as a magnet hospital requires a significant investment of time and financial resources. Nonetheless, 69 health care organizations had received this prestigious recognition in 2003 (ANCC, 2003). Providing a strong nursing support system pays off. In spite of a national nursing shortage, magnet hospitals

are successful in retaining and recruiting nurses (Aiken, Havens, & Sloane, 2000).

Generational Differences

Managing employees from different generations will be discussed more fully in succeeding chapters, but it bears noting here that such differences can significantly affect the organization's culture (Hersey, Blanchard, & Johnson, 2001). Generation G is known as the "gray generation." Age 54 and older, these workers are nearing retirement time, have a strong work ethic, and have a sustained commitment to their job.

Generation B, ages 35 to 53, are the "baby boomers." They are idealistic and ambitious and their identities are shaped by their work. Generation X, ages 23 to 34, desire a positive work environment and for their work to have worth. They want independence, fun, and to balance work with other important areas of their lives, including personal relationships, child rearing, and pleasurable pursuits. Generation Y, ages 12 to 22, are the workers of tomorrow. They are technically savvy, responsible, and competent. Already experts in connecting online, they may someday be the workers who participate in structures such as heterarchy described by Porter-O'Grady (Porter-O'Grady & Malloch, 2002).

In summary, organizations that require decision-making ability and empower nurses to participate in determining their practice environment will retain nurses who desire a substantial degree of autonomy. Systems involving participatory management and shared governance create organizational climates that reward decision making, creativity, independence, and autonomy. These organizations retain and recruit independent, accountable professionals. In response to consumer demands for fast attention to concerns and questions, organizations that empower nurses to make decisions will better meet consumer requests. As the health care environment continues to evolve, more and more organizations are adopting consumer-sensitive cultures that require accountability and decision making from nurses.

What You Know Now

- The schools of organizational theory are classical theory, neoclassical theory, systems theory, contingency theory, and chaos theory.
- Organizations can be viewed as social systems consisting of people working in a predetermined pattern of

relationships who strive toward a goal. The goal of health care organizations is to provide a particular mix of health services.

- Traditional organizational structures are functional, service-integrated, hybrid, matrix, and parallel structures.

- Relationship-oriented structures are shared governance, heterarchy, and self-organizing.

- The organizational structure determines the formal communication system and guides organizational activities. This structure can be either horizontal or vertical.

- Concepts of shared governance provide the framework for empowerment and partnership and are leading nursing organizations into stronger partnerships with other disciplines and with the health care organization.

- Organizations develop strategic plans based on the values, philosophy, and mission of the organization and the vision of its leaders.

- Organizational climate and culture define the environment of the organization.

- The magnet hospital recognition program identifies hospitals that provide a supportive environment for nursing.

- Generational differences must be considered when managing an organization's workforce.

Questions to Challenge You

1. Secure a copy of the organizational chart from your employment or clinical site. Would you describe the organization the same way the chart depicts it? If not, redraw a chart to illustrate how you see the organization.

2. What organizational structure would you prefer? Think about how you might go about finding an organization that meets your criteria.

3. Organizational theories explain how organizations function. Which theory or theories describes your organization's functioning? Do you think it is the same theory your organization's administrators would use to describe it? Explain.

4. Have you been involved in strategic planning? If so, explain what happened and how well it worked in directing the organization's activities.

5. What is the culture of your organization (school or work)? What would you change about the culture? Do generational differences affect its culture?

Explore 🌐 MediaLink

NCLEX review questions, essay activities, group activities, and other interactive resources for this chapter can be found on the Web site at http://www.prenhall.com/sullivan-decker. Click on "Chapter 2" to select activities for this chapter.

References

Aiken, L. H., Havens, D., & Sloane, D. (2000). The magnet nursing services recognition program: A comparison of two groups of magnet hospitals. *American Journal of Nursing, 100*(3), 26–35.

Aiken, L. H., Clarke, S. P., Sloane, D. M., Sochalski, J., & Silber, J. H. (2002). Hospital nurse staffing and patient mortality, nurse burnout, and job dissatisfaction. *Journal of the American Medical Association, 288*(16), 1987–1993.

American Hospital Association. (1995). *AHA guide to the health care field* (1995–1996 ed.). Chicago: Author.

American Nurses Credentialing Center. (2003). *Magnet recognition program.* Retrieved from September 30, 2003, http://www.nursingworld.org/ancc/magnet/Magnet2.htm

Barnard, C. I. (1938). *The functions of the executive.* Cambridge, MA: Harvard University Press.

Cannon, E. (Ed.). (1925). *Adam Smith, An inquiry into the nature and causes of the wealth of nations* (4th ed.). London: Methuen. (Original work published 1776).

Cooke, R. A., & Lafferty, J. L. (1989). *Organizational culture inventory.* Plymouth, MI: Human Synergistics.

Connors, H. R., Weaver, C., Warren, J., & Miller, K. L. (2002, September-October). An academic-business partnership for advancing clinical informatics. *Nursing Education Perspectives*, 228–233.

DeBaca, V., Jones, K., & Tornebini, J. (1993). A cost-benefit analysis of shared governance. *Journal of Nursing Administration, 23*(7/8), 50–57.

Fitzpatrick, M. J., McElroy, M. J., & DeWoody, S. (2001). Building a strong nursing organization in a merged, service-line structure. *Journal of Nursing Administration, 31*(1), 24–32.

Galbraith, J. R. (1977). *Organizational design.* Reading, MA: Addison-Wesley.

Gellinas, L. S., & Manthey, M. (1997). The impact of organizational redesign on nurse executive leadership. *Journal of Nursing Administration, 27*(10), 35–42.

Hersey, P., Blanchard, K. H., & Johnson, D. E. (2001). *Management of organizational behavior.* Upper Saddle River, NJ: Prentice Hall.

Katz, D., & Kahn, R. (1978). *The social psychology of organizations*. New York: Wiley.

Kellert, S. (1994). *In the wake of chaos*. Chicago: University of Chicago Press.

Kovner, C., & Gergen, P. J. (1998). Nurse staffing levels and adverse events following surgery in U.S. hospitals. *Image: Journal of Nursing Scholarship, 30*(4), 315–321.

Longest, B. B., Rakich, J. S., & Darr, K. (2000). *Managing health services organizations and systems* (4th ed.). Baltimore: Health Professions Press.

March, J. G., & Simon, H. (1958). *Organizations*. New York: Wiley.

McConnell, C. R. (2000). The manager and the merger: Adaptation and survival in the blended organization. *Health Care Manager, 19*(1), 1–11.

McDaniel, C., & Stumpf, L. (1993). The organizational culture. *Journal of Nursing Administration, 23*(4), 54–60.

Mintzberg, H. (1989). *Mintzberg on management: Inside our strange world of organizations*. New York: Free Press.

Newhouse, R. P., & Mills, M. E. (1999). Vertical systems integration. *Journal of Nursing Administration, 29*(10), 22–29.

Porter-O'Grady, T. (1994). Re-engineering the nursing profession. *Aspen's Advisor for the Nurse Executive, 9*(7), 7–8.

Porter-O'Grady, T., & Tornebini, J. (1993). Outcomes of shared governance: Impact on the organization. *Seminars for Nurse Managers, 1*(2), 63–73.

Porter-O'Grady, T., & Malloch, K. (2002). *Quantum leadership: A textbook of new leadership*. Gaithersburg, MD: Aspen.

Robbins, S. P. (1983). *Organizational theory*. Englewood Cliffs, NJ: Prentice-Hall.

Shortell, S., Rousseau, D., Gillies, R., Devers, K. J., & Simons, T. L. (1991). Organizational assessment in intensive care units (ICUs): Construction, development, reliability and validity of the ICU nurse-physician questionnaire. *Medical Care, 29*(8), 709–726.

Tetenbaum, T. J. (1998). Shifting paradigms: From Newton to chaos. *Organizational Dynamics, 26*(4), 21–32.

Wheatly, M. J. (1992). *Leadership and the new science: Learning about organization from an orderly universe*. San Francisco: Berrett-Koehler.

Weber, M. (1958). *From Max Weber: Essays in sociology*. H. Gerth & C. W. Mills (Eds.). New York: Oxford University Press.

How Nursing Care Is Delivered

Types of Nursing Care Delivery Systems

Functional Nursing
Team Nursing
Total Patient Care
Primary Nursing
Practice Partnerships
Case Management
Critical Pathways
Differentiated Practice
Patient-Centered Care

Looking Ahead

Previous chapters have focused on understanding the environment in which nurses work, from the fundamental infrastructure of organizations to the effects of changes in health care on the roles of nurses and nurse managers. This chapter focuses on the way nursing care is delivered. Different types of nursing care delivery systems exist to provide structure to nursing care delivery. As the health care industry changes and restructuring occurs, nurses face the challenge of modifying existing methods to use fewer resources effectively.

Objectives

In this chapter, you will learn

- How the delivery system structures nursing care.
- What types of nursing care delivery systems exist.
- What the positive and negative aspects of different systems are.
- What new types of delivery systems have emerged.
- What skills are required to use the system effectively.

MediaLink www.prenhall.com/ sullivan-decker

Additional resources for this chapter can be found on the Companion Website at www.prenhall.com/ sullivan-decker. Click on "Chapter 3" to select the activities for this chapter.

- NCLEX Review
- Critical Thinking Activities
- Current Events
- MediaLinks
- *Nursing Leadership & Management in Action*: Comparing Nursing Care Delivery Systems

One of the significant issues challenging nursing is the way in which nursing care is delivered. The essence of providing nursing care revolves around the work environment and culture, the type of nursing care delivery system, and staffing and scheduling practices, especially as they relate to the results of workload calculations from patient classification systems. Pressures from many sources, all centered on an overall expectation to reduce the cost of care, enhance efficiency, and maintain quality, affect the organization of nursing care. This chapter describes how nursing care is organized to ensure quality care in an era of cost containment.

Types of Nursing Care Delivery Systems

The purpose of a nursing care delivery system is to provide a structure that enables nurses to deliver nursing care to a specified group of patients. The delivery of care includes assessing care needs, formulating a plan of care, implementing the plan, and evaluating the patient's responses to interventions.

Since World War II, nursing care delivery systems have undergone continuous and significant changes (Box 3-1). Over the years, various nursing care delivery systems have been critiqued. Debates regarding the pros and cons of each method have focused on identifying the perfect delivery system for providing nursing care to patients with varying needs of intensity of care. This ongoing evaluation has been spurred by changes in availability of nursing personnel, reductions in reimbursement for patient care and hospital revenue, changes in acuity levels of patients, shorter lengths of stay, demands by health care consumers for quality care at a reduced rate, and demands by nurses, physicians, and other health care professionals for more effective delivery systems. The major challenges of any nursing care delivery system include effectiveness, cost efficiency, quality, and the needs of consumers and practitioners.

No delivery system is perfect. Most organizations use a combination or modification of various nursing care delivery systems to meet the unique demands of different patient care units. Before adopting any nursing care delivery system, the nursing organization must consider its goals, characteristics, and needs; the demands placed on it; and the cost of the nursing care delivery system.

Functional Nursing

Functional nursing, also called task nursing (Figure 3-1), began in hospitals in the mid-1940s in response to a national nursing shortage. The number of registered nurses (RNs) serving in the armed forces during World

(sidebar, left margin:) MEDIALINK ◆ American Nurses Association

(sidebar, left margin:) MEDIALINK ◆ Comparing Nursing Care Delivery Systems

---

Box 3-1   Job Description of a Floor Nurse (1887)

Developed in 1887 and published in a magazine of Cleveland Lutheran Hospital.

In addition to caring for your 50 patients, each nurse will follow these regulations:

1. Daily sweep and mop the floors of your ward, dust the patients' furniture and window sills.

2. Maintain an even temperature in your ward by bringing in a scuttle of coal for the day's business.

3. Light is important to observe the patient's condition. Therefore, each day fill kerosene lamps, clean chimneys, and trim wicks. Wash windows once a week.

4. The nurse's notes are important to aiding the physician's work. Make your pens carefully. You may whittle nibs to your individual taste.

5. Each nurse on day duty will report every day at 7 A.M. and leave at 8 P.M., except on the Sabbath, on which you will be off from 12 noon to 2 P.M.

6. Graduate nurses in good standing with the Director of Nurses will be given an evening off each week for courting purposes, or two evenings a week if you go regularly to church.

7. Each nurse should lay aside from each pay a goodly sum of her earnings for her benefits during her declining years, so that she will not become a burden. For example, if you earn $30 a month you should set aside $15.

8. Any nurse who smokes, uses liquor in any form, gets her hair done at a beauty shop, or frequents dance halls will give the Director of Nurses good reason to suspect her worth, intentions, and integrity.

9. The nurse who performs her labor, serves her patients and doctors faithfully and without fault for a period of five years will be given an increase by the hospital administration of five cents a day providing there are no hospital debts that are outstanding.

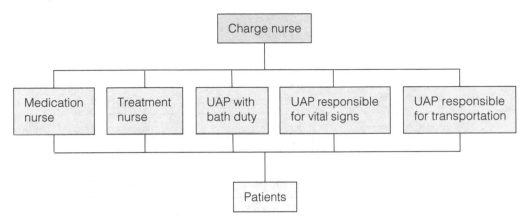

Figure 3-1   Functional nursing.

War II depleted the supply of nurses at home. As a result of this loss of RNs, the composition of nursing staffs in hospitals changed; staffs composed almost entirely of RNs gave way to widespread use of licensed practical nurses (LPNs) and unlicensed assistive personnel (UAPs) to deliver nursing care.

In functional nursing, the needs of a group of patients are broken down into tasks. Tasks are assigned to RNs, LPNs, or UAPs so that the skill and licensure of each caregiver is used to the best advantage. An RN assesses patients whereas others give baths, make beds, take vital signs, administer treatments, and so forth.

The advantage of this system is that all employees, even UAPs, become very efficient and effective at performing their regular assigned tasks. However, these personnel are likely to be less effective and efficient if assigned to another task.

Other disadvantages of functional nursing include

- Uneven continuity of care,
- Absence of a holistic view of the patient,
- Time-consuming communications, and
- Problems with follow-up.

Today, functional nursing care is used infrequently in acute care facilities and only occasionally in long-term–care facilities.

Team Nursing

Team nursing (Figure 3-2) remains the most common nursing care delivery system in the United States in acute as well as long-term–care settings. Historically, team nursing evolved from functional nursing and has remained popular since the middle to late 1940s. Under this system, a team of nursing personnel provides total patient care to a group of patients. In some instances, a team may be assigned a certain number of patients; in others, the assigned patients may be grouped by diagnoses or provider services.

Modular nursing is a modification of team nursing that tries to enhance the effectiveness of the team concept by assigning a module that is confined to a limited geographic area. The size of the module varies according to physical layout of the unit, patient acuity, and nursing skill mix. The team or module is led by an RN and may include other RNs, LPNs, and UAPs. Team members provide patient care under the direction of the team (module) leader. The team, acting as a unified whole, has a holistic perspective of the needs of each patient. The team speaks for each patient through the team (module) leader.

Typically, the team (module) leader's time is spent in indirect patient care activities, such as

- Developing or updating nursing care plans,
- Resolving problems encountered by team (module) members,
- Conducting nursing care conferences, and
- Communicating with physicians and other health care personnel.

KEY TERMS

Functional nursing   A nursing care delivery system in which the needs of patients are broken down into tasks and assigned to caregivers.

Team nursing   The most common delivery system; nursing staff are divided into teams, which are responsible for the care of a group of patients.

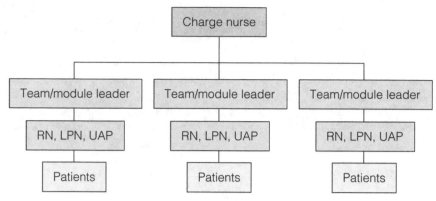

Figure 3-2   Team/modular nursing.

With team or modular nursing, the unit nurse manager consults with team leaders, supervises patient care teams, and may make rounds with all physicians. To be effective, team nursing requires that all team members have good communication skills. A key aspect of team nursing is the nursing care conference, where the team leader reviews with all team members each patient's plan of care and progress. An advantage of team nursing is that it allows the use of less prepared staff members (LPNs and UAPs) to carry out some functions (e.g., making beds, transporting patients, collecting some data) that do not require the expertise of an RN. Another advantage of team nursing is that it allows patient care needs requiring more than one staff member, such as patient transfers from bed to chair, to be easily coordinated.

Team or modular nursing has several negative features. First, a large amount of time is required for the team leader to maintain effective communication for team planning, supervising, and coordinating the care provided by all team members. Second, continuity of care may be diminished because of day-to-day changes in team members and leaders, as well as the group of patients assigned to the team. Third, because each member of the team is assigned specific tasks for the patient and no one considers the total patient, team or modular nursing does not allow for a holistic view of the patient.

Role confusion and resentment are other potential problems. The UAPs and licensed team members may view the role of the team leader as more focused toward paperwork and less directed at the physical or real needs of the patient.

Skills in delegating, communicating, and problem solving are essential for a team leader to be effective. Open communication between team leaders and the nurse manager also is important to avoid duplication of effort, overriding of delegated assignments, or competition for control or power. Problems in delegation and communication are the most common reasons why team nursing is less effective than it theoretically could be.

Although the geographical boundaries of modular nursing help save steps and time, these same boundaries pose an additional problem: Nurses have decreased control over their assignments. As a result, the assignments may be unequal if they are based on patient acuity or monotonous if nurses continuously care for patients with similar conditions (e.g., all patients with hip replacements).

Total Patient Care

The original model of nursing care delivery was **total patient care,** also called case method (Figure 3-3), in which a registered nurse was responsible for all aspects of the care of one or more patients. During the 1920s, total patient care was the typical nursing care delivery system. Student nurses often staffed hospitals, whereas RNs provided total care to the patient at home. In total

---

KEY TERMS

Total patient care   The original model of nursing care delivery, in which one RN is responsible for all aspects of one or more patients' care.

Primary nursing   A nursing care delivery system in which one nurse is responsible and accountable for the nursing care of specific patients for the duration of their stay.

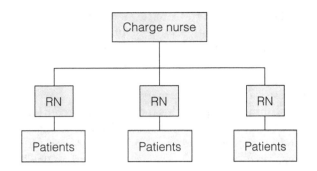

Figure 3-3   Total patient care.

patient care, RNs work directly with the patient, family, physician, and other health care staff in implementing a plan of care.

The goal of this delivery system is to have one nurse give all care to the same patient(s) for the entire shift. Total patient care delivery systems are typically used in areas requiring a high level of nursing expertise, such as in critical care units or postanesthesia recovery areas.

The advantages of a total patient care system include

- Continuous, holistic, expert nursing care;
- Total accountability for the nursing care of the assigned patient(s) for that shift; and
- Continuity of communication with the patient, family, physician(s), and staff from other departments.

The disadvantage of this system is that RNs spend some time doing tasks that could be done more cost-effectively by less skilled persons. This inefficiency adds to the expense of using a total patient care delivery system.

Primary Nursing

Conceptualized by Marie Manthey and implemented during the late 1960s after two decades of team nursing, **primary nursing** (Figure 3-4) was designed to place the registered nurse back at the patient's bedside (Manthey, 1980). Decentralized decision making by staff nurses is the core principle of primary nursing, with responsibility and authority for nursing care allocated to staff nurses at the bedside. Primary nursing recognized that nursing was a knowledge-based professional practice, not just a task-focused activity.

In primary nursing, the RN maintains a patient load of primary patients. A primary nurse designs, implements, and is accountable for the nursing care of patients in the patient load for the duration of the patient's stay on the unit. Actual care is given by the primary nurse and/or associate nurses (other RNs).

Primary nursing advanced the professional practice of nursing significantly because it provided

- A knowledge-based practice model;
- Decentralization of nursing care decisions, authority, and responsibility to the staff nurse;
- 24-hour accountability for nursing care activities by one nurse;
- Improved continuity and coordination of care; and
- Increased nurse, patient, and physician satisfaction.

Disadvantages also exist. Primary nursing requires excellent communication between the primary nurse and associate nurses. Primary nurses must be able to hold associate nurses accountable for implementing the nursing care as prescribed. Because of transfers to different units, critically ill patients may have several primary care nurses, disrupting the continuity of care inherent in the model.

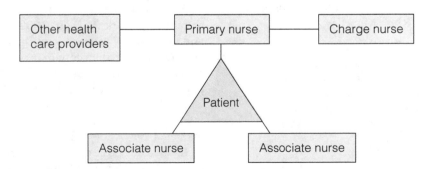

Figure 3-4   Primary nursing.

Although the concept of 24-hour accountability is worthwhile, it is a fallacy. Staff nurses are neither compensated nor legally responsible for patient care outside their hours of work. Another difficulty is the unwillingness of associates to take direction from the primary nurse. Lastly, when primary nursing was first implemented, many organizations perceived that it required an all RN staff. This practice was viewed as not only expensive but also ineffective because many tasks could be done by less skilled persons. As a result, many hospitals discontinued the use of primary nursing. Other hospitals successfully implemented primary nursing by identifying one nurse who was assigned to coordinate care and with whom the family and physician could communicate, and other nurses or unlicensed assistive personnel assisted this nurse in providing care.

Practice Partnerships

The **practice partnership** (Figure 3-5) is a more recent concept also introduced by Marie Manthey (1989). Practice partnerships can be applied to primary nursing and used in other nursing care delivery systems, such as team nursing, modular nursing, and total patient care. As organizations downsized and reduced salary budgets, practice partnerships offered an efficient way of using the skills of a mix of professional and nonprofessional staff with differing levels of expertise.

In the practice partnership model, an RN and an assistant—UAP, LPN, or less experienced RN—agree to be practice partners. The partners work together with the same schedule and the same group of patients. The senior RN partner directs the work of the junior partner within the limits of each partner's skill set and the limits in the state's nurse practice act.

The relationship between the senior and junior partner is designed to create synergistic energy as the two work in concert with patients. The senior partner performs selected patient care activities but delegates less specialized activities to the junior partner. The partners can achieve the workload or outcomes that previously were achieved by two RNs (Manthey, 1989).

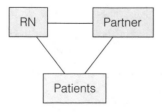

Figure 3-5   Practice partnerships.

When compared to team or modular nursing, practice partnerships offer more continuity of care and accountability for patient care. When compared to total patient care or primary nursing, partnerships are less expensive for the organization and more satisfying professionally for the partners.

One disadvantage of this model is that organizations tend to increase the number of UAPs and decrease the ratio of professional nurses to nonprofessional staff. If, for example, one UAP is assigned to more than one RN, the UAP must follow the instructions of several people, making a synergistic relationship with any one of them difficult. Another problem is the potential for the junior member of the team to assume more responsibility than appropriate. Senior partners must take caution not to delegate inappropriate tasks to junior partners.

Case Management

Following the introduction and impact of prospective payment, nursing case management, used for decades in community and psychiatric settings, was adopted for acute inpatient care. Nursing **case management** (Figure 3-6) is a model for identifying, coordinating, and monitoring the implementation of services needed to achieve desired patient care outcomes within a specified period of time (Zander, 1988). Nursing case management organizes patient care by major diagnoses or diagnosis-related groups (DRGs) and focuses on attaining predetermined patient outcomes within specific time frames and resources.

The essential elements of nursing case management are

- Collaboration of all health care members,
- Identification of expected patient outcomes with time frames,
- Use of principles of continuous quality improvement (CQI) and variance analysis, and
- Promotion of professional practice.

Case management has been particularly successful with disability management, helping injured employees to return to work (Salazar, 2000). Likewise home care and ambulatory settings lend themselves to case management as well. The case manager, who may be called a care coordinator, usually does not provide direct patient care but rather supervises the care provided by licensed and unlicensed nursing personnel. Patient involvement and participation is key to successful case management (Aliotta, 2002).

In an acute care setting the case manager has a caseload of 10 to 15 patients and follows patients' progress through the system from admission to discharge,

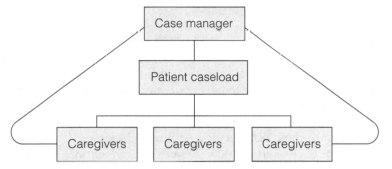

Figure 3-6   Case management.

accounting for variances from expected progress. One or more nursing case managers on a patient care unit may coordinate, communicate, collaborate, problem solve, and facilitate patient care for a group of patients. Ideally, nursing case managers have advanced degrees and considerable experience in nursing.

After a specific patient population is selected to be "case managed," a collaborative practice team is established. The team, which includes clinical experts from appropriate disciplines (e.g., nursing, medicine, physical therapy) needed for the selected patient population, defines the expected outcomes of care for the patient population. Based on expected patient outcomes, each member of the team, using his or her discipline's contribution, helps determine appropriate interventions within a specified time frame.

To initiate case management, specific patient diagnoses that represent high-volume, high-cost, and high-risk cases are selected. High-volume cases are those that occur frequently, such as total hip replacements on an orthopedic floor. High-risk cases include patients or case types who have complications, stay in a critical care unit longer than 2 days, or require ventilatory support. Patients also may be selected because they are treated by one particular physician who supports case management. Whatever patient population is selected, base-line data must be collected and analyzed first. These data provide the information necessary to measure the effectiveness of case management. Essential base-line data include length of stay, cost of care, and complication information.

Five elements are essential to successful implementation of case management. These are

- Support by key members of the organization (administrators, physicians, nurses),
- Selection of a qualified nurse case manager,
- Collaborative practice teams,
- A quality management system, and
- Established critical pathways.

In case management, all professionals are equal members of the team; thus, one group does not determine interventions for other disciplines. All members of the collaborative practice team agree on the final draft of the critical pathways, take ownership of patient outcomes, and accept responsibility and accountability for the interventions and patient outcomes associated with their discipline. The emphasis must be on managing interdisciplinary outcomes and building consensus with physicians. In addition, outcomes must be specified in measurable terms.

Case management has contributed to a reduction in complications (Taunton, Kleinbeck, Stafford, Woods, & Bott, 1994), reduced cost (Cohen, 1991; Mahn, 1993), increased collaboration (Baggs, Ryan, Phelps, Richeson, & Johnson, 1992; Kimball, 1993), and improved quality of care (Lumsdon & Hagland, 1993).

Critical Pathways

Successful case management relies on **critical pathways** to guide care. The term *critical path* refers to the expected outcomes and care strategies developed by

---

KEY TERMS

Practice partnership   A nursing care delivery system in which senior and junior staff members share patient care responsibilities.

Case management   A model for identifying, coordinating, and monitoring the implementation of services needed to achieve desired patient care outcomes within a specified period of time.

Critical pathways   Tools or guidelines that direct care by identifying expected outcomes.

the collaborative practice team. Again, interdisciplinary consensus must be reached and specific, measurable outcomes determined.

Critical paths provide direction for managing the care of a specific patient during a specified time period. Critical paths are useful because they accommodate the unique characteristics of the patient and the patient's condition. Critical paths use resources appropriate to the care needed and, thus, reduce cost and length of stay (Middleton & Roberts, 2000; Rohrbach, 1999). Critical paths are used in every setting where health care is delivered (National Association of Clinical Nurse Specialists [NACNS], 1998).

A critical path quickly orients the staff to the outcomes that should be achieved for the patient for that day. Nursing diagnoses identify the outcomes needed. If patient outcomes are not achieved, the case manager is notified and the situation analyzed to determine how to modify the critical path.

Altering time frames or interventions is categorized as a variance, and the case manager tracks all variances. After a time, the appropriate collaborative practice teams analyze the variances, note trends, and decide how to manage them. The critical pathway may need to be revised or additional data may be needed before changes are made.

Some features are included on all critical paths, such as specific medical diagnosis, the expected length of stay, patient identification data, appropriate time frames (in days, hours, minutes, or visits) for interventions, and patient outcomes. Interventions are presented in modality groups (medications, nursing activity, and so on). The critical path must include a means to identify variances easily and to determine whether the outcome has been met.

Table 3-1 is an example of a collaborative critical path for patients having a total hip replacement. Normally a patient would be expected to be discharged on the sixth day after surgery. This path describes expectations for days 1 through 3.

A recent evolution of critical paths is the incorporation of actual and potential nursing diagnoses with specific time frames into the critical pathway (the lower section of Table 3-1). Education paths are also excellent tools for planning patient and family education (Table 3-2). A copy of this form is given to the patient and the family, and the nurse reviews the

---

Table 3-1   Critical Path with Actual/Potential Nursing Diagnoses for Total Hip Replacement

Collaborative Critical Path
Case Type: Total Hip Replacement

Patient Name: _____

Record Number: _____

DRG: <u>209</u>

Expected LOS: <u>6 days</u>

	Day 1 / OR	Y/N	Day 2 / Postoperative Day 1	Y/N	Day 3 / Postoperative Day 2	Y/N
Patient Activity	Bed rest	—	Begin mobility plan;	—	Cont mobility plan	—
	T-DB q2h	—	T-DB q2h	—	T-DB q2h	—
	Initiate skin protection protocol	—	Cont skin protection protocol	—	Cont skin protection protocol	—
Nursing	VS qh × 4, then q4h	— —	VS q4h	—	VS q8h	—
	Assess cir/neuro legs qh × 4, then q4h	— —	Assess cir/neuro q4h	—	D/C assessment	—
	Check drainage/ Hemovac qh × 4, then q4h;	— —	Check drainage/ Hemovac q4h	—	D/C Hemovac; Check drainage q8h	—
	I & O (Foley/ Hemovac) q8h;	—	I & O (Foley/ Hemovac) q8h	—	I & O q8h	—
	Thigh-hi elastic hose	—	Cont elastic hose	—	D/C Foley; urinates within 8h	—
					Cont elastic hose	—

Table 3-1   Continued

	Day 1		Day 2		Day 3	
Medications	Antibiotic	—	Cont antibiotic	—	Cont antibiotic	—
	Pain control:		Cont pain control	—	PO pain control	—
	PCA pump	—				
	Stool softener	—	Cont stool softener	—	Cont stool softener	—
	Cont home Rx;	—	Cont home Rx	—	Cont home Rx	—
	IVs	—	IVs cont	—	IV to heparin lock	—
			Coumadin	—	Cont coumadin	—
			Sleeping Rx	—	Sleeping Rx	—
Physical Therapy	Preop instructions	—	Evaluate mobility progress	—	Evaluate mobility progress	—
Diagnostic Tests	H & H 2h postop	—	H & H	—	Prothrombin time	—
			Prothrombin time	—		
Nutrition	NPO—Cl liq as tol	—	Diet as tolerated	—	Diet as tolerated	—
Teaching	*Preop:* Pain control	—	Repeat teaching		Repeat teaching	
	Use of assist devices	—	if nec	—	if nec	—
	Gait control	—				
	Incentive spirometry	—				
	Mobility plan	—				
	Pt/family crit plan given & reviewed	—	Review pt/family crit plan if nec	—	Review pt/family crit plan if nec	—
Discharge Plan	SNU evaluation	—			Review transfer discharge needs	—
	Home Health evaluation	—				

Patient Problems and Outcomes for Total Hip Replacement

Nursing Diagnosis	Day 1 / OR	Y/N	Day 2 / Postoperative Day 1	Y/N	Day 3 / Postoperative Day 2	Y/N
Knowledge deficit: medications; use of assistive devices; treatments	Appropriately uses: PCA pump, incentive spirometry, assistive devices; Verbalizes mobility plan	— — —	Uses all devices appropriately	—	Verbalizes additions to care	—
Pain related to surgery, physical injury	Pain managed	—	Pain managed	—	Pain managed	—
Risk for infection related to invasive procedures, immobility	Remains afebrile No skin breakdown	— —	Remains afebrile No skin breakdown	— —	Remains afebrile	—
Impaired physical mobility related to surgery, prosthesis	Verbalizes mobility plan Verbalizes role of staff providing assistance	— —	Meeting mobility expectations	—	Participates in transfer/discharge plans, decisions	—
Risk for injury related to altered tissue perfusion, altered mobility, and prosthesis	Explains need for frequent assessments Verbalizes need for early mobility and hose	— —	Circulation to extremities good Leg maintained in proper alignment	— —	Circulation to extremities normal; Leg in proper alignment	—

Table 3-2   Patient/Family Education Path for Total Hip Replacement

	Day 1 / OR	Day 2 / Postoperative Day 1	Day 3 / Postoperative Day 2
Unit	Admission process; surgery & recovery areas; then Orthopedic Unit	Orthopedic Unit	Orthopedic Unit (Possible transfer next day to SNU or Rehab Unit)
Patient Activity and Safety Issues	Bed rest first 24 h; leg exercises qh (q4h); T-DB q2h; explain skin protection plan; give copy of mobility plan; assist c̄ bath; thigh-hi elastic support hose	Up in chair c̄ help; Leg exercises q2h; T-DB q2h; cont skin protect plan; cont mobility plan; assist c̄ bath; cont thigh-hi elastic support hose	Up in chair and walking as outlined in mobility plan; T-DB q2h; cont skin protection plan; assist c̄ bath; cont thigh-hi elastic support hose
Nursing Care	Frequency of taking vital signs (BP-P-R-T); check drainage on dressing; check circulation and sensations to legs; intake & output measured q8h; Foley and Hemovac in for 48 h	Vital sign checks q4h; dressing, circulation, and sensation checks to legs q4h; I & O (Foley and Hemovac) measured q8h	Vital sign checks q8h; D/C Foley and Hemovac; I & O q8h; urinate within 8 h; D/C dressing, circulation, and sensation checks to legs
Medications	Verify list of home Rx so physician can order; pain medication and PCA pump; IVs and need for arm restraint; other drugs that will be ordered (e.g., antibiotics; stool softener)	Cont pain management c̄ PCA pump; IVs; cont arm restraint; cont antibiotic and other drugs (sleeping assistance)	Oral pain management; IV to heparin lock; cont antibiotic and other drugs
Diet	NPO before OR; clear liquids, ice chips	Diet as tolerated	Diet as tolerated
Tests	Blood test: Hemoglobin and hematocrit 2 h after OR	Blood tests: H & H and prothrombin time	Blood test: prothrombin time
Teaching	Pain management; use of assistive devices (trapeze, walker) and incentive spirometry; mobility plan reviewed: how to transfer from bed to chair, and so on	Clarify questions	Clarify questions
Discharge Plan	Discuss purpose of Skilled Nursing Unit and Rehab Unit; identify need for Home Health Service after discharge	Cont with discussion of SNU, Rehab, and Home Health Services	Clarify questions and needs with transfer/discharge plans

information with them. Thus, both the patient and the family know what to expect during an anticipated, uncomplicated hospitalization.

Differentiated Practice

Differentiated practice is a method that maximizes nursing resources by focusing on the structure of roles and functions of nurses according to their education, experience, and competence. Differentiated practice is designed to identify distinct levels of nursing practice based on defined abilities that are incorporated into job descriptions.

In differentiated practice, the responsibilities of RNs (mainly those with bachelor's and associate degrees) differ according to the competence and training associated with the two education levels as well as the nurses' experience and preferences. The scope of nursing practice and level of responsibility are specifically defined for each level. Some organizations differentiate roles, responsibilities, and tasks for professional nurses, licensed practical nurses, and unlicensed assistive personnel, which are incorporated into their respective job descriptions.

Differentiated practice models have been used in a variety of inpatient, acute care settings as well as in home care and clinics. Differentiated practice improves patient care and contributes to patient safety, allows for the most effective and efficient use of scarce resources, offers increased satisfaction for nurses, and provides opportunity to compensate nurses fairly based on their expertise, contributions, and productivity (American Association of Colleges of Nursing [AACN], 2002). Differentiated practice is especially important to maintain quality of care, ensure patient outcomes, and address personnel budget concerns.

Patient-Centered Care

Patient-centered care is a model of nursing care delivery in which the role of the nurse is broadened to coordinate a team of multifunctional unit-based caregivers (Redman & Jones, 1998). In patient-centered care, all patient care services are unit-based, including admission and discharge, diagnostic and treatment services, and support services, such as environmental and nutrition services and medical records. The focus of patient-centered care is decentralization, the promotion of efficiency and quality, and cost control.

In this model of care the number of caregivers at the bedside is reduced, but their responsibilities are increased so that service and waiting times are decreased. A typical team in a unit providing patient-centered care consists of

- Patient care coordinators (RNs);
- Patient care associates or technicians who are able to perform delegated patient care tasks;

- Unit support assistants who provide environmental services and can assist with hygiene and ambulation needs;
- Administrative support personnel who maintain patient records, transcribe orders, coordinate admission and discharge, and assist with general office duties; and
- A nurse manager (Redman & Jones, 1998).

The patient-centered care model also may be used in outpatient and home care settings. Patients with chronic conditions are appropriate candidates for patient-centered care approaches, including the use of complementary and alternative medicine therapies (Parkman, 2000).

This model greatly affects the role of the nurse manager. Staff and management issues consume a greater proportion of the manager's time. No longer is the manager doing rounds and assisting with patient care. Instead, being responsible for a staff that is more diverse with fewer professional RN staff demands a strong leader proficient in interviewing, hiring, training, and motivating. Some organizations share assistive staff between units, also increasing the need for more communication and coordination with other managers.

What You Know Now

- Nursing care delivery systems provide a structure for nursing care. Most organizations use a combination of nursing care delivery systems or modify one or more systems to meet their own needs.
- The most commonly used nursing care delivery systems are team nursing, total patient care, and primary nursing.
- Case management is a collaborative patient care system that uses case managers (RNs) who are responsible for facilitating patient interventions and achieving patient outcomes from admission to discharge.
- Critical paths are used to designate specific patient outcomes within specified time frames.
- Differentiated practice and patient-centered care are two systems that use nurses and support personnel based on expertise of staff and needs of patients.

Questions to Challenge You

1. Describe the patient care delivery system(s) at your place of work or clinical placement site. How functional is it? Can you suggest a better system?
2. Pretend that you are designing a new nursing care

delivery system. Select the system or combination of systems you would use. Explain your rationale.

3. As a manager, which system would you prefer? Why?

Explore ⊕ MediaLink

NCLEX review questions, essay activities, group activities, and other interactive resources for this chapter can be found on the Web site at http://www.prenhall.com/sullivan-decker. Click on "Chapter 3" to select activities for this chapter.

References

Aliotta, S. (2002). Direct outcomes of case management: Involvement/participation, empowerment, and knowledge. *Case Manager, 13*(4), 67–71.

American Association of Colleges of Nursing. (2002). Hallmarks of the professional nursing practice environment. *Journal of Professional Nursing, 18*(5), 295–304.

Baggs, J. G., Ryan, S. A., Phelps, C. E., Richeson, J. F., & Johnson, J. E. (1992). The association between interdisciplinary collaboration and patient outcomes in a medical intensive care unit. *Heart & Lung, 21*(1), 18–24.

Cohen, E. L. (1991). Nursing case management: Does it pay? *Journal of Nursing Administration, 21*(4), 20–25.

Kimball, L. (1993). Collaborative care: A quality improvement and cost reduction tool. *Journal of Hospital Quarterly, 15*(4), 6–9.

Lumsdon, K., & Hagland, M. (1993). Mapping care. *Hospitals & Health Networks, 67*(20), 34–40.

Mahn, V. A. (1993). Clinical nurse case management: A service-line approach. *Nursing Management, 24*(9), 48–50.

Manthey, M. (1980). *The practice of primary nursing.* St. Louis: Mosby.

Manthey, M. (1989). Practice partnerships: The newest concept in care delivery. *Journal of Nursing Association, 19*(2), 33–35.

Middleton, S., & Roberts, A. (2000). *Integrated care pathways: A practical approach to implementation.* Oxford: Butterworth Heinemann.

National Association of Clinical Nurse Specialists. (1998). *Statement on clinical nurse specialist practice and education.* Glenview, IL: Author.

Parkman, C. A. (2000). The patient-centered plan of care. *Case Manager, 11*(6), 25–27.

Redman, R., & Jones, K. (1998). Effects of implementing patient-centered care models on nurse and non-nurse managers. *Journal of Nursing Administration, 28*(11), 46–53.

Rohrbach, J. I. (1999). Critical pathways as an essential part of a disease management program. *Journal of Nursing Care Quality, 14*(1), 11–15.

Salazar, M. K. (2000). Maximizing the effectiveness of case management service delivery. *Case Manager, 11*(3), 58–63.

Taunton, R. L., Kleinbeck, S. V. M., Stafford, R., Woods, C. Q., & Bott, M. J. (1994). Patient outcomes: Are they linked to registered nurse absenteeism, separation, or work load? *Journal of Nursing Administration, 24*(4S), 48–55.

Zander, K. (1988). Nursing case management. *Nursing Clinics of North America, 23*(3), 503–520.

Leading and Managing

Looking Ahead

What is the relationship between leaders and managers? What are the differences and similarities? How does leadership fit into these roles? This chapter provides an in-depth look at theories of leadership and general management functions. Building on these concepts, the chapter explores the roles and functions of nurses in management and describes the various levels of management.

Objectives

In this chapter, you will learn

- Why every nurse is a manager and can be a leader.

- What the difference between leaders and managers is.
- How different theories explain leadership.
- How different theories explain management.
- How levels of management interact.

MediaLink 🌐 www.prenhall.com/sullivan-decker

Additional resources for this chapter can be found on the Companion Website at www.prenhall.com/sullivan-decker. Click on "Chapter 4" to select the activities for this chapter.

- NCLEX Review
- Critical Thinking Activities
- Current Events
- MediaLinks
- *Nursing Leadership & Management in Action:* Recognizing Contemporary Leadership Styles; Contrasting Management Responsibilities in Nursing; Identifying Nurse Manager Functions

Managers are essential to any organization. A manager's functions are vital, complex, and frequently difficult. They must be directed toward balancing the needs of patients, the health care organization, employees, physicians, and self. Nurse managers need a body of knowledge and skills distinctly different from those needed for nursing practice, yet few nurses have the education or training necessary to be managers. Frequently, managers depend on experiences with former supervisors, who also learned supervisory techniques "in the trenches." Often a gap exists between what managers know and what they need to know.

Today, all nurses are managers, not in the formal organizational sense but in practice. They direct the work of nonprofessionals and professionals in order to achieve desired outcomes in patient care. As such, all nurses need to learn leadership and management skills to be more efficient and effective.

This chapter delineates the difference between leaders and managers, explains leadership and management theories, describes management levels in nursing, and discusses the roles and functions of nursing management.

Leaders and Managers

Manager, leader, supervisor, and *administrator* are often used interchangeably, yet they are not the same. A **leader** is anyone who uses interpersonal skills to influence others to accomplish a specific goal. The leader exerts influence by using a flexible repertoire of personal behaviors and strategies. The leader is important in forging links—creating connections—among an organization's members to promote high levels of performance and quality outcomes. Antrobus and Kitson (1999) found that leaders are skilled in empowering others, creating meaning and facilitating learning, developing knowledge, thinking reflectively, communicating, solving problems, making decisions, and working with others. Leaders generate excitement; they clearly define their purpose and mission. Leaders understand people and their needs; they recognize and appreciate differences in people, individualizing their approach as needed.

Leaders also have the capacity to earn and hold trust. They have a genuine concern for others and help others achieve their potential (Kerfoot, 2000). Leadership is relationship management. The organizational structure heterarchy, described by Porter-O'Grady and Malloch (2002) and displayed in Figure 2-13 (see Chapter 2), exemplifies the importance of the leader's relationship skills.

Leadership requires attending to and acknowledging others and being personally authentic and accountable (Lewin & Regine, 2000). The leader must have enthusiasm, energy, and commitment, but most of all, the leader must be able to inspire others to commit to the goals of the organization.

The functions of a leader are to achieve a consensus within the group about its goals, maintain a structure that facilitates accomplishing the goals, supply necessary information that helps provide direction and clarification, and maintain group satisfaction, cohesion, and performance.

A **manager**, in contrast, is an individual employed by an organization who is responsible and accountable for efficiently accomplishing the goals of the organization. Managers focus on coordinating and integrating resources, using the functions of planning, organizing, supervising, staffing, evaluating, negotiating, and representing. Interpersonal skill is important, but a manager also has authority, responsibility, accountability, and power defined by the organization. The manager's job is to

- Clarify the organizational structure,
- Choose the means by which to achieve goals,
- Assign and coordinate tasks, developing and motivating as needed, and
- Evaluate outcomes and provide feedback.

All good managers are also good leaders—the two go hand in hand. However, one may be a good manager of resources and not be much of a leader of people. Likewise, a person who is a good leader may not manage well. Both roles can be learned; skills gained can enhance either role.

Leadership

Leadership may be formal or informal. Leadership is **formal** when practiced by a nurse with legitimate authority conferred by the organization and described in a job description (e.g., nurse manager, supervisor, coordinator, case manager). Formal leadership also depends on personal skills, but it may be reinforced by organizational authority and position. Insightful formal leaders recognize the importance of their own informal leadership activities and the informal leadership of others who affect the work in their areas of responsibility.

Leadership is **informal** when exercised by a staff member who does not have a specified management role. A nurse whose thoughtful and convincing ideas substantially influence the efficiency of work flow is exercising leadership skills. Informal leadership depends primarily on one's knowledge, status (e.g., advanced practice nurse, quality improvement coordinator, education specialist, medical director), and personal skills in persuading and guiding others.

Leadership Theories

Most students of leadership find the search for definitive explanations of leadership effectiveness both fascinating and puzzling. Research on leadership has a long history, but the focus has shifted over time from personal traits to behavior and style, to the leadership situation, to change agency (the capacity to transform), and to other aspects of leadership. Each phase and focus of research has contributed to managers' insights and understandings about leadership and its development. This chapter discusses four categories of leadership theories: trait theories, behavioral theories, contingency theories, and contemporary theories.

Trait Theories

Studies conducted during the first seven decades of the 1900s were leader-centered and focused on defining what leaders are. Researchers sought to identify inborn traits of successful leaders. Attempts to specify a universal set of leadership characteristics produced ambiguous results. However, Stogdill (1974) developed a profile of successful leaders and traits.

Bass (1990) added more traits, which he classified into three categories: intelligence, personality, abilities. Gilbert (1975), in examining the personalities of nursing graduate students, found that potential leaders were more likely to exhibit traits such as dominance, aggressiveness, ambition, high capacity to attain status, poise, self-confidence, tolerance for others' views, high need to achieve, orderly thinking, sensitivity to others, and flexibility. Although inconclusive, these early attempts to specify unique leadership traits provided benchmarks by which most leaders continue to be judged.

Behavioral Theories

Research on leadership in the early 1930s focused on the abilities and behaviors of leaders, that is, what leaders do. In the behavioral view of leadership, personal traits provide only a foundation for leadership; real leaders are made through education, training, and life experiences.

Leadership Styles Behavior-based theories assume that effective leaders acquire a pattern of learned behaviors. Initial studies of teams of teenage boys identified three patterns or *styles* of leadership: autocratic, democratic, and laissez-faire (Lewin & Lippit, 1938; Lewin, Lippit, & White, 1939). The **autocratic leadership** style assumes that individuals are motivated by external forces, such as power, authority, and need for

---

KEY TERMS

Leader Someone who uses interpersonal skills to influence others to accomplish specific goals.

Manager An individual employed by an organization who is responsible for efficiently accomplishing the goals of the organization.

Formal leadership Leadership that is exercised by an individual with legitimate authority conferred by position within the organization.

Informal leadership Leadership that is exercised by an individual who does not have a specified management role.

approval; the leader makes all the decisions and uses coercion, punishment, and direction to change followers' behavior and achieve results.

The **democratic leadership** style assumes that individuals are motivated by internal drives and impulses, want active participation in decisions, and want to get the task done; the leader uses participation and majority rule in setting goals and working toward achievement. The **laissez-faire leadership** style also assumes that individuals are motivated by internal drives and impulses and that they need to be left alone to make decisions about how to complete the work; the leader provides no direction or facilitation.

Jenkins and Henderson (1984) added a fourth style, the **bureaucratic leadership** style. The bureaucrat assumes that employees are motivated by external forces. This leader trusts neither followers nor self to make decisions and therefore relies on organizational policies and rules to identify goals and direct work processes. Table 4-1 compares the four leadership styles.

By the early 1950s, leadership styles in work settings began to be explored (Katz & Kahn, 1952; Stogdill & Coons, 1957). Two major dimensions of behavioral style were identified: initiating structure and consideration. *Initiating structure* refers to the behaviors that managers use to organize and define the goals of work, work patterns and methods, channels of communication, and roles. For example, administration develops a manual of

---

KEY TERMS

Autocratic leadership   A leadership style that assumes individuals are motivated by external forces; therefore, the leader makes all the decisions and directs the followers' behavior.

Democratic leadership   A leadership style that assumes individuals are motivated by internal forces; leader uses participation and majority rule to get work done.

Laissez-faire leadership   A leadership style that assumes individuals are motivated by internal forces and should be left alone to complete work; leader provides no direction or facilitation.

Bureaucratic leadership   A leadership style that assumes individuals are motivated by external forces; leader trusts neither followers nor self to make decisions and therefore relies on organizational policies and rules.

Table 4-1   Comparison of Leadership Styles

Leadership Style	Assumed Employee Motivators	Leader Characteristics
Authoritarian (autocratic)	External forces, e.g., power and authority, needs for approval	• Concerned with task accomplishment rather than relationships • Uses directive behavior • Makes decisions alone • Expects respect and obedience of staff • Lacks group support generated by participation • Exercises power with coercion • Proves useful (even necessary) in crisis situations
Democratic (participative)	Internal drives and impulses	• Is primarily concerned with human relations and teamwork • Fosters communication that is open and usually two-way • Creates a spirit of collaboration and joint effort that results in staff satisfaction
Permissive (laissez-faire)	Internal drives and impulses	• Tends to have few established policies; abstains from leading • Is not generally useful in highly structured organizations (e.g., health care institutions)
Bureaucratic	External forces	• Lacks a sense of security and depends on established policies and rules • Exercises power by applying fixed, relatively inflexible rules • Tends to relate impersonally to staff • Avoids decision making without standards or norms for guidance

job descriptions, personnel policies, and procedures for granting time off, implementing a new policy on intravenous tubing changes, or family visiting.

Consideration, the employee-centered dimension, refers to behavior that conveys mutual trust, respect, friendship, warmth, and rapport between the manager and the staff. When the leader is considerate, the employee learns to expect that the manager will hear a concern openly and without reprisal, will involve employees in decision making, and will attend to the needs of the work group as a whole. The manager is alert to employees' responses to stress, the effects of personal crises on their work, and the social dynamics of the work group.

Despite the substantial contributions of the structure/consideration concepts to the development of leadership theory, research has produced confounding results. Followers' and managers' perceptions of managers' leadership style often differ; attempts to enhance a manager's style in one area or the other do not necessarily result in higher employee performance or improved goal achievement; equally effective leaders might possess strength in consideration or structure or both.

With the realization that different combinations of leader behaviors might produce different effects, researchers began searching for an optimal mix of behaviors that would produce optimal employee performance. As these models evolved, researchers began to recognize the complexity and range of the approaches managers use to produce results in organizations.

System 4 Management Likert (1967) developed the System 4 model of management based on the premise that involving employees in decisions about work is central to effective leadership. The model is composed of four dimensions based on increasing levels of employee involvement. *Autocratic leaders* have little trust in employees and systematically exclude them from decision making. *Benevolent leaders* are kind to employees but still do not involve them in decision making. *Consultative leaders* seek employees' advice about decisions. *Participative* or *democratic leaders* value employee involvement, teamwork, and team building; they also have high levels of confidence in employees and seek consensus in decision making. In doing so, the participative leader shares power.

The Managerial Grid Another model for depicting leadership along a continuum is the managerial grid (Figure 4-1). Five leadership styles are plotted in four quadrants of a two-dimensional grid. The grid depicts various degrees of leader concern for production (structure) and concern for people (consideration). Leadership styles are labeled "impoverished" (low concern for both production and people), "authority compliance" (high concern for production, low concern for people), "country club" (high concern for people, low concern for production), "middle of the road" (moderate concern for both production and people), and "team" (high concern for both production and people).

Continuum of Leadership Behavior Leadership behavior also is depicted as occurring along a continuum. This model focuses specifically on the decision-making style of managers. As displayed in Figure 4-2, the left end of the continuum reflects a manager-centered style. Managers are autocratic and directive and simply make and announce decisions. At the right end of the continuum, managers are employee-centered; they use a laissez-faire style and permit employees to set their own goals and function within established parameters. No single leadership style is correct or appropriate for every management situation.

The numerous variations of the multidimensional, behavioral approach have contributed significantly to our understanding of managers' performance and effectiveness. Nurse managers may use these perspectives as a basis for analyzing the leadership styles of others and analyzing and developing their own styles.

Contingency Theories

Contingency approaches suggest that managers adapt their leadership styles in relation to changing situations. According to contingency theory, leadership behaviors range from authoritarian to permissive and vary in relation to current needs and future probabilities. A nurse manager may use an authoritarian style when responding to an emergency situation such as a cardiac arrest but use a participative style to encourage development of a team strategy to care for patients with multiple system failure. The manager might delegate to a highly competent and eager follower group decision making and task completion in designing a new patient intake form. The most effective leadership style for a nurse manager is the one that best complements the organizational environment, the tasks to be accomplished, and the personal characteristics of the people involved in each situation. Numerous contingency models have been developed. Four are discussed in this chapter: Fiedler's contingency theory, situational leadership theory, Vroom–Yetton expectancy model, and House–Mitchell path–goal theory.

Fiedler's Contingency Theory Fiedler (1967) proposed that a leader is most effective when he or she matches leadership style (relationship-oriented or task-

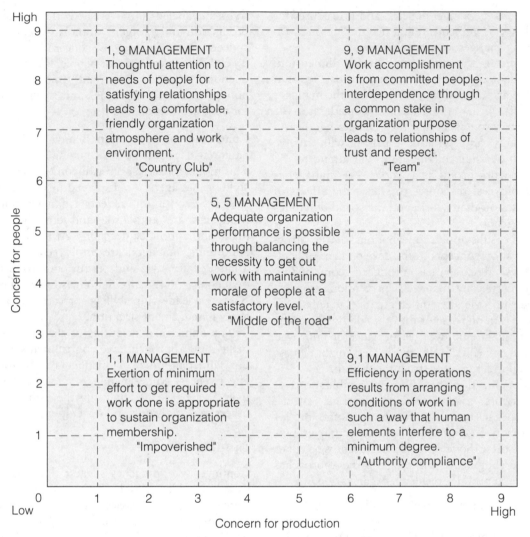

Figure 4-1 **The managerial grid. From *Leadership Dilemmas—Grid Solutions,* by R. R. Blake and A. A. McCanse, 1991, Austin, TX: Grid International. Reprinted with permission.**

oriented) to situational factors. Fiedler described three situational factors of leadership, which are listed in decreasing order of importance:

- Manager–follower relationship (good to poor)
- Task structure (high to low)
- Manager power (strong to weak)

Manager–follower relations reflect the degree to which the leader enjoys the loyalty and support of subordinates. Task structure is the degree to which the task or result is clearly described and/or standard operating procedures guarantee successful completion and evaluation of the quality of the task. Position power is the degree to which leaders are able to administer rewards and punishment by virtue of their positions (that is, legitimate power).

Figure 4-3 illustrates how the task-motivated leader will be more effective under high and low structures and the relationship-motivated leader will have greater effectiveness under in-between situations.

Situational Leadership Theory Hersey, Blanchard, and Johnson (2001) expanded Fiedler's contingency model by considering the followers' readiness and willingness to perform the assigned tasks. In their theory of situational leadership, four distinct leadership styles (S) are prescribed according to the readiness and ability of followers (R) (Figure 4-4).

Leaders use a telling style (S1—high task, low relationship) with followers who are unable and unwilling or insecure about performing the task (R1). Leaders use a selling style (S2—high task, high relationship) with

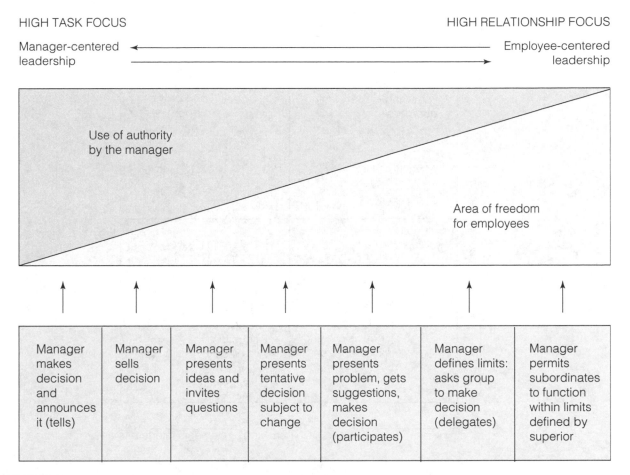

HIGH TASK FOCUS

HIGH RELATIONSHIP FOCUS

Manager-centered
leadership

Employee-centered
leadership

Use of authority
by the manager

Area of freedom
for employees

| Manager makes decision and announces it (tells) | Manager sells decision | Manager presents ideas and invites questions | Manager presents tentative decision subject to change | Manager presents problem, gets suggestions, makes decision (participates) | Manager defines limits: asks group to make decision (delegates) | Manager permits subordinates to function within limits defined by superior |

Figure 4-2 **Continuum of leadership behavior. From "How to Choose a Leadership Pattern," by R. Tannenbaum and W. H. Schmidt, 1973, *Harvard Business Review, 51*, p. 164. Reprinted by permission. Copyright © 1973 by the Harvard Business School Publishing Corporation; all rights reserved.**

Figure 4-3 **Fiedler's situational variables and their preferred leadership styles. From *Organizational Behavior*, 8th ed. (p. 291), by J. R. Schermerhorn, Jr., J. G. Hunt, and R. N. Olson, 2003, New York: Wiley. This material is used by permission of John Wiley & Sons, Inc.**

Leader behavior

(High)

S3
Share ideas
and facilitate
in making
decisions

S2
Explain your
decisions
and provide
opportunity for
clarification

PARTICIPATING

SELLING

Hi. Rel.
Low Task

Hi. Task
Hi. Rel.

Relationship behavior
(Supportive behavior)

Low Rel.
Low Task

Hi. Task
Low Rel.

DELEGATING

TELLING

S4
Turn over
responsibility
for decisions and
implementation

S1
Provide
specific
instructions
and closely
supervise
performance

(Low) ←——— Task behavior ———→ (High)
(Directive behavior)

Follower readiness

High	Moderate		Low
R4	R3	R2	R1
Able and willing or motivated	Able but unwilling or insecure	Unable but willing or motivated	Unable and unwilling or insecure

Figure 4-4 Situational Leadership® model. From *Management of Organizational Behavior*, 8th ed. (pp. 189, 196), by P. Hersey, K. H. Blanchard, and D. E. Johnson, 2001, Upper Saddle River, NJ: Prentice Hall. © Copyrighted material. Adapted with permission of Center for Leadership Studies, Escondido, CA 92025. All rights reserved.

followers who are unable but are willing or confident in performing the task (R2). Leaders use a participating style (S3—low task, high relationship) with followers who are able but unwilling or lacking in confidence in performing the task (R3). Finally, leaders use a delegating style (S4—low task, low relationship) with followers who are both able and willing and have confidence in performing the task (R4).

Vroom–Yetton Expectancy Model Vroom and Yetton (1973) developed a prescriptive model for determining the amount of participation leaders should seek from employees in decision making. This model, depicted in Figure 4-5, helps managers decide how to make a decision contingent on the task to be accomplished and needs of both managers and employees.

Manager has all of the information
needed to make the decision

Figure 4-5   **Variables affecting use of participation in leadership.**

Three questions guide the manager's selection of an appropriate leadership style and the extent of participation employees should have in decision making.

1. Is all the information available to make the decision?
2. Is the staff's acceptance of the decision required for effective implementation?
3. Would the group make a decision the leader could live with?

Vroom and Yetton (1973) identified five leadership styles: tell, sell, consult, join, and delegate. Here are their guidelines to decide which leadership style to use:

Use a telling style to assess a problem, make a decision independently, and inform followers.

Use a selling style to gather information from followers about a problem, make a decision independently, and persuade followers to implement it.

Use a consultative style to seek advice from followers individually, make the decision independently, and inform followers.

Use a joining style to join the group, seek suggestions, independently make a decision, and inform followers.

Use a delegation style to work with followers in developing solutions to the problem and facilitate con-

sensus-building toward a group solution, which generally is accepted and implemented as the group wishes.

Consider the example of decision making shown in Box 4-1.

The manner in which managers make decisions directly reflects their leadership style. A model or framework that addresses the many contingencies in a decision-making situation helps managers analyze how to make decisions successfully. It also helps managers demonstrate a consistent, predictable decision-making style, which enables co-workers to anticipate the manager's expectations and perform accordingly.

House–Mitchell Path–Goal Theory   Path–goal theory applies a theory of human motivation and task performance to leadership effectiveness (House & Mitchell, 1974). Because a primary function of leadership is to motivate others to attain goals, path–goal theory proposes that removing obstacles to goal attainment, coaching, and providing personal rewards for achievement will result in high levels of performance and productivity. The leader affects performance by influencing employees' perceptions of their work and personal goals and facilitating the process by which employees achieve goals.

The motivational functions of leadership derive directly from the expectancy theory of motivation (Porter & Lawler, 1968; Vroom, 1964; also see Chapter 19). Employees work for rewards they find attractive and that result from successful performance.

Three concepts are central to expectancy theory:

Expectancy is the perceived probability that effort will result in successful performance.

KEY TERMS

Expectancy   The perceived probability that effort will result in successful performance.

Box 4-1 Example of Vroom–Yetton Model of Decision Making

Administration wants to pilot a model of self-directed teams on one unit in the hospital. One of the nurse managers, Martina Duchek, volunteers. She analyzes the staff's responses. Martina addresses the following questions:

1. Is the information needed to make the decision available? The manager needs to know, for example, how much the staff know about self-directed teams, how they feel about them, and what they would need by way of training and development to implement them. The answer to question 1 is no.

2. Is the staff's acceptance required for implementation? In this case, the answer to question 2 is clearly yes.

3. If the decision to adopt self-directed work teams is delegated to the staff, will they make a decision acceptable to Martina? She thinks not and realizes that it is the manager's responsibility to make a final decision with extensive staff involvement. Therefore, the answer to question 3 is no.

Martina could participate with the staff in a meeting to consider the costs and benefits of moving to self-directed teams, facilitate group decision making about what might be required to implement them, and create an implementation plan. Alternatively, she could discuss the pros and cons of implementing self-directed teams with individual staff members, gather information, analyze potential costs and other possible consequences to the unit, seek staff recommendations, and then make a decision.

Instrumentality is the perceived probability that performance will lead to desired outcomes.

Valence is the probability that the desired outcomes will lead to a valued reward.

The manager exercises leadership by defining and clarifying expectancies, instrumentalities, and valences associated with specific tasks and employees' personal goals.

Path–goal theory specifies four leader behaviors (House, 1971):

Directive leadership involves telling employees what is expected, giving specific guidance, ensuring adherence to rules and procedures, and scheduling and coordinating work efforts. This type of leadership is most effective for employees who are marginally trained or prepared and are performing partially routine and ambiguous tasks.

Supportive leadership focuses on the needs of employees, displays concern for their well-being, and creates a friendly climate in the work environment. Supportive leadership behavior is most effective for employees who are performing routine work or are very experienced with the work.

Participative leadership involves consultation with subordinates and requests for opinions and suggestions, which the leader takes into consideration when making decisions. This style works best for employees who have moderate skill levels and are performing somewhat ambiguous work. Involvement of employees encourages mutual clarification of objectives and specification of mutually helpful work processes.

Achievement-oriented leadership includes setting challenging goals, seeking performance improvements, emphasizing excellence in performance, and showing confidence that employees will attain high levels of performance. It is indicated for employees who are skilled and perform highly innovative and ambiguous work. By setting challenging goals and pointing out valued rewards, managers fulfill a strong motivating role.

Staff members interpret and respond to leader behavior in different ways, depending on personal characteristics and characteristics of the task and environment. Specifically, employees' needs for achievement, affiliation, power, competence, autonomy, and personality traits form a context within which leaders function. As in situational leadership, the effect of leadership behavior on employee satisfaction and effort depends on the task and the work situation.

Path–goal theory is interesting because it suggests that there are substitutes for direct leader–follower interaction. On the one hand, the manager can influence employee performance directly by clarifying the route to desired goals. On the other hand, actions that clarify objectives, specify roles, increase the value of rewards, provide needed support to complete tasks successfully, and facilitate performance might be viewed as substitutes for direct leadership activity.

The application of any contingency theory to leadership practice requires continuous monitoring of employees' expectancies, abilities, and motivations and an understanding of the task and options for completing it. Managers must also thoroughly consider the consequences of their actions on employee performance. For every leader's action, a predictable employee reaction is likely to occur. A nurse manager must carefully observe the cause-and-effect relationships that exist between leader behavior and employee response and continuously take into account the multitude of environmental factors that influence leader–employee interactions.

Contemporary Theories

Leaders in today's health care environment place increasing value on collaboration and teamwork in all aspects of the organization. They recognize that as health systems become more complex and require integration, personnel who perform the managerial and clinical work must cooperate, coordinate their efforts, and produce joint results. Leaders must use additional skills, especially group and political leadership skills, to create collegial work environments.

Quantum Leadership

Trait, behavioral, and contingency theories represent conventional approaches to leadership and have provided important foundations for leadership. Current views of leadership are neither complete reformulations nor simple refinements of conventional perspectives. Evolved from the principles of quantum mechanics, effective leadership today reflects a remarkable fusion of trait, behavior, and contingency approaches.

Quantum leadership is based on the concepts of chaos theory (see Chapter 2). Reality is constantly shifting, and levels of complexity are constantly changing. Movement in one part of the system reverberates throughout the system. Roles are fluid and outcome oriented. It matters little what you did; it only matters what outcome you produced. Within this framework, employees become directly involved in decision making as equitable and accountable partners, and managers assume more of an influential facilitative role, rather than one of control (Porter-O'Grady & Malloch, 2002).

Quantum leadership demands a different way of thinking about work and leadership. Change is expected. In fact, the leader's role is to encourage employees to "close the door on receding practices and challenge them to simply turn around and squarely confront the opportunities and challenges of emerging practice" (Porter-O'Grady, 2003, p. 177).

KEY TERMS

Instrumentality   The perceived probability that performance will lead to desired outcomes.

Valence   The probability that desired outcomes will lead to a valued reward.

Directive leadership   A leadership style that involves telling employees expectations, giving guidance, ensuring adherence to rules, and scheduling work efforts.

Supportive leadership   A leadership style that focuses on the needs of employees.

Participative leadership   A leadership style that involves consultation with subordinates in decision making.

Achievement-oriented leadership   A leadership style that includes goal setting and maintaining high levels of performance in order to motivate employees.

Quantum leadership   A leadership style based on the concepts of chaos theory.

Charismatic leadership   Leadership based on valued personal characteristics and beliefs.

Informational power, previously the purview of the leader, is now available to all. Patients and staff alike can access untold amounts of information. The challenge, however, is to assist patients, uneducated about health care, how to evaluate and use the information they have. Because staff have access to information only the leader had in the past, leadership becomes a shared activity, requiring the leader to possess excellent interpersonal skills.

Charismatic Leadership

Charismatic leadership is based on personal qualities such as charm, persuasiveness, personal power, self-confidence, extraordinary ideas, and strong (often unconventional) convictions. The leader's personality arouses great affection and emotional commitment, first to the leader and secondarily to the beliefs and causes the leader espouses. Few leaders possess genuine charisma. Those who do often use their powerful personalities to advance revolutionary goals.

Transactional Leadership

Transactional leadership is similar to the path–goal view of leadership and is based on the principles of social exchange theory (Homans, 1958; Thibaut & Kelley, 1959). The primary premise of social exchange theory is that individuals engage in social interactions expecting to give and receive social, political, and psychological benefits or rewards. The exchange process between leaders and followers is viewed as essentially economic. Once initiated, a sequence of exchange behavior continues until one or both parties finds that the exchange of performance and rewards is no longer valuable. The nature of these transactions is determined by the participating parties' assessments of what is in their best interests; for example, staff respond affirmatively to a nurse manager's request to work overtime in exchange for granting special requests for time off. Leaders are successful to the extent that they understand and meet the needs of followers and use incentives to enhance employee loyalty and performance. Transactional leadership is aimed at maintaining equilibrium, or the status quo, by performing work according to policy and procedures, maximizing self-interests and personal rewards, emphasizing interpersonal dependence, and routinizing performance.

Transformational Leadership

Transformational leadership goes beyond transactional leadership. Transformational leadership emphasizes the importance of interpersonal relationships (Ward, 2002). Transformational leadership is not concerned with the status quo, but with effecting revolutionary change in organizations and human service. Whereas traditional views of leadership emphasize the differences between employees and managers, transformational leadership focuses on merging the motives, desires, values, and goals of leaders and followers into a common cause. The goal of the transformational leader is to generate employees' commitment to the vision or ideal rather than to themselves.

Transformational leaders appeal to individuals' better selves rather than these individuals' self-interests. They foster followers' inborn desires to pursue higher values, humanitarian ideals, moral missions, and causes. Transformational leaders also encourage others to exercise leadership. The transformational leader inspires followers and uses power to instill a belief that followers also have the ability to do exceptional things. The effectiveness of this leadership style depends on the leader's ability to stimulate the growth and development of others and discourage dependence.

> ### KEY TERMS
>
> ***Transactional leadership*** A leadership style based on principles of social exchange theory in which social interaction between leaders and followers is essentially economic, and success is achieved when needs are met, loyalty is enhanced, and work performance is enhanced.
>
> ***Transformational leadership*** A leadership style focused on effecting revolutionary change in organizations through a commitment to the organization's vision.
>
> ***Relational (connective) leadership*** A leadership style that values collaboration and teamwork; interpersonal skills are used to promote collegiality in achieving organizational goals.
>
> ***Shared leadership*** An organizational structure in which several individuals share the responsibility for achieving the organization's goals.
>
> ***Servant leadership*** The premise that leadership originates from a desire to serve; a leader emerges when others' needs take priority.

Transformational leaders may be a natural model for nursing managers, because nursing has traditionally been driven by its social mandate and its ethic of human service. Transformational leadership can be used effectively by nurses with clients or co-workers at the bedside, in the home, in the community health center, and in the health care organization.

Relational Leadership

Relational leadership, also known as relationship-oriented leadership or connective leadership, recognizes that today we are all connected and that relationships form the cornerstone of contemporary leadership. Klakovich (1994) proposed a connective leadership paradigm for nursing. This paradigm acknowledges the need for more flexible systems in health care that empower employees, their interdisciplinary colleagues, clients, and families. Klakovich explains that contemporary nursing leadership skills should include the ability to create interconnections between and across caregiving settings and among multiple constituencies.

The purpose of relational leadership is to better coordinate and integrate patient care services in a caring, non-competitive manner. The focus is to link professionals, communities, governing groups, and voluntary agencies to improve patient-centered care. Connective leaders use their interpersonal skills to broker alliances, encourage collaboration, and integrate systems. Klakovich stresses the importance of collegiality among health care professionals in achieving patient care and organizational goals.

The nurse manager applies relational leadership principles when convening a group of physicians, administrators, nursing staff, and representatives of other disciplines to plan a new patient care program, for example, or bring nursing staff members together to develop a staff orientation program or seek the assistance of an external expert to help in the professional development of the nursing staff. Hierarchical relationships break down and leadership develops at all levels in the organization.

Relational leadership requires both content and process skills (such as the task and relationship skills discussed earlier). Both power and political tactics may be needed (see Chapter 6). The ability to manage groups and team interactions is essential. (Teams and team building are discussed in Chapter 15.) In addition, leaders must recognize that integrating the activities of diverse participants in health care involves creating connections that extend beyond well-defined groups.

The process of developing relationships and creating connections requires the leader to

- Identify actual and potential collaborators,
- Communicate and sell a potential shared vision to those in varied settings and under disparate conditions,
- Describe the value each collaborator could bring to the endeavor, both to the individual and others,
- Facilitate communication by sharing information, preparing for interactions, and following up on communications exchanges,
- Build and maintain social interaction and comfort,
- Define and sell roles and assignments,
- Track and reward contributions, and
- Formalize an integrated effort at the right time.

Shared Leadership

Reorganization, decentralization, and the increasing complexity of problem solving in health care have forced administrators to recognize the value of **shared leadership,** which is based on the empowerment principles of participative and transformational leadership. Essential elements of shared leadership are relationships, dialogues, partnerships, and understanding boundaries (McCrea, 1998). The application of shared leadership assumes that a well-educated, highly professional, dedicated workforce is comprised of many leaders. It also

assumes that the notion of a single nurse as the wise and heroic leader is unrealistic and that many individuals at various levels in the organization must be responsible for the organization's fate and performance.

Different issues call for different leaders, or experts, to guide the problem-solving process. A single leader is not expected always to have knowledge and ability beyond that of other members of the work group. Appropriate leadership emerges in relation to the current challenges of the work unit or the organization. Individuals in formal leadership positions and their colleagues are expected to participate in a pattern of reciprocal influence processes. Examples of shared leadership in nursing include

- *Self-directed work teams.* Work groups manage their own planning, organizing, scheduling, and day-to-day work activities.
- *Shared governance.* The nursing staff are formally organized at the service area and organizational levels to make key decisions about clinical practice standards, quality assurance and improvement, staff development, professional development, aspects of unit operations, and research. Decision making is conducted by representatives of the nursing staff who have been authorized by the administrative hierarchy and their colleagues to make decisions about important matters.
- *Co-leadership.* Two people work together to execute a leadership role. This kind of leadership has become more common in service-line management, where the skills of both a clinical and administrative leader are needed to successfully direct the operations of a multidisciplinary service. For example, a nurse manager provides administrative leadership in collaboration with a clinical nurse specialist, who provides clinical leadership. The development of co-leadership roles depends on the flexibility and maturity of both individuals, and such arrangements usually require a third party to provide ongoing consultation and guidance to the pair.

Servant Leadership

Servant leadership is based on the premise that leadership originates from a desire to serve and that in the course of serving, one may be called to lead. According to Greenleaf (1991), servant leadership occurs when other people's needs take priority, when those being served "become healthier, wiser, freer, more autonomous, and more likely themselves to become servants" (p. 7). The servant leader must address the question of whether the least advantaged in society benefit from the leader's service. The concept of servant leadership may have some substantive appeal for nursing leadership because nursing is founded on principles of caring, service, and the growth and health of others. Nurse leaders serve many constituencies, often quite selflessly, and consequently bring about change in individuals, systems, and organizations.

Health care environments require innovations in care delivery and therefore innovative leadership approaches. Quantum, charismatic, transactional, transformational, relational, shared, and servant leadership comprise a new generation of leadership styles that have emerged in response to the need to humanize working environments and improve organizational performance. Traditional perspectives, especially participative leadership, also offer nurse managers leadership concepts that may be emulated, learned, modeled, and refined in management practice. In practice, leaders tap a variety of styles culled from diverse leadership theories.

Management Functions

Classical Description

In 1916, French industrialist Henri Fayol first described the functions of management as planning, organizing, directing, and controlling. These are still relevant today.

Planning   **Planning** is a four-stage process to

- Establish objectives (goals),
- Evaluate the present situation and predict future trends and events,
- Formulate a planning statement (means), and
- Convert the plan into an action statement.

Planning is important on both an organizational and a personal level and may be an individual or group process that addresses the questions of what, why, where, when, how, and by whom. Decision making and problem solving are inherent in planning. Numerous computer software programs and databases are available to help facilitate planning.

Organization-level plans, such as determining organizational structure and staffing or operational budgets, evolve from the mission, philosophy, and goals of the organization. The nurse manager plans and develops specific goals and objectives for her or his area of responsibility.

Antonio, the nurse manager of a home care agency, plans to establish an in-home phototherapy program, knowing that part of the agency's mission is to meet the

health care needs of the child-rearing family. To effectively implement this program, he would need to address

- *How the program supports the organization's mission,*
- *Why the service would benefit the community and the organization,*
- *Who would be candidates for the program,*
- *Who would provide the service,*
- *How staffing would be accomplished,*
- *How charges would be generated, and*
- *What those charges should be.*

Planning can be contingent or strategic. **Contingency planning** refers to the identification and management of the many problems that interfere with getting work done. Contingency planning may be reactive, in response to a crisis, or proactive, in anticipation of problems or in response to opportunities. What would you do if two registered nurses called in sick for the 12-hour night shift? What if you were a manager for a specialty unit and received a call for an admission, but had no more beds? Or what if you were a pediatric oncology clinic manager and a patient's sibling exposes a number of immunocompromised patients to chickenpox? Planning for crises such as these are examples of contingency planning.

Strategic planning refers to defining and prioritizing long-term objectives of the organization and developing

---

KEY TERMS

Planning   A four-stage process that includes decision making and problem solving in order to achieve specific goals.

Contingency planning   The reactive or proactive identification and management of problems that arise.

Strategic planning   The process of defining and prioritizing long-term objectives of an organization and developing strategies for implementation.

Organizing   The process of coordinating the work to be done within an organization.

Directing   The process of getting the work within an organization done.

Controlling   The process of establishing standards of performance, determining the means to be used in measuring performance, evaluating performance, and providing feedback.

strategies for implementation. Strategic planning is future oriented, focusing on plans for the next 2 to 5 years (see Chapter 2). Its purpose is to create an image of the desired future and design ways to make those plans a reality. To do so involves a systematic process of assessing the internal and external environment, identifying strengths, recognizing demands, acknowledging sources of competition, and assessing available means by which to achieve the desired end. Examples of strategic plans might include an acute care hospital's addition of home health care services or a health department's initiative to provide public health nurses with notebook computers.

Organizing Organizing is the process of coordinating the work to be done. Formally, it involves identifying the work of the organization, dividing the labor, developing the chain of command, and assigning authority. It is an ongoing process that systematically reviews the use of human and material resources. In health care, the mission, formal organizational structure, delivery systems, job descriptions, skill mix, and staffing patterns form the basis for the organization. *In organizing the home phototherapy project, Antonio develops job descriptions and protocols, determines how many positions are required, selects a vendor, and orders supplies.*

Directing Directing involves the process of getting the organization's work done. Power, authority, and leadership style are intimately related to a manager's ability to direct. Communication abilities, motivational techniques, and delegation skills also are important. In today's health care organization, professional staff are autonomous, requiring guidance rather than direction. The manager is more likely to sell the idea, proposal, or new project to staff rather than tell them what to do. The manager coaches and counsels to achieve the organization's objectives. In fact, it may be the nurse who assumes the traditional directing role when working with unlicensed personnel. *In directing the home phototherapy project, Antonio assembles the team of nurses to provide the service, explains the purpose and constraints of the program, and allows the team to decide how they will staff the project, giving guidance and direction when needed.*

Controlling Controlling functions involve establishing standards of performance, determining the means to be used in measuring performance, evaluating performance, and providing feedback. The efficient manager constantly attempts to improve productivity by incorporating techniques of quality management, evaluating outcomes and performance, and instituting change as necessary.

Today, managers share many of the control functions with the staff. In organizations using a formal quality improvement process, such as continuous quality improvement (CQI), staff participate in and lead the teams. Some organizations use peer review to control quality of care. *When Antonio introduces the home phototherapy program, the team of nurses involved in the program identify standards regarding phototherapy and their individual performances. A subgroup of the team routinely reviews monitors designed for the program and identifies ways to improve the program.*

Planning, organizing, directing, and controlling reflect a systematic, proactive approach to management. This approach is used widely in all types of organizations, health care included. Timmereck (2000) found that health care managers used these classic functions extensively.

Mintzberg's Behavioral Description

A newer model is based on a behavioral approach to management. Mintzberg (1973) believed that much of a manager's activity involves human relations, a premise that is supported by the contemporary leadership theories discussed previously. Mintzberg also believed managers were more reactive than proactive. As a result of these two premises, he identified three categories of managerial roles: interpersonal roles, informational roles, and decisional roles.

Interpersonal Roles Mintzberg describes three interpersonal roles that reflect the formal authority inherent in the manager's position: the figurehead, the leader, and the liaison. The *figurehead role* reflects the ceremonial performance of duties, such as welcoming new employees at orientation or attending social events. As a *leader,* the manager defines the work environment of the organization and is responsible for the work of associates—motivating, training, and disciplining as needed. The manager, as a leader, determines the mission and objectives of the organization and sees that they are accomplished efficiently. The third interpersonal role, *liaison,* deals with expanding the manager's information sources and networks outside the organization. National conferences, local coalitions, and professional meetings are valuable resources for obtaining information and expanding networks.

Informational Roles Mintzberg also describes three informational roles. As a *monitor,* the manager informally seeks information about the organization through internal networks, gossip, and observations.

MediaLink Mintzberg on Management

Tours of the organization, as well as formal and informal meetings, provide the manager with information about the needs and functions of the organization. In the *disseminator* role, managers either share information between work units or share information from outside the organization. Information is a source of power; sharing information empowers employees and improves job satisfaction. As a *spokesperson*, the manager shares information with individuals outside the organization and provides visibility for the organization. Attending community meetings, offering continuing education, and participating in professional organizations are examples of ways in which the manager serves as a spokesperson.

Decisional Roles   Mintzberg describes four decisional roles. The *entrepreneur* constantly seeks ways to solve problems and make improvements in the organization.

Reorganization of supplies, staff redesign, and creation of new roles are all examples of entrepreneurship. The *disturbance handler* responds to unforeseen circumstances, such as replacement of staff for sick call, nosocomial outbreaks, or missing equipment. As *resource allocators*, managers schedule their own time, determine division and coordination of work, and authorize the timing and implementation of major decisions. Finally, the *negotiator* deals with outside forces mediating resources and decisions, such as resolving labor disputes or making business acquisitions.

A Contemporary Model of Managerial Work

Mintzberg (1994) proposed a new model to describe managerial functions depicted in Figure 4-6. In this model, managerial work is envisioned as occurring on three levels represented by concentric circles: *infor-*

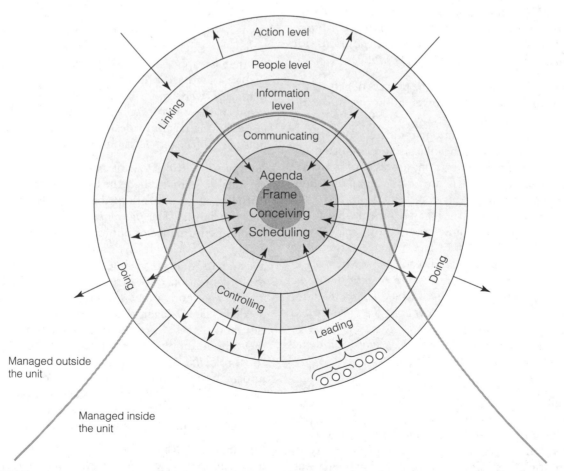

Figure 4-6   A model of managerial work. From "Managing as blended care" by H. Mintzberg, 1994, *Journal of Nursing Administration, 24,* p. 30.

mation, people, and *action.* The manager, in the center, brings to the position a set of values, experiences, knowledge, and competencies. The manager conceives the frame, which includes the purpose of the job, the work needed, and how it should be done. Managing involves

- Communicating and controlling at the information level,
- Leading and linking at the people level, and
- Doing at the action level.

The first level of work, informational processing, is the most abstract and includes communicating and controlling. *Communicating* involves receiving and sharing information with others, whereas controlling is using information to manage the work of others.

The second level of managerial work involves leading and linking people in order to encourage people to take action. *Leading* involves encouraging and enabling of others—individually, as a team, or as an entire organization—to take effective action. *Linking* is the manager's establishment of networks outside the unit in order to relay needs and exchange influence.

At the third and most concrete level, the focus is on managing action by doing. *Doing* includes taking supervisory actions—directing change, handling disturbances, and negotiating external agreements.

Using this framework for an analysis of nursing management, Mintzberg (1994) found that the roles previously described are blended into an intricate, caring management style.

Roles and Functions of Nursing Managers

The American Organization of Nurse Executives (AONE) is an organization for the top nursing administrators in hospitals. AONE describes six roles and functions of the nurse manager (1992):

1. *The nurse manager is accountable for excellence in the clinical practice of nursing and the delivery of patient care on a selected unit or area within the health care institution.* This function is the primary focus of the nurse manager. To meet this responsibility, the nurse manager has the authority to plan and implement strategies and programs consistent with the organization's policies, goals, and objectives, as well as with professional standards and governmental rules and regulations. The manager is responsible for maintaining a safe and caring environment that promotes health teaching and maintenance. The manager is responsible for assessing patient and family response to nursing care as well as evaluating the effectiveness and quality of the care and services and their consistency with identified regimens. Supporting research and ensuring that research findings are incorporated into practice are also the responsibility of the manager.

2. *The nurse manager is accountable for managing human, fiscal, and other resources needed to manage clinical nursing practice and patient care.* With heightened awareness of the cost of health care, managers face a difficult task. Because nurses are the primary providers of patient care, nursing accounts for use of most of the resources. Therefore, nurse managers are accountable for efficient use of personnel, equipment, and supplies. Skill mix is important in meeting patient needs. Consequently, managers must prepare, monitor, and maintain budgets consistent with health care policy and economics. The nurse manager also must ensure that the staff are proficient in providing care and in using available equipment and resources wisely. It is the manager's responsibility to communicate to the staff constraints regarding resources and to coach and mentor the staff appropriately.

3. *The nurse manager is accountable for facilitating development of licensed and unlicensed nursing and health care personnel.* To maintain excellence in nursing practice and patient care, the staff must be competent to perform delegated roles and responsibilities. The manager is responsible for seeing that competency levels are maintained and that staff acquire new skills as needed. The nurse manager also plays an important role in providing a supportive environment for nursing and other health profession students.

4. *The nurse manager is accountable for ensuring institutional compliance with professional, regulatory, and government standards of care.* The provision of excellent nursing practice and patient care also involves compliance with standards of care. The nurse manager must be informed and be able to translate pertinent standards of care for staff and to implement required programs.

5. *The nurse manager is accountable for strategic planning as it relates to the unit(s) or area(s), department, and organization as a whole.* The manager is responsible for communicating input

from the staff to the clinical director and chief nurse executive. The nurse manager also is responsible for developing and implementing a strategic plan for the unit that supports the department's and organization's plan. Finally, the manager is responsible for facilitating staff support for the strategic plan and modifying the plan as needed in response to changes in the environment.

6. *The nurse manager is accountable for facilitating cooperative and collaborative relationships among disciplines/departments to ensure effective quality patient care delivery.* Today, more than ever, cooperative and collaborative relationships are necessary to deliver efficient, cost-effective care. The nurse manager plays an important role in developing collegial relationships based on mutual respect and support. To do so, the manager must play an active role in interdisciplinary committees responsible for developing patient-focused programs.

The Association of Community Health Nursing Educators (ACHNE) is another group of administrators who work in community health settings. Information may be found on their Web site at www.uncc.edu/achne.

Mathena (2002) studied nurse managers, asking them to name which skills they thought were most important to success in their roles. Communication, negotiation, critical thinking, balance between work and home, and conflict management were most often listed. Then the managers were asked to identify those skills for which they needed professional development. The results revealed that managers needed development for a different skill set. Situational analysis, data management, cost–benefit analysis, financial projections, and financial analysis were most often named.

Levels of Management

Whereas managers direct the work of a specified area, product line, or service, administrators (sometimes called executives) focus on establishing goals and on integrating work units to achieve the organization's mission. Generally, three levels of management are used in nursing: first (nurse manager), middle (director), and upper (executive) (Figure 4-7), although the tendency today is to continually push management decisions to lower and lower levels.

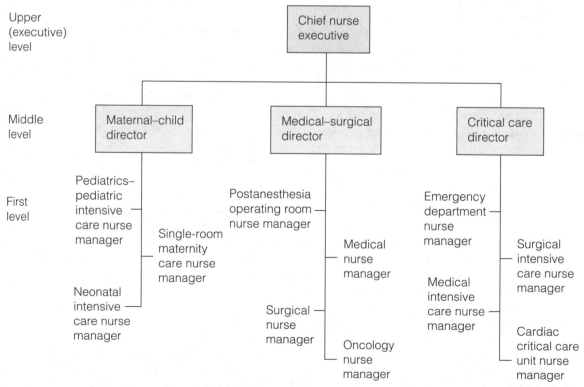

Figure 4-7 **Levels of management for an inpatient setting.**

First-Level Management

The **first-level manager,** also known as a *first-line manager,* is responsible for supervising the work of non-managerial personnel and the day-to-day activities of a specific work unit or units. The manager is responsible for clinical nursing practice; patient care delivery; use of human, fiscal, and other resources; personnel development; compliance with regulatory and professional standards; fostering interdisciplinary, collaborative relationships; and strategic planning (AONE, 1992). With primary responsibility for motivating the staff to achieve the organization's goals, the first-level manager represents staff to upper administration, and vice versa. Nurse managers have 24-hour accountability for the management of a unit(s) or area(s) within a health care organization. In the hospital setting, the first-level manager is usually the head nurse, nurse manager, or an assistant. In other settings, such as an ambulatory care clinic or a home health care agency, a first-level manager may be referred to as a coordinator. Box 4-2 describes a first level manager's day.

Middle-Level Management

The **middle-level manager** supervises a number of first-level managers, usually within related specialties or in a given geographic area. Middle-level managers are responsible for the people and activities within the departments they supervise, and they too have 24-hour responsibility for their defined area. Typically, middle-level managers act as a liaison between upper management and first-level managers. A middle manager may be referred to as a supervisor, director, or assistant or associate director of nursing. Graduate education often is required for this position.

A typical day in the life of a middle-level manager is seen in Box 4-3.

Many changes are continuing to occur in first- and middle-level management in hospitals and other health care organizations today. In some, middle management positions are being consolidated and/or eliminated. Rather than holding the position of director of maternal–child nursing overseeing three managers and their subsequent units, the middle manager may hold the title of director of clinical services, with responsibility spanning all medical–surgical services. In addition, departments previously under separate management, such as laboratory and respiratory therapy, now may be under the direction of nursing. Conversely, nursing practice may be divided under the supervision of nonclinical managers in service-line organizational structures.

These changes reflect attempts at cost containment as well as movement toward a more participatory style of decentralized management. Not only does the organization benefit, but so do the patients, staff, and individual managers. Savings in management salaries can be used to meet cost-containment goals, purchase more equipment, or hire more caregivers. Decentralization empowers the manager and the staff, increasing job satisfaction and improving the quality of care.

Upper-Level Management

Upper-level management, or *executive-level management,* refers to top executives (administrators) such as the vice president for nursing or chief nurse executive, to whom middle managers report. This administrator is primarily responsible for establishing organizational goals and strategic plans for the entire division of nursing, integrating work units to achieve the organization's mission, and buffering the effects of the external environment on nurses within the organization. Some chief nurse executives have responsibilities for other departments, such as the respiratory therapy, housekeeping, or dietary departments. Nurses also are assuming systemwide administrative roles as directors of education, informatics, and quality (Krejci, 1999).

According to the American Organization of Nurse Executives (1990), "A nurse executive is a registered nurse who is part of the executive management team and as such is responsible for the management of the nursing organization and the clinical practice of nursing throughout the organization" (p. 1). At this level, a graduate degree and a record of progressively increased management experience are necessary.

KEY TERMS

First-level manager   The manager responsible for supervising nonmanagerial personnel and day-to-day activities of specific work units.

Middle-level manager   A manager who supervises first-level managers within a specified area and is responsible for the people and activities within those areas; generally acts as liaison between first-level and upper-level management.

Upper-level management   The top level to whom middle management reports; primarily responsible for establishing organizational goals and strategic plans for entire division of nursing.

Box 4-2   A Day in the Life of a First-Level Manager

As the manager for a surgical intensive care unit (SICU), Jamal Johnson is routinely responsible for supervising patient care, trouble shooting, maintaining compliance with standards, and giving guidance and direction as needed. In addition, he has fiscal and committee responsibilities and is accountable to the organization for maintaining its philosophies and objectives. The following exemplifies a typical day.

As Jamal came on duty, he learned that there had been a multiple car accident and that three of the victims were currently in surgery and destined for the unit. The assistant manager for nights had secured more staff for days: two part-time SICU nurses and a staff nurse from the surgical floor. However, she had not had time to arrange for two more patients to be moved out of the unit. From their assigned nurses, Jamal obtained an update on the patients who were candidates for transfer and, in consultation with his assistant, made the appropriate arrangements for the transfers.

Other staffing problems were at hand: In addition to the nurse who had been pulled from the floor, there were two orientees, and the staff needed to attend a safety in-service. As soon as the charge nurse came in, Jamal apprised her of the situation. Together, they reviewed the operating room schedule and identified staffing arrangements. Fortunately, Jamal had only one meeting today and would be available for backup staffing. In the meantime, he would work on evaluations.

After his discussions with the charge nurse, Jamal met with each of the night nurses to get an update on the status of the other patients. Then he went to his office to review his messages and plan his day. Tamera, an RN, had just learned she was pregnant, but she stated that she planned to work until delivery. Jamal learned that his budget hearing had been scheduled for the following Monday at 10 A.M. A pharmaceutical representative wanted to provide an in-service for the unit. Fortunately, there were no immediate crises.

Jamal called his supervisor to inform her of the status of affairs on the unit and learned that two other individuals in the accident had been transported to another hospital; one had since died. They discussed the ethical and legal ramifications. Jamal would need to review the policies on relations with the press and law enforcement and to update his staff.

As the first patient returned from surgery, Jamal went to help admit the patient and receive a report. Learning that the patient was stable, he informed Lucinda, the charge nurse, that the patient they had just received was likely to be charged with manslaughter and reviewed media and legal policies with her. They also discussed how the staff were doing. There were some equipment problems in room 2110; Lucinda had temporarily placed the patient on a transport monitor and was waiting for a biomedical technology staff member to check the monitor. Could Jamal follow up? Jamal agreed and commended Lucinda for her problem solving. She reminded Jamal they would need backup for lunch and in-services.

As Jamal returned to his office, he noted that the alarms were turned off on one of the patients. He pulled aside the nurse assigned to the patient and reminded her of the necessity to keep the alarms on at all times. Finally, back in his office he called biomedical technology to ascertain their plans to check the monitor and made notes regarding the charge nurse's problem-solving abilities and the staff nurse's negligence.

He reviewed staffing for the next 24 hours and noted that an extra nurse was needed for both the evening and night shifts because of the increased workload. After finding staff, he was able to finish one evaluation before covering for the in-services and lunch and then attending the policy and procedure team meeting.

Teresa is an example of an upper-level manager (see Box 4-4).

Charge Nurse

In health care, a number of roles that do not fit the traditional levels of management have evolved. The **charge nurse** is one of these. In some organizations, the position may be permanent and assigned and thus a part of the formal management team; in other organizations, the job may be rotated among experienced staff. In still other organizations, the assistant head nurse may perform the functions usually relegated to the charge nurse. In some organizations, a differential

KEY TERM

Charge nurse   An expanded staff nurse role with increased responsibility and the function of liaison to the nurse manager.

Box 4-3   A Day in the Life of a Middle-Level Manager

Kirsten Knudsen is a middle-level manager. She is the director of maternal–child nursing at a large hospital. Within her division are the pediatric unit, pediatric intensive care unit (PICU), newborn intensive care unit (NICU), and the single-room maternity care (SRMC) area. Three nurse managers report to her. Kirsten routinely meets with her managers each day to identify patient or employee issues. She assists the managers in decision making and problem solving. She facilitates interdepartmental collaboration. In fact, much of her day is spent in meetings. A typical day might look like this.

Kirsten usually starts her day with personal organization, noting what meetings she has scheduled and planning when she will meet with her managers. From the bed census reports she notes that both the pediatric and PICUs are full; the newborn intensive care unit and single-room maternity care area have low censuses.

Today, the first thing on Kirsten's agenda is an interdisciplinary meeting with the obstetricians. As Kirsten enters the meeting, she thinks about the issues involved. Kirsten wants to know what plans her institution has for the residency program in light of another local hospital's closure of its obstetrical units. Will more residents be placed at her institution? What will be the impact on census and, subsequently, staffing? What, if any, fiscal effects will be noted? A great deal of discussion in the meeting revolves around the topic. Additional topics discussed are current quality improvement measures, departmental statistics, and recently released new care guidelines.

Following the interdisciplinary meeting, Kirsten meets with the SRMC nurse manager. They discuss the impact of an increase in residents. Kirsten suggests that the manager envision the direction the unit will take and present a plan for growth and development. They also discuss the status of the patients and staff. Since census is down in SRMC, the pediatric unit could use more staff. The manager informs Kirsten about a high-risk patient; her infant was admitted to NICU for a septic workup.

Kirsten next meets with the manager of NICU. She makes a point to get a report on the new infant. In addition, she learns that two transport teams are out getting babies and that there is a potential for a third. The manager also identifies a need to set a meeting time to discuss the educational conference she proposed the hospital would offer that fall. The appointment is set, and Kirsten suggests that the manager be prepared to identify a team to handle the arrangements.

A meeting with the pediatric/PICU manager is brief because she is busy helping the staff. Kirsten learns the booming census is due to a number of respiratory illnesses. Because all patients are stable, she asks if some of the adolescents can be moved to adult units to make more room for smaller children. Kirsten agrees to make the arrangements and informs the manager that staffing assistance is available from SRMC.

Kirsten returns to her office, arranges for adolescent transfers to medical and surgical units, reads her mail, and returns phone calls. A distributor wants to talk about a new product, a nursing school faculty member wants to discuss new clinical opportunities, a graduate student wants to examine the potential for research, Dr. Pacheco wants to explore the possibility of implementing a new procedure, and the director of the laboratory wants to discuss a problem with maintaining hazard precautions with placentas.

After a quick lunch, Kirsten heads to the continuous quality improvement meeting, which she chairs. The quarterly nurse council meeting is next. She returns the phone calls she received earlier before heading home for the day.

---

amount of compensation is paid to the person performing charge duties; in others, no differential is paid because the position is shared equally among staff or represents a higher rung of a career ladder (possibly the first rung of a management ladder).

Although the job description varies from organization to organization, the charge nurse position is an expanded staff nurse role with increased responsibility. The charge nurse functions as a liaison to the nurse manager, assisting in shift-by-shift coordination and promotion of quality patient care as well as efficient use of resources. The charge nurse often troubleshoots problems and assists other staff members in decision making. Role modeling, mentoring, and educating are additional roles that the charge nurse often assumes. Therefore, the charge nurse usually has extensive experience, skills, and knowledge in clinical practice and is familiar with the organization's standards and practices.

There are numerous ways in which the charge nurse's job differs from that of the first-level manager. First, the charge nurse's responsibilities are confined to a specific shift or task, whereas the first-level manager has 24-hour responsibility and accountability for all unit activities. Second, the charge nurse has limited

---

Box 4-4   Example of a Chief Nurse Executive

Theresa Mickelson is a chief nurse executive (CNE) in charge of nursing at a 500-bed hospital. As such, she is intimately involved with the administration of the hospital. Theresa completed a graduate program in nursing administration.

On any given day she may meet with other administrators or executives. She also may meet with community or professional leaders. Theresa spends much of her time gathering and sharing information.

Theresa has ultimate responsibility for the quality and cost effectiveness of the nursing care provided in the organization. As CNE, she is mutually responsible for establishing and maintaining a safe, caring environment for nursing practice and patient care. This involves an assessment of the internal and external environment. Internal factors include patient mix; nursing staff mix, skills, and knowledge; research and education activities; available resources; and established health care outcomes. External factors include bioethical standards, legislation and regulations, public and health policy, community needs and expectations, economic climate, and technology.

Theresa also needs to be able to forecast trends, participate in strategic planning, and interpret the role of nursing to other disciplines. She then develops and implements policies and programs based on available resources that support nursing practice and the mission of the organization. These policies and procedures address not only patient care issues but also the development of education and research programs. She also is responsible for evaluating nursing policies, programs, and services for effectiveness and consistency with the organization's mission, goals, and objectives. Another important role is the mentoring and career development of other nurse managers.

Through role modeling, meetings, and education, Theresa provides examples of leadership and professionalism.

---

authority; the charge nurse functions as an agent of the manager and is accountable to the manager for any actions taken or decisions made. Although often involved in planning and organizing the work to be done, the charge nurse has a limited scope of responsibility, usually restricted to the unit for a specific time period. In the past, the charge nurse had limited involvement in the formal evaluation of performance, but in today's climate of efficiency, the charge nurse may be involved in evaluations as well. With the trend toward participative management, charge nurses are assuming more of the roles and functions traditionally reserved for the first-level manager.

A charge nurse usually has considerable influence with the staff and may actually have more informal power than the manager. Therefore, the charge nurse is an important leader and can benefit by developing the skills considered necessary for a manager. Acting as charge nurse is often the first step toward a formal management position.

Staff Nurse

Although not formally a manager, the staff nurse working with other professionals and assistive personnel is also a manager who needs management and leadership skills. Management responsibilities involve supervising others to ensure safe, quality patient care. Communication, delegation, and motivation skills are indispensable.

In some organizations, shared governance has been implemented and traditional management responsibilities are allocated to the work team. In this case, staff nurses have considerable involvement in managing the unit. More information about shared governance and other innovative management methods is provided in Chapter 2.

What You Know Now

- A leader employs specific behaviors and strategies to influence individuals and groups to attain goals.
- Managers are responsible for efficiently accomplishing the goals of the organization.
- Leadership approaches are not static; they can be adapted for different situations, tasks, individuals, and future expectations.
- Trait theories attempt to identify the inborn characteristics of successful leaders whereas behavioral theorists focus on learned leadership abilities and behaviors.
- Contingency theorists contend that leaders should adapt their style in relation to changing situations.
- Contemporary theorists assert that reality is fluid, complex, and interrelated and that interpersonal relationships are core to successful leadership.

- Traditional management functions include planning, organizing, directing, and controlling.
- Contemporary management requires communication, leadership, and action.
- All nurses are managers and, in addition, nurses hold management positions at all levels in health care organizations.

Questions to Challenge You

1. Think about people you know in management positions. Are any of them leaders as well? Describe the characteristics that make them leaders.
2. Think about people you know who are not in management positions but are leaders nonetheless. What characteristics do they have that make them leaders?
3. Describe the manager to whom you report. (If you are not employed, use the first-level manager on a clinical placement site.) Evaluate this person using the functions of management described in the chapter.
4. Think about yourself as a manager whether you are in a management position or not. What skills do you possess that help you? What skills would you like to improve?
5. Evaluate yourself as a leader. How would you like to improve?

Explore MediaLink

NCLEX review questions, essay activities, group activities, and other interactive resources for this chapter can be found on the Web site at http://www.prenhall.com/sullivan-decker. Click on "Chapter 4" to select activities for this chapter.

References

American Organization of Nurse Executives. (1990). The role and function of the hospital nurse executive. In *American Hospital Association Advisory*. Chicago: American Hospital Association.

American Organization of Nurse Executives. (1992). The role and functions of the hospital nurse manager. In *American Hospital Association Advisory*. Chicago: American Hospital Association.

Antrobus, S., & Kitson, A. (1999). Nursing leadership: Influencing and shaping health policy and nursing practice. *Journal of Advanced Nursing, 29*(3), 746–753.

Bass, B. (1990). *Bass and Stogdill's handbook of leadership: Theory, research and managerial applications* (3rd ed.). New York: Free Press.

Fiedler, F. E. (1967). *A theory of leadership effectiveness.* New York: McGraw-Hill.

Gilbert, M. A. (1975). Personality profiles and leadership potential of medical-surgical and psychiatric nursing graduate students. *Nursing Research, 24,* 125–130.

Greenleaf, R. K. (1991). *The servant as leader.* Indianapolis: The Robert K. Greenleaf Center.

Hersey, P., Blanchard, K. H., & Johnson, D. E. (2001). *Management of organizational behavior.* Upper Saddle River, NJ: Prentice Hall.

Homans, G. (1958). Social behavior as exchange. *American Journal of Sociology, 63*(6), 597–606.

House, R. J. (1971). A path–goal theory of leader effectiveness. *Administrative Science Quarterly, 16*(3), 321–338.

House, R. J., & Mitchell, T. R. (1974). Path–goal theory of leadership. *Journal of Contemporary Business, 3,* 81–98.

Jenkins, R. L., & Henderson, R. L. (1984). Motivating the staff: What nurses expect from their supervisors. *Nursing Management, 15*(2), 13–14.

Katz, D., & Kahn, R. L. (1952). Some recent findings in human relations research. In G. E. Swanson, E. M. Newcomb, & R. E. Hartley (Eds.), *Readings in social psychology.* New York: Holt, Rinehart & Winston.

Kerfoot, K. (2000). On leadership: Leading from the inside out. *Nursing Economics, 18*(6), 6–7.

Klakovich, M. D. (1994). Connective leadership for the 21st century: A historical perspective and future directions. *Advances in Nursing Science, 16*(4), 42–54.

Krejci, J. W. (1999). Changing roles in nursing: Perceptions of nurse administrators. *Journal of Nursing Administration, 29*(3), 21–29.

Lewin, K., & Lippitt, R. (1938). An experimental approach to the study of autocracy and democracy: A preliminary note. *Sociometry, 1,* 292–300.

Lewin, K., Lippitt, R., & White, R. K. (1939). Patterns of aggressive behavior in experimentally created social climates. *Journal of Social Psychology, 10,* 271–301.

Lewin, R., & Regine, B. (2000). *The soul at work: Listen. Respond. Let go.* New York: Simon & Schuster.

Likert, R. (1967). *The human organization: Its management and value.* New York: McGraw-Hill.

Mathena, K. A. (2002). Nursing manager leadership skills. *Journal of Nursing Administration, 32*(3), 136–142.

McCrea, M. (1998). Personal reflections on early learning in shared leadership. *Seminars for Nurse Managers, 6*(2), 83–88.

Mintzberg, H. (1973). *The nature of managerial work.* New York: Harper & Row.

Mintzberg, H. (1994). Managing as blended care. *Journal of Nursing Administration, 24,* 29–36.

Porter, L. W., & Lawler, E. E. (1968). *Managerial attitudes and performance.* Homewood, IL: Irwin-Dorsey.

Porter-O'Grady, T. (2003). A different age for leadership, Part 2: New rules, new roles. *Journal of Nursing Administration, 33*(3), 173–178.

Porter-O'Grady, T., & Malloch, K. (2002). *Quantum leadership: A textbook of new leadership.* Gaithersburg, MD: Aspen.

Stogdill, R. M. (1974). *Handbook of leadership: A survey of the literature.* New York: Free Press.

Stogdill, R. M., & Coons, A. E. (Eds.). (1957). *Leadership style: Its description and measurement.* Research Monograph O. 88. Columbus, OH: Bureau of Business Research, Ohio State University.

Thibaut, J. W., & Kelley, H. H. (1959). *The social psychology of groups.* New York: Wiley.

Timmereck, T. C. (2000). Use of the classical functions of management by health services midmanagers. *Health Care Manager, 19*(2), 50–67.

Vroom, V. H. (1964). *Work and motivation.* New York: Wiley.

Vroom, V. H., & Yetton, P. W. (1973). *Leadership and decision making.* Pittsburgh: University of Pittsburgh Press.

Ward, K. (2002). A vision for tomorrow: Transformational nursing leaders. *Nursing Outlook, 50*(3), 121–126.

Understanding Legal and Ethical Issues

Laws and Ethics

Ethical Decision Making

Autonomy
Beneficence and Nonmaleficence
Distributive Justice

The Legal System

Sources of Law
Types of Law
Liability

Legal Issues in Nursing

Nursing Licensure
Patient Care Issues
Management Issues
Employment Issues

Looking Ahead

Chapter 5 outlines the legal and ethical issues facing nurses, beginning with a discussion of the principles of ethical decision making and followed by an overview of the legal system and a more specific examination of legal issues in nursing.

Objectives

In this chapter, you will learn

- What ethical principles are.
- What is involved in ethical decision making.
- What types of laws exist.
- How nurses and nurse managers are liable for their actions.
- What legal issues nurses face.

MediaLink 🌐 **www.prenhall.com/ sullivan-decker**

Additional resources for this chapter can be found on the Companion Website at www.prenhall.com/ sullivan-decker. Click on "Chapter 5" to select the activities for this chapter.

- NCLEX Review
- Critical Thinking Activities
- Current Events
- MediaLinks
- *Nursing Leadership & Management in Action*: Identifying Malpractice

Today's health care system presents many ethical and legal dilemmas for nurses. Advanced technology, escalating health care costs, a growing elderly population, and social and economic pressures are just a few of the factors posing ethical dilemmas. As the role of the professional nurse expands to include increased expertise, specialization, autonomy, and accountability, so does the number of legal issues involving nurses. This chapter provides an overview of ethical decision making and the legal system to help nurses and nurse managers manage common ethical and legal dilemmas in nursing.

Laws and Ethics

Laws are rules of conduct, established and enforced by authority, which prohibit extremes in behavior so that one can live without fear for oneself or one's property. **Ethics** is a science that deals with principles of right and wrong, good and bad; it governs our relationships with others. Ethics are based on personal beliefs and values that guide the decision-making process. Each ethical dilemma is subject to philosophical, moral, and individual interpretations by all the involved parties.

Everyone has a system of right and wrong that guides decision making. Although the definitions of law and ethics may seem clear, there is a fine line between ethics and law, and the two may overlap in some health care encounters. In some cases, the overlap may be congruent; in others, conflictual. For example, what is ethical may not be legal, and what is legal may not be ethical. Making this distinction between ethics and law is important because the outcomes are very different. When you violate legal principles, you may be held liable for your actions. When you violate ethical principles, you may feel badly because of the results of your actions.

The American Nurses Association's Code of Ethics, found in Box 5-1, makes explicit the profession's values and standards of conduct. This document was adopted originally in 1950 and is revised periodically to reflect changes in the profession and society. It serves to inform the nurse and the public of the profession's expectations in ethical matters. It also provides a decision-making framework for solving ethical problems. Although the code of ethics is not legally enforceable, violation of these standards often results in violation of laws that have been enacted to ensure protection of the public; for example, violation of guidelines in the code regarding issues of confidentiality and incompetent practice also constitutes violation of law.

Ethical Decision Making

Several key principles play a role in solving ethical dilemmas. The principles most directly related to nursing management are the principles of autonomy, beneficence, and distributive justice.

Autonomy

Autonomy is the right of individuals to take action for themselves. It includes respect for individuals and the right of individuals to make decisions for and about themselves, even if those decisions are not congruent with others' goals. To respect autonomy is to respect others. It requires recognizing the uniqueness of others and listening to and understanding another person in a way that allows you to put yourself in that other person's position.

People engaged in autonomous and self-determining actions must have the capability of self-governance, operate from a stable and internalized set of principles, and view themselves as capable of implementing autonomous decisions. Inherent in this principle is the understanding that a person acts with intention and with knowledge and without external control or influence. Like most rights, autonomy is not an absolute right: Under certain circumstances, the individual's rights do not prevail over the rights of others. Individual autonomy does not prevail, for example,

---

KEY TERMS

Laws   Rules of conduct, established and enforced by authority, which prohibit extremes in behavior so that one can live without fear for oneself or one's property.

Ethics   The science that deals with the principles of right and wrong, good and bad; it governs our relationships with others and is based on personal beliefs and values.

Autonomy   The right of individuals to take action for themselves.

Beneficence/nonmaleficence   The duty to help others by doing what is best for them without inflicting evil or harm.

Distributive justice   Giving a person that which is deserved.

Box 5-1   Code of Ethics for Nurses

The nurse, in all professional relationships, practices with compassion and respect for the inherent dignity, worth, and uniqueness of every individual, unrestricted by considerations of social or economic status, personal attributes, or the nature of health problems.

The nurse's primary commitment is to the patient, whether an individual, family, group, or community.

The nurse promotes, advocates for, and strives to protect the health, safety, and rights of the patient.

The nurse is responsible and accountable for individual nursing practice and determines the appropriate delegation of tasks consistent with the nurse's obligation to provide optimum patient care.

The nurse owes the same duties to self as to others, including the responsibility to preserve integrity and safety, to maintain competence, and to continue personal and professional growth.

The nurse participates in establishing, maintaining, and improving health care environments and conditions of employment conducive to the provision of quality health care and consistent with the values of the profession through individual and collective action.

The nurse participates in the advancement of the profession through contributions to practice, education, administration, and knowledge development.

The nurse collaborates with other health professionals and the public in promoting community, national, and international efforts to meet health needs.

The profession of nursing, as represented by associations and their members, is responsible for articulating nursing values, for maintaining the integrity of the profession and its practice, and for shaping social policy.

From *Code of ethics for nurses with interpretive statements*, 2001. Reprinted with permission from American Nurses Association, © 2001 American Nurses Publishing, American Nurses Association, Washington, DC.

when it interferes with the rights, health, or well-being of another. For example, a nurse has the right to refuse to render care to a patient because of religious beliefs; however, if the safety of the patient is jeopardized because of that lack of care, the nurse may suffer legal consequences if care is not provided. In addition, the nurse has an ethical obligation to be sure the patient has adequate care.

Beneficence and Nonmaleficence

Beneficence is the duty to help others by doing what is best for them. This belief also implies the principle of **nonmaleficence,** or to "do no harm." One has the duty not only to do good, but also not to inflict evil or harm or to risk harm to others. A beneficent nurse manager acts with empathy for the patients and staff and without resentment or malice. A manager who acts in bad faith or out of ill will or who makes false accusations concerning a patient or employee violates the principle of beneficence.

In many instances, the demands of beneficence and the functions required in a health care setting come into conflict. Sometimes, for example, treatment decisions are viewed as harmful from the patient's perspective. When an individual does not

desire what others determine to be in that person's best interest—such as when a patient refuses treatment—the principles of beneficence and autonomy conflict. Generally speaking, in conflict situations involving patient care decisions, the principle of autonomy overrides the principle of beneficence, and this has been affirmed by the courts (Furrow, Johnson, Jost, & Schwartz, 1991).

Distributive Justice

Distributive justice is giving a person that which he or she deserves. It implies that benefits and burdens ought to be distributed equally and fairly, regardless of race, gender, religion, or socioeconomic status so that no one person bears a disproportionate share of benefits or burdens. As health care technology increases and health care costs soar, nurse managers find themselves entrenched in conflicts between cost containment and the equal distribution of finite health care resources regardless of the patient's ability to pay.

Allocation (macroallocation) and **rationing** (microallocation) of scarce resources are the most important ethical issues facing nurse managers today. Allocation is a decision society makes regarding how many of its resources will be devoted to a particular effort, for example, organ transplants. Rationing is a decision regarding who gets the transplant and who does not. Allocation and rationing decisions require that some societal values take precedence over some individual values.

The goal-driven or patient-centered model of care, which was traditionally taught to nurses in the past, does not suffice in the current health care delivery system, in which resources are finite. The traditional model stressed nurses' commitment to the patient regardless of the person's ability to pay or the cost of the person's care to society. Resource allocation was viewed as an absolute individual right that allowed individuals to make unlimited claims on societal resources. Ideally, nurses were taught to identify goals and then find the resources to meet those goals. Frequently, nurses did a good job with limited resources, but they did not feel right about the care they provided because it was less than ideal. In the current resource-driven model, nurses must learn to use finite resources efficiently and to be satisfied that resources were used wisely. Allocation of scarce resources is not an issue that can be addressed by individual nurses or even by the nursing profession alone. It requires cooperative efforts and interdisciplinary understanding among a variety of participants, including policymakers and economists, as well as a new perspective on nursing ethics. Resource allocation cannot be discussed without looking at the process by which resources are made available, the constraints on decision makers who must allocate those resources, and the comparative values of health care and other goods of society.

The Legal System

Law comes from a variety of sources. Understanding the sources of law and the various types of laws helps determine their impact on nursing practice. Nurses must understand the changing legal climate and their responsibilities as viewed by the public and the legal system.

Sources of Law

Three branches of government contribute to the creation of law. They, in conjunction with the Constitution, form the basis of the judicial system of this country. The Constitution is the supreme law of the land. It defines the structure, power, and limits of the government and guarantees people certain fundamental rights as individuals. Influences of the legislative, judicial, and executive branches of government are reflected in statutory law, common law, and administrative law.

Statutory Law **Statutory laws** are enacted by the legislative branch of government. They are designed to declare, command, or prohibit something. Licensing laws for health care providers, including nurses, are examples of statutory laws, which are designed to protect the public from incompetent practitioners. Other statutory laws affecting nursing practice are guardianship codes, statutes of limitation, informed consent, living will legislation, and protective and reporting laws.

Common Law **Common law** is judge-made law. This type of law is derived from earlier decisions made by courts. Common law establishes a custom or tradition by which other similar cases are judged; this custom is referred to as legal precedent. Common law is not absolute; earlier decisions can be and frequently are overruled. As time and circumstances change, court decisions become obsolete and may require a different opinion. Each state has its own body of common law related to the delivery of health care within that state. These laws should be reviewed by health professionals as a basis for accountability, quality, and risk management within their professional practice. As the number of malpractice suits involving nurses increases, the body of common law regulating nursing practice also increases. Awareness of this law assists nurses to function within the boundaries of their role and to advocate for nursing practice when necessary.

Administrative Law **Administrative laws** are made by administrative agencies. According to certain statutes, administrative agencies are granted authority to enact rules and regulations that will carry out specific intentions of the statute. This allows the legislature to delegate to an administrative agency of experts in the field the authority to create rules and regulations governing a specific area of practice. For example, state boards of nursing are authorized by nurse practice acts (statutory law) to write rules and regulations governing the practice of nursing. These rules and regulations are incorporated into the nurse practice act and are as binding as the statutory law itself. Another example of administrative law is the attorney general's opinion regarding the interpretation of a law, which also is binding.

Types of Law

Law also can be categorized according to specific types. The two basic types of law are public law and private law (civil law). **Public law** consists of constitutional law, administrative law, and criminal law. **Private law** is further classified into tort law, contract law, and protecting and reporting law; however, the latter sometimes falls under the category of criminal law. All these have an impact on nursing practice; however, the most common law affecting nursing practice is that of torts.

Tort Law   Tort law is divided into two categories—unintentional and intentional. Negligence and malpractice (professional negligence) fall under the category of unintentional torts.

Unintentional Torts.   **Negligence** is defined as the failure of an individual not to perform an act (omission) or to perform an act (commission) that a reasonable, prudent person would or would not perform in a similar set of circumstances. **Malpractice** is professional negligence; it evolves from negligence law and the premise that all individuals are responsible for the consequences of their actions or inactions. It refers to any misconduct or lack of skill in carrying out professional responsibilities. For malpractice to exist, four elements must be present: duty, breach of duty, causation, and injury. If there is not a preponderance of evidence that demonstrates negligence, then the malpractice claim may be dismissed.

Intentional Torts.   In **intentional torts,** the intent to harm is present. Assault, battery, false imprisonment, invasion of privacy, libel, slander, and defamation of character are examples of actions considered to be intentional torts.

Liability

To understand malpractice, one must understand the various types of liability. As individuals, nurses are responsible and accountable for their own actions or inactions. This is referred to as **personal liability.** In addition, the law ascribes negligence to certain parties who may not be negligent themselves but whose negligence is assumed because of association with the negligent person. This is called **vicarious liability.** It is based on the legal principle of **respondeat superior,** which means "let the master speak." This doctrine allows the courts to hold the employer responsible for the actions of the employee when the employee is performing services for the organization.

   All too frequently, nurses have a false sense of security concerning the doctrines of respondeat superior and vicarious liability. Employees sometimes believe that the organization's responsibility protects them

---

KEY TERMS

Allocation   The decision of a society about how much of its resources will be devoted to a particular effort.

Rationing   The process by which decisions are made about who will get the resources and who will not.

Statutory laws   Laws enacted by the legislative branch of government.

Common law   Laws derived from earlier decisions made by courts.

Administrative laws   Laws made by administrative agencies.

Public law   The domains of constitutional law, administrative law, and criminal law.

Private law   The domains of tort law, contract law, and protecting and reporting law.

Tort law   A law that addresses wrongful acts, whether unintentional or intentional, against a person or property.

Negligence   The unintentional failure of an individual to perform or not perform an act that a reasonable person would or would not perform in a similar set of circumstances.

Malpractice   Professional negligence that refers to any misconduct or lack of skill in carrying out professional responsibilities.

Intentional torts   Action in which the intent to harm was present.

Personal liability   The responsibility and accountability of individuals for their own actions or inactions.

Vicarious liability   The assignment of negligence to certain parties, whose negligence is assumed due to their association with a negligent person.

Respondeat superior   The legal principle that allows the court to hold an employer responsible for the actions of an employee when performing services for the organization.

---

from being sued as individuals; this is not the case. Patients have the right to sue both the employee and the organization when they have suffered an injury as a result of substandard care. Also, the organization

MEDIALINK   Identifying Malpractice

has the right to sue the employee for damages incurred as a result of the nurse's substandard care. This is why it is important for nurses to carry their own personal liability insurance. Nurse managers are not responsible for the actions of others but are responsible for their own acts of delegation and supervision of others. Failure to delegate and supervise properly can result in liability for the nurse manager. This is not a result of vicarious liability, but an issue of personal liability.

Corporate liability holds that the organization is responsible for its own wrongful conduct. The health care organization has the responsibility of maintaining an environment conducive to quality health care for its consumers. Corporate liability includes (a) the duty to hire, supervise, and maintain qualified, competent, and adequate staff; (b) the duty to provide, inspect, repair, and maintain reasonably adequate equipment; and (c) the duty to maintain safety in the physical environment. Responsibility to achieve these goals is delegated to managers even though the organization is ultimately responsible. For example, the organization has a responsibility to have a mechanism in place for reporting incompetent, unethical, and illegal practice; however, if the nurse manager is aware of such practice but does not report it, the nurse manager also is liable. Many states have statutory laws regarding mandatory reporting of legal and ethical problems.

Legal Issues in Nursing

Nursing Licensure

Licensure is a type of credential provided for by state statutes that authorizes qualified individuals to perform designated skills and services. In nursing, these statutes are referred to as **nurse practice acts**. Nurse practice acts establish boards of nursing, whose members are granted the authority to set and enforce rules and regulations pertaining to the practice of nursing. Currently, each state's board of nursing establishes requirements for licensure in that state. Licensure protects the use of the titles, registered or practical nurse, and establishes educational, examination, and behavioral standards intended to protect the health, safety, and welfare of the public.

Because each state controls and maintains its own database of licensees, mobility for nurses is hampered. To practice in a state other than the one where the nurse is already licensed, the nurse must apply for a reciprocal license from the state. Although all nurses

take the same licensure exam, not all states' policies regarding nursing practice are alike.

Uniform Licensure Requirements One remedy proposed by the National Council of State Boards of Nursing (NCSBN) is to develop uniform licensure requirements among the states that would not only facilitate nurse mobility, but also ensure public access to qualified practitioners (Box 5-2). The framework for these requirements is competence—competence in development, assessment, and conduct (NCSBN, 1999).

Multistate Licensure Another initiative by the NCSBN is multistate licensure. **Multistate licensure** is a process similar to obtaining a driver's license. Each state that agrees to the interstate compact would mutually recognize the nurse's license, allowing practice in more than one state. As of March 2002, fifteen states had entered an interstate compact to allow multistate licensure privilege (NCSBN, 2002a). The state of residence is considered the home state. All other states in the contract are remote states. The nurse is still responsible for meeting the standards set forth by the nurse practice acts where practice occurs. Disciplinary actions may be taken by both the home and remote state (NCSBN, 1998).

KEY TERMS

Corporate liability The responsibility of an organization for its own wrongful conduct.

Licensure A credential provided for by state statute that authorizes qualified individuals to perform designated skills and services.

Nurse practice acts State statutes that authorize individuals to perform designated skills and services.

Multistate licensure A licensure process whereby more than one state mutually recognizes licensure.

Model nursing practice act The model act that defines nursing practice and that states can use to increase consistency among states and improve mobility for nurses while protecting the public.

Invasion of privacy The right to be left alone without being subjected to unwarranted or uninvited publicity and to make personal choices without interference.

Box 5-2   Uniform Core Licensure Requirements

I. Competence Development: Nursing education—registered nurses (RN)

- Graduation from or verification of completion and eligibility for graduation from state-approved registered nursing program.

II. Competence Assessment: Assessment of U.S. candidates—RN

- Nursing Knowledge, Skills and Abilities
- NCLEX-RN® examination, unlimited attempts

III. Competence Conduct:

Criminal convictions—RN and LPN/VN

- Self-report regarding all felony convictions.

- Conviction of lesser-included offenses arising from felony arrests.
- Local/state and federal background checks using current technology (i.e., fingerprinting) to validate self-reports.

Chemical dependency—RN and LPN/VN

- Self-report regarding any drug-related behavior that affects the candidate's ability to provide safe and effective nursing care.

Functional abilities—RN and LPN/VN

- Self-report regarding any functional ability deficit that would require accommodation to perform essential nursing functions.

From "Uniform core licensure requirements for initial licensure of RNs and LPN/VNs," by National Council State Boards of Nursing, 1999, *Issues, 20*(3), pp. 1–2.

Model Nurse Practice Act   The NCSBN also has developed a **model nursing practice act** (NCSBN, 2002b). The model act defines nursing, its scope of practice, titles, advanced practice nursing standards, educational requirements, and violations and penalties. Improved uniformity among states would result if states adopt the model act.

Patient Care Issues

Patient's Rights   When individuals enter the health care system, they retain their basic fundamental rights ascribed to individuals by the Constitution and courts of law. These rights are spelled out in the Patient's Bill of Rights (American Hospital Association [AHA], 1992), a document frequently given to individuals when they enter the health care system. Although not always legally binding, this document frequently is used as a standard for judging the nursing care rendered. Some argue that a bill of rights for patients is not necessary because it simply reiterates the basic rights already recognized; however, this document is designed to protect the rights of the individual at a time when he or she is most vulnerable to abuse. The Patient's Bill of Rights is designed to protect such basic rights as privacy, confidentiality, informed consent, and refusal of treatment.

Privacy Rights   The tort **invasion of privacy** is the violation of a person's right to be left alone without being subjected to unwarranted or uninvited publicity and to make personal choices without interference. Information

disclosed by patients is confidential and as such is available to authorized personnel only. Patients can sue for invasion of privacy when confidential information is revealed to any unauthorized person. Similarly, a patient can sue for invasion of privacy when unauthorized personnel, directly or indirectly, observe the patient without permission. Authorized personnel are those involved in the diagnosis, treatment, and related care of the patient. Generally speaking, these are members of the health care team.

Nurses, as well as others, cannot use photographs, videotapes, or research data without the explicit permission of the involved patient. Also, the nurse should be discreet about the release of information over the telephone regarding the patient's status because it is difficult, if not impossible, to identify the caller accurately over the telephone. The nurse must even obtain the patient's permission to release information to family members and close friends.

Other cases regarding invasion of privacy involve the freedom to make choices without interference. Patients have the right to make informed choices, such as contraception use, abortion, and the right to refuse treatment, and they should be assured that these decisions will be respected and upheld even if they are not the same decisions or choices the health professional may make. Nurses often serve as advocates to safeguard these rights.

Health Information Portability and Accountability Act. The Health Information Portability and Accountability Act of 1996 (HIPAA) was implemented in the spring of

MEDIALINK Patient's Bill of Rights

2003. HIPAA requires health care providers, including individuals and organizations, to take far more stringent measures to ensure their patients' privacy than were required previously. Communication between providers requires a release from the patient. Offices and public places in health care agencies must prevent names and identifying information to be overheard or seen. Providers must be certain that mail, fax, e-mail, and phone messages are accessible only by the patient. Complying with the requirements for HIPAA has involved a major overhaul of most health care systems, and the success of these efforts remains to be seen (Maddox, 2002).

Confidentiality. **Confidentiality** is the right to privacy of records. Individuals have the right to believe that information disclosed to health professionals is to be used strictly for the purpose of diagnosis and treatment and will not be released to others without permission of the individual. This is considered protected information by the privilege doctrine. According to this doctrine, people who have protected relationships cannot be forced to reveal communication between them unless the person who would benefit from the relationship agrees to it. Confidentiality assurances have been strengthened under the regulations of HIPAA. Under certain circumstances, the nurse can lawfully disclose confidential information about the patient, such as when the welfare of a person or a group is at stake or when a personal injury or workers' compensation claim is being filed.

Informed Consent   To provide treatment without the patient's consent, except in an emergency situation, could result in liability for unauthorized touching, or battery. Three basic requirements are necessary for **informed consent**: capacity, voluntariness, and information.

Individual *capacity* to consent is determined by age and competence. Generally, one must be an adult in the technical and legal sense in order to consent to treatment. The legal age for adult status is established by state statute and varies from state to state. Based on state statute, minors may consent to certain types of treatment, such as abortion and substance abuse treatment. Adults are considered competent when they can make choices and understand the consequences of their choices.

Individuals act *voluntarily* when they exercise freedom of choice without force, fraud, deceit, duress, or any other form of coercion. Consent that is compelled by threats or provoked by fraud is legally considered to

be no consent at all. Because patients are exceptionally vulnerable when they need medical care, they may believe, or be led to believe, that they must comply with the recommendations of health care professionals. Often patients believe that if they don't comply they may get less than adequate care or no care at all. All too frequently, nurses and other health professionals take it for granted that because a patient is under their care, the patient will agree to whatever care is deemed necessary. Nurses have an obligation to create an atmosphere that avoids any indication of coercion or manipulation.

The third element of informed consent is *information.* Information must be supplied to patients in a manner that is understandable to them. Lay terminology is preferred to professional terminology. The information must include the following:

- An explanation of the treatment to be performed and the expected results
- A description of the anticipated risks and discomforts
- A list of potential benefits
- A disclosure of possible alternatives
- An offer to answer the patient's questions
- A statement that the patient may withdraw his or her consent at any time

The legal responsibility to provide the necessary information for informed consent rests with the individual who will perform the treatment. When a nurse asks a patient to sign a consent form, the nurse is merely attesting to the fact that there is reason to believe that the patient is informed regarding the impending treatment and is witnessing the signature. If the nurse asks the patient to sign a consent form knowing that the patient has had no prior explanation of the treatment, the consent is invalid.

Right to Refuse Treatment   Just as competent adults have the right to consent to treatment, they also have the right to refuse treatment. In addition, guardians of incompetent adults have the right to refuse treatment for them. The right of competent adults to refuse treatment is guaranteed by the Constitution and has been tested in court with several landmark cases (*Quinlan v. New Jersey,* 1976; *Cruzan v. Director, Missouri Department of Health,* 1990). In recent years, most states have adopted statutory laws to protect these rights and to protect the health care provider who agrees to not treat even when treatment could be considered medically indicated. These laws are referred to as living wills, durable power of attorney, and advance directives.

In 1990, Congress enacted the **Patient Self-Determination Act.** This is a federal law that requires every health care facility that receives Medicare or Medicaid funds to provide written information to adult patients concerning their right under state law to make health care decisions. These decisions include the right to accept or refuse treatment and the right to formulate advance directives (Omnibus Budget Reconcillation Act [OBRA], 1990).

An **advance directive** is a document that allows the competent patient to make choices prior to the need for medical treatment. Examples include decisions such as refusing treatment, being placed on life support, and stopping treatment. The two most common advance directives are the living will and the durable power of attorney for health care (Figure 5-1).

With the **living will,** the competent adult signs a form indicating what health care the person wants done in the future. These decisions will be upheld should that adult's decision-making capacity be lost.

The **durable power of attorney for health care decisions** permits a competent adult to appoint a surrogate or proxy to make decisions for that person in the event that he or she becomes incompetent. The health care provider must follow the expressed wishes as stated in these documents. Difficulties arise when the patient is incompetent and does not have an advance directive or the directive is vague. In these cases, the health provider often relies on family members to make these decisions. In most states, however, family members do not have the legal authority to make such decisions unless they are the legally appointed guardians or parents.

Freedom from Restraint Another potential area of liability is the use of restraints. The Omnibus Budget Reconciliation Act (OBRA) of 1987 provides patients the right to be free from any physical or chemical restraint imposed for the purpose of discipline or convenience and not required to treat medical symptoms. These regulations apply to nursing homes, state and federal agencies, and other health care organizations that receive Medicare and Medicaid funds. According to these rules, health professionals are required to assess the need for restraints and consider the use of alternative measures. When restraints are deemed necessary, a physician's order specifying duration and circumstances is required. No orders for as-needed (PRN) restraints are permitted. When restraints are used, the patient must be monitored closely and reassessed periodically to evaluate the continued need for restraints. In addition to federal regulations, most states have laws governing the use of restrictive devices.

Federal mandates also call for the judicious use of psychotropic drugs, which are frequently used as chemical restraints. Psychotropic drugs no longer may be used for the purpose of controlling behavior; they may be prescribed only for diagnosis-related conditions. The intention is to prevent indiscriminate use of psychotropic drugs that frequently cause patients to become deeply sedated, agitated, or combative.

In July 1992, the Food and Drug Administration (FDA) issued a warning to health care providers concerning the potential hazards associated with the use of physical restraint devices. Nurses frequently believe that restraints protect the patient from injury to self or others, yet there is no proof that restraints actually prevent injury. On the contrary, there is more evidence that restraints cause injury: The FDA (1992) estimates at least 100 deaths or injuries per year are associated with the use of restraints.

The use of restraints should be based on the principles of informed consent. If patients are unable to consent, then reliable proxy consent should be obtained with full disclosure of risks and benefits. Restraining

---

KEY TERMS

Confidentiality The right to privacy of records.

Informed consent The consent for treatment given by a patient after three requirements are met: the individual has the capacity to consent, consent is voluntary, and the individual receives information regarding treatment in a manner that is understandable to him or her.

Patient Self-Determination Act A federal law requiring every health care facility receiving Medicare or Medicaid to provide written information to adult patients concerning their right to make health care decisions.

Advance directive A document that allows the competent patient to make choices regarding health care prior to its need.

Living will An advance directive that indicates what an individual wants done regarding treatment or lifesaving measures in the future.

Durable power of attorney for health care decisions A document that permits an individual to give a surrogate or proxy the authority to make decisions for that person in the event that she or he becomes incompetent.

This is a Durable Power of Attorney for Health Care Decisions, and the authority of my agent shall not terminate if I become incapacitated. I grant my agent full authority to make decisions for me regarding my health care. In exercising this authority, my agent shall follow my desires as stated in my Health Care Treatment Directive or otherwise known to my agent. My agent's authority to interpret my desires is intended to be as broad as possible and any expenses incurred should be paid by my resources. My agent may not delegate the authority to make decisions. My agent is authorized as follows to:

> If there is a statement in paragraphs 1 through 6 below with which you do not agree, draw a line through it and add your initials.

1. Consent, refuse or withdraw consent to any care, treatment, service or procedure (including artificially supplied nutrition and/or hydration/tube feeding) used to maintain, diagnose or treat a physical or mental condition;
2. Make decisions regarding organ donation, autopsy and the disposition of my body;
3. Make all necessary arrangements for any hospital, psychiatric hospital or psychiatric treatment facility, hospice, nursing home or similar institution; to employ or discharge health care personnel (any person who is licensed, certified or otherwise authorized or permitted by the laws of the state to administer health care) as the agent shall deem necessary for my physical, mental and emotional well being;
4. Request, receive and review any information, verbal or written, regarding my personal affairs or physical or mental health including medical and hospital records and to execute any releases of other documents that may be required in order to obtain such information;
5. Move me into or out of any state for the purpose of complying with my Health Care Treatment Directive or the decisions of my agent;
6. Take any legal action reasonably necessary to do what I have directed.

I appoint the following person to be my agent to make health care decisions for me WHEN AND ONLY WHEN I lack the capacity to make or communicate a choice regarding a particular health care decision and my Health Care Treatment Directive does not adequately cover circumstances. I request that the person serving as my agent be my guardian if one is needed.

> If you do not wish to name an agent, write "None" in the space provided below.

Agent's Name: _____ Telephone: _____

Address: _____

_____

If my agent is not available or not willing to make health care decisions for me, or if my agent is my spouse and is legally separated or divorced from me, I appoint the person or persons named below (in the order named if more than one listed) as my agent: (It is not necessary to name an alternate agent.)

First Alternate Agent   Second Alternate Agent

Name: _____   Name: _____

Address: _____   Address: _____

Telephone: _____   Telephone: _____

Protection of Persons Who Rely on My Agent: I and my estate hold my agent and my caregivers harmless and protect them against any claim for following this durable power of attorney.

Severability: If any part of this document is held to be unenforceable under law, I direct that all of the other provisions of the document shall remain in force and effect.

Date: _____ X Signature _____

Witness _____ Date _____ Witness _____ Date _____

Figure 5-1   **Sample durable power of attorney for health care decisions. This Advance Directive Document, consisting of a Health Care Treatment Directive and a Durable Power of Attorney for Health Care Decisions, is a product of the Advance Directive Community Project operated by Midwest Bioethics Center, Kansas City, MO.**

Health Care Treatment Directive

I _____ make this Health Care Treatment Directive to exercise my
Print Name
right to determine the course of my health care and to provide clear and convincing proof of my treatment decisions when I lack the capacity to make or communicate my decisions and there is no realistic
hope that I will regain such capacity.

If my physician believes that a certain life prolonging procedure or other health care treatment
may provide me with comfort, relieve pain or lead to a significant recovery, I direct my physician to try the
treatment for a reasonable period of time. However, if such treatment proves to be ineffective, I direct
treatment be withdrawn even if so doing may shorten my life.

I direct I be given health care treatment to relieve pain or to provide comfort even if such treatment might shorten my life, suppress my appetite or my breathing, or be habit-forming.

> I direct all life prolonging procedures be withheld or withdrawn when there is no hope of significant
> recovery, and I have:
> - a terminal condition; or
> - a condition, disease or injury without reasonable expectation that I will regain an
>   acceptable quality of life; or
> - substantial brain damage or brain disease which cannot be significantly reversed.
>
> 1. When any of the above conditions exist, I DO NOT WANT the life prolonging procedures which
>   I have initialed below. (You should assume any treatments not initialed may be administered
>   to you.)
>   - surgery . . . . _____ initials
>   - heart-lung resuscitation (CPR) . . . . _____ initials
>   - antibiotics . . . . _____ initials
>   - dialysis . . . . _____ initials
>   - mechanical ventilator (respirator) . . . . _____ initials
>   - tube feedings (food and water delivered through a tube in the vein,
>   nose, or stomach) . . . . _____ initials
>   - other _____ _____ initials
> 2. I make other instructions as follows: (You may describe what a minimally acceptable quality of
>   life is for you.)
>   _____
>   _____
>   _____
>   _____

> If you do not wish to name an agent as referred to on the reverse side, initial here _____ ,
> write "None" in the space provided for agent's name, sign and have witnessed and/or notarized.

Figure 5-1   **Sample durable power of attorney for health care decisions.** (*continued*)

Notarization

> Notarization of the Durable Power of Attorney is required in some states (e.g., Missouri but not Kansas). If this document is both witnessed and notarized, it is more likely to be honored in other states.

On this _____ day of _____, _____, before me personally appeared the aforesaid declarant, to me known to be the person described in and who executed the foregoing instrument and acknowledged that he/she executed the same as his/her free act and deed. IN WITNESS WHEREOF, I

have hereunto set my hand and affixed my official seal in the County of _____,

State of _____ , the day and year first above written.

_____   _____
Notary Public   My Commission Expires

Acceptance: (Optional) I have discussed this document with the person making this durable power of attorney and I accept the responsibility designated to me as stated above.

Date _____   Agent _____

Figure 5-1   Sample durable power of attorney for health care decisions. (*continued*)

patients without consent or sufficient justification may be interpreted as false imprisonment. In addition to legal rights, the use of restraints clearly involves ethical issues such as autonomy and beneficence.

Management Issues

Delegation and Supervision With the redesign of health care delivery systems and the use of more unlicensed workers, the professional nurse's responsibility has increased. Now, more than ever, nurses must understand the legal responsibilities they assume when delegating and supervising unlicensed assistive personnel.

Nursing management encompasses supervision of nursing care and the personnel who provide that care. Nurses are personally liable for the reasonable exercise of their delegation and supervision activities. They must be aware of the staff's knowledge, skills, and competencies when delegating tasks and should supervise appropriately. Nurses have a legal duty to ensure that staff members under their supervision are performing in a manner consistent with the desired standard of practice. If a nurse makes an assignment to an individual who the nurse knows is not competent to perform that assignment, the nurse will be liable if the patient is injured (see Chapter 10.)

Staffing According to established standards, the organization must provide adequate staffing with qualified personnel (Joint Commission on the Accreditation

of Healthcare Organizations [JCAHO], 2003). The organization that fails to retain the level of nursing personnel required to provide safe, quality care may be held liable under the doctrines of respondeat superior and corporate liability if an injury occurs related to short staffing. The responsibility of the organization to maintain an adequate staffing level is the nurse manager's. What constitutes adequate personnel is not specified in JCAHO guidelines because what is satisfactory under one set of circumstances may not be satisfactory under another.

Although retaining appropriate nursing personnel is the responsibility of the organization, if it can be shown that the staff nurse acted unreasonably under the circumstances, the individual nurse also can be held liable for acts of omission or commission. In other words, inadequate staff is no excuse for negligent acts; however, if the nurse acts reasonably under the circumstances, the individual may not be found culpable for malpractice. And if the hospital can demonstrate that it has taken appropriate actions to alleviate the staffing crisis, then it may not be held liable.

Staffing an organization is not as clear-cut as it may seem. Although the organization has some guidelines to follow, such as those mandated by federal and state regulatory bodies, these guidelines are broad and require a certain amount of judgment. Other factors involved in providing adequate staff are somewhat subjective and the responsibility of the organization. Patient classification systems help provide an objective measure of the number of staff needed; however, they do not take into consideration whether the staff are experienced or inexperienced. They also do not take into consideration whether adequate equipment is accessible, appropriate policies exist, and sufficient supervision is available, all of which are helpful adjuncts during a staffing crunch.

Job Reassignment   The hospital has a legal duty to ensure that all areas of the hospital are adequately staffed. With fluctuating patient census, this often places the hospital in a position in which reassigning nurses' duties is the only way to balance the needs of the unit and the safety of patients. **Job reassignment** (floating) is the process of pulling nurses from one area of the hospital to another. This practice is commonplace in today's health care organization, but concerns are raised by both staff and administration. Floating nurses to unfamiliar areas, especially specialty areas, increases the chance of error and may increase the nurse's anxiety, which in turn may affect job satisfaction and morale.

Reassigning hospital personnel is a necessary evil that in many instances cannot be avoided. Nurses have no legal ground to refuse to float unless it has been previously specified in their contract, or unless the organization has policies and procedures to the contrary. The nurse who refuses to float may face the possibility of discharge on the grounds of insubordination. Nurses must realize they have a professional responsibility to serve in the best interest of the patient. Open communication regarding limitations and concerns, creative problem solving, and cross-training are some solutions to the problem of reassignment.

Policies and Procedures   When the nurse is responsible for performing procedures that require judgments beyond the usual scope of nursing practice, a standardized procedure, or protocol, is necessary. These procedures must be written and authorized by the organization. Routinely, the standardized protocol must specify

- Functions the nurse may perform under specific circumstances;
- Requirements that must be followed in performing the function;
- Education, experience, and training requisites of the nurse performing the procedures; and
- Method for evaluating the competence of the nurse performing the practice.

Policies and procedures are required for all health care organizations. These documents serve to stan-

dardize care, set standards, and guide practices. They should be well delineated, clearly stated, and based on current and actual practice.

Release of Information   The same guiding principles regarding release of information about patients also apply to release of information about employees. Information regarding employees is considered confidential and must not be released outside the organization without the explicit consent of the employee except to verify employment or to comply with legal investigation. The Privacy Act of 1974 outlines stringent requirements for handling personnel matters related to privacy issues. The nurse manager needs to be familiar with this law, especially as it relates to giving references and recommendations.

Incompetent Practice   The "due care" standard requires nurse managers to confront unsafe practice. It is important for the nurse manager to be familiar with both the organization's procedures for addressing safety and professional conduct and the state boards of nursing guidelines. Many states have instituted mandatory reporting of unsafe practices to safeguard public health. Mandatory reporting is a complex process involving both legal and ethical parameters. The vast majority of the complaints and disciplinary actions are for impairment or drug diversion. Chapter 23 provides more information about impaired nursing practice.

National Practitioner Data Bank   The **National Practitioner Data Bank** (NPDB) was created as a follow-up to the Health Care Quality Improvement Act of 1986. The NPDB serves as an information clearinghouse regarding adverse actions, such as licensure sanctions, against health care professionals, including physicians and nurses. Federal regulations require health care institutions, license boards, professional societies, and malpractice payers to report any actions taken against professionals (Sheehan, 2001).

KEY TERMS

Job reassignment   The process of pulling or floating nurses from one area of the hospital to another.

National Practitioner Data Bank   An information clearinghouse for reporting adverse action against health care professionals.

Employment Issues

Increasingly, nurse managers are responsible and liable for employment decisions within health care organizations. For this reason, the nurse manager needs to be familiar with the growing body of antidiscrimination laws. These statutes have a profound effect on hiring, advancement, and termination practices of the employer. Matters of employee rights have been pronounced since the passage of the Civil Rights Act of 1964. Today, we continue to see increased activity related to discrimination of various kinds, and many states have enacted laws governing civil rights and antidiscrimination.

Civil Rights Act of 1964   Title VII of the 1964 Civil Rights Act (CRA) bars discrimination on the basis of race, color, sex, or national origin. It governs all public and private agencies with 15 or more employees and addresses all aspects of employment (e.g., hiring, promotion, discipline, supervision, performance appraisal, dismissal). The Equal Employment Opportunity Commission (EEOC) is the federal agency that administers and enforces Title VII. In 1978, the CRA was extended to include discriminatory treatment of pregnant women; as a result, employers who require mandatory maternity leave without regard to the employee's ability to work are in violation of Title VII. Two exceptions are the bona fide occupational qualifications (BFOQ) and bona fide seniority or merit system. The BFOQ states that it is lawful to make employment decisions on the basis of national origin, religion, and sex (but not race or color) if this is necessary for the job. Proof of necessity may be difficult to verify. The bona fide seniority or merit system contends that it is permissible to make decisions about promotions and layoffs based on seniority.

Sexual Harassment   In 1980, the EEOC established guidelines stating that sexual harassment in the workplace violates Title VII. Under these guidelines, the employer can be held liable for acts of sexual harassment committed by employees whether or not the employer had any prior knowledge of the reported acts. For these reasons, employers frequently establish proactive policies to sensitize employees to the problem and to help prevent instances of sexual harassment in the workplace. The guidelines define sexual harassment to include conduct in which

- Submission to sexual advances is explicitly or implicitly a term or condition of an individual's employment,

- Submission to or rejection of sexual advances is used as a basis for employment decisions, and
- The nature of the sexual advances has the purpose or effect of interfering with work performance or creating an intimidating, hostile, or offensive work environment.

Age Discrimination in Employment Act   Passage of the Age Discrimination in Employment Act (ADEA) in 1967 made it unlawful for employers to discriminate against older men and women in decisions regarding all phases of employment. In 1986, this act was extended to prohibit discrimination against individuals over the age of 40, and mandatory retirement for persons at any age is prohibited. The ADEA applies to public and private organizations with 20 or more employees. Again, as with Title VII, an employer may exercise bona fide occupational qualifications (BFOQ) and the bona fide seniority system as exemptions.

Americans with Disabilities Act   Title I of the Americans with Disabilities Act (ADA, 1990), which became effective July 1992, is designed to eliminate discrimination against disabled persons in employment by enforcing equal access to jobs and accommodations. In general, no employer, public or private, with 15 or more employees may discriminate against a qualified individual with a disability because of the disability.

The ADA (1990) broadly defines disability as

- A physical or mental impairment that substantially limits one or more of the major life activities,
- A record of such impairment, and
- Regarded as having such impairment.

These guidelines apply to all phases of the employment process, including hiring, advancement, compensation, training, discharge, or other conditions of employment. Furthermore, the ADA not only prohibits discrimination but also requires employers to provide reasonable accommodations for disabled employees, which includes employees who have been identified as recovering from alcohol or drug addiction. (See Chapter 23 for more on employees with substance abuse problems.)

Reasonable accommodations might include providing leaves of absence with or without pay, job reassignment, and job restructuring. The exact recommendations for providing these accommodations are not yet clear. Other suggestions from the courts include keeping disabled employees informed of other, more suitable, job openings within the agency, allowing the employee to work at home, and assigning another employee to work with the disabled employee as part of a team. Until such time when there are enough consistent data from the test cases, the nurse manager should be open-minded, flexible, and creative when it comes to making reasonable accommodations for disabled employees.

Just as what constitutes making accommodations is vague, so are the definition itself and the EEOC's implementation regulations. Therefore, many alleged violations are being decided by the courts on a case-by-case basis. As these court decisions are handed down, the working definition of "disability" as well as key issues and answers surrounding this act are becoming clearer. Nurse managers are urged to keep abreast of these latest court decisions.

Family and Medical Leave Act The Family and Medical Leave Act (FMLA) of 1993 provides eligible employees with a leave of up to 12 weeks during any 12-month period for the employee's own serious illness, the birth or adoption of a child, the placement of a foster child into the household, or the care of a seriously ill child, spouse, or parent. Knowledge of this act, which is described in more detail in Chapter 23, provides guidance for leave issues.

Occupational Safety and Health Act The Occupational Safety and Health Act (OSHA) of 1970 was established to ensure a safe and healthful work environment for employees and to preserve human resources. OSHA standards are sets of rules designed to minimize specific on-the-job risks to employees. These risks include exposure to toxic chemicals, infectious agents, hazardous waste, and hazardous equipment. When OSHA deems agencies to be in violation of these standards, severe penalties are assessed. This act created three administrative bodies to carry out its mission:

1. The Occupational Safety and Health Administration (OSHA) is primarily responsible for creating and enforcing standards and procedures to enhance employee safety and health.
2. The National Institute of Occupational Safety and Health (NIOSH) engages in safety research and makes recommendations to OSHA.
3. The Occupational Safety and Health Review Committee (OSHRC) reviews contested actions made by employers following citations for noncompliance.

With the increased awareness of AIDS and the dangers of hepatitis infections, OSHA published regulations in 1991 designed to reduce occupational risks of infection from blood-borne pathogens. This standard is the most pervasive regulation imposed by OSHA on health care organizations. It applies to all occupational exposure to blood and other body fluids. Although most health care organizations comply with the Center for Disease Control and Prevention's universal precautions, OSHA regulations mandate several additional guidelines.

- Develop an exposure control plan to eliminate or minimize exposure.
- Make hepatitis B vaccine available to all employees at risk for exposure.
- After an exposure, ensure that the employee is tested and provided with follow-up treatment and counseling.
- Implement certain engineering and work practice controls to eliminate or minimize on-the-job risks.
- Store or maintain sharps or contaminated materials in accordance with regulations.
- Communicate to employees and the public the nature of contaminated waste by affixing appropriate labels bearing biohazard symbols.
- Provide training programs for all employees at the time of initial employment and annually thereafter.
- Maintain accurate and confidential records related to personnel training, vaccination, and management of exposures.

OSHA (2001) revised the regulations in 2001 requiring employers to

- Select safer needle devices as they become available,
- Involve employees in identifying and choosing the devices, and
- Maintain a log of injuries from contaminated sharps.

Although the number of guidelines regarding patient care, management, and employment may seem overwhelming, it is important to realize the improvements these guidelines have contributed to the work environment. They have helped to improve the quality of care and minimize risks. In addition, they have helped make efforts to eliminate discrimination successful.

Learn how one nurse manager handled an employee's injury, applying the appropriate regulations (see Case Study 5-1).

CASE STUDY 5-1: Legal and Ethical Issues

Denise Martinez is a nurse manager for a stand-alone surgical center, which is part of a 10-facility, not-for-profit health care system. She has management responsibilities for outpatient scheduling, operating room, postanesthesia care unit (PACU), and pain clinic.

John Robertson is a part-time registered nurse in the PACU, generally working 16 hours per week. He notifies Denise that he sustained a shoulder injury during his last work shift, 3 days ago. As a nurse manager, Denise's immediate responsibilities are for proper notification of injury (Occupational Safety and Health Act and Workers' Compensation) and ensuring that John receives appropriate and authorized medical treatment for his workplace injury.

If John's injury is serious enough to warrant extended leave from the surgical center, he will be eligible for temporary workers' compensation benefits. However, since John is a part-time employee and has not worked more than 1,250 hours at the surgical center in the past 12 months, he is not eligible for Family and Medical Leave (FMLA) nor is the surgical center required to guarantee reinstatement once he is released to return to work.

Denise assures John that she will work closely with him and follow up with the human resources department regarding his case.

Manager's Checklist

The nurse manager is responsible for

- Properly notifying OSHA and Workers' Compensation,
- Understanding and following the organization's policies regarding workplace injury and medical leave,
- Understanding eligibility of the employee for FMLA,
- Effectively communicating accurate information to the injured employee regarding his or her employment status,
- Following up with the human resource department and the employee regarding eligible benefits (e.g., health insurance, leave status, and return to work), and
- If necessary, making appropriate accommodations for the employee upon return to work.

What You Know Now

- Both ethical and legal principles guide the practice of nurses and nurse managers.
- Ethics deals with principles of right and wrong, good and bad; are based on personal beliefs and values; and govern our relationships with others.
- The Code of Ethics for Nurses explicitly defines the profession's values and standards of conduct.
- Laws are rules of conduct, established and enforced by authority, that prohibit extremes in behavior so that one can live without fear for self or property.
- Negligence is the failure of an individual to perform or not perform an act that a reasonably prudent person under the same circumstances would or would not perform.
- Liability may be personal, vicarious (as in the principle of respondeat superior), or corporate.
- Liability issues that directly concern nurse managers are delegation and supervision, staffing, floating, policies and procedures, unsafe practice, and employment regulations.
- Nurse managers must be knowledgeable about OSHA standards and regulations as well as the

laws regarding antidiscrimination and sexual harassment.

Questions to Challenge You

1. Study the Code of Ethics for Nurses. Do you agree with it? Explain your reasons.

2. Have you been faced with an ethical dilemma? Are you satisfied with the way you handled your part? How did it turn out? Would you handle a similar situation differently now?

3. You are manager of the home care division of a health care organization. What regulations might apply in the following situations?

   a) An employee's husband has just been diagnosed with cancer

   b) An employee who has been on sick leave returns to announce that she's been treated for alcohol dependency

   c) An employee reports a needle stick injury and you discover the organization is not using the latest needle safety equipment

4. How would you handle each of the above situations?

5. Have you been involved in a legal action or threat of one in health care? How was the situation handled and what was the outcome?

Explore 🌐 MediaLink

NCLEX review questions, essay activities, group activities, and other interactive resources for this chapter can be found on the Web site at http://www.prenhall.com/sullivan-decker. Click on "Chapter 5" to select activities for this chapter.

References

Alexander, Hawes & Audet, LLP. (2003). The Americans with disabilities act: Questions and answers. Retrieved July 2003, from http://consumerlawpage.com/brochure/disab.shtml

American Hospital Association (AHA). (1992). *A patient's bill of rights*. Chicago: Author.

American Nurses Association (ANA). (2001). *Code of ethics for nurses*. Washington, DC: Author.

Americans with Disabilities Act of (1990), Pub. L. No. 101-336, 42 U.S.C. Subsection 12101 (1991).

Cruzan v. Director, Missouri Department of Health, 110 S. Ct. 2841 (1990).

Food and Drug Administration. (1992). *FDA safety alert: Potential hazards with restraint devices*. Rockville, MD: Department of Health and Human Services.

Furrow, B., Johnson, S., Jost, T., & Schwartz, R. (1991). *Bioethics: Health care law and ethics*. St. Paul, MN: West.

Joint Commission on the Accreditation of Health Care Organizations [JCAHO]. (2003). *Staffing effectiveness.*

Retrieved July 2003, from http://www.jcaho.org/accredited+organizations/hospitals/standards/hospital+faqs/manage+human+res/planning/staffing+effectiveness.htm

Maddox, P. J. (2002). HIPAA: Update on rule revisions and compliance requirements. *Nursing Economics, 20*(2), 88–92.

National Council of State Boards of Nursing [NCSBN]. (1998). Mutual recognition model for nursing regulation: Frequently asked questions. *Issues, 19*(1), 1–4.

NCSBN. (1999). Uniform core licensure requirements for initial licensure of RNs and LPN/VNs. *Issues, 20*(3), 1–2.

NCSBN. (2002a). *State compact bill status*. Retrieved July 2003, from http://www.ncsbn.org/public/nurselicensure compact/mutual_recognition_nurse.htm and http://www.ncsbn.org/public/news/news_interstate_compact_for_nursing.htm

NCSBN. (2002b). *Model nursing practice act*. Retrieved July 2003, from http://www.ncsbn.org/public/regulation/nursing_practice_model_practice_act.htm

Occupational Safety and Health Act of 1970, Pub. L. No. 91-596, 29 U.S.C. 651-678 (1970).

Occupational Safety and Health Administration. (2001). Occupational Injury and Illness Recording and Reporting Requirements 29 CFR Parts 1904 and 1952.

Omnibus Budget Reconciliation Act (OBRA), Pub. L. No. 100-203 Sec. 420(a), 421(a) (1987).

Omnibus Budget Reconciliation Act (OBRA). Pub. L. No. 101-508, Sec. 4206, 4751 (1990).

Quinlan v. New Jersey, 355 A. 2d 647 (NJ 1976).

Sheehan, J. P. (2001). Double-check data bank reporting. *Nursing Management, 32*(5), 22–23.

Understanding Power and Politics

Looking Ahead

What is power? How can power help reshape and improve nursing? What do politics mean to our everyday existence? How can political action influence the environment in which we live and work? In this turbulent time in health care, these are important questions for nurses to consider. Chapter 6 defines the role of politics in nursing and management, providing a framework of political action. In addition, the chapter addresses the relationship of power to leadership and image and provides an in-depth look at how political action in combination with power can have an impact on the future of health care.

Objectives

In this chapter, you will learn

- What power is.
- How power is used.
- How image is a source of power.
- How to increase your power.
- What politics means.
- How political action affects policy.
- How to use political action for professional goals.

MediaLink www.prenhall.com/sullivan-decker

Additional resources for this chapter can be found on the Companion Website at www.prenhall.com/sullivan-decker. Click on "Chapter 6" to select the activities for this chapter.

- NCLEX Review
- Critical Thinking Activities
- Current Events
- MediaLinks
- *Nursing Leadership & Management in Action*: Identifying the Personal Sources of Power; Identifying the Impact of Power; Differentiating the Types of Power

MEDIALINK Identifying the Impact of Power

As a nurse, do you want power? Do you need power? Do you have power? Are you politically savvy? Should you be more involved in the politics of nursing and health care? These are essential questions for nurses to consider. Although many nurses believe their work should be apolitical, failure to recognize the politics of patient care and nursing management can result in poor quality of care for the patient and frustration for the nurse.

This chapter identifies sources and uses of power, discusses the principles of power and politics, discusses strategies for effective political action, and applies these principles to the practice of the staff nurse, the role of the nurse manager, and the role of nurse leaders in the community.

Why Power?

Power emerges in every human encounter, whether you choose to acknowledge it or not. Often, the content, meaning, and purpose of power use or abuse are misunderstood or ignored. Power needs to be your ally, and you must seek to understand its dynamic qualities.

Power is the potential ability to influence (Hersey, Blanchard, & Johnson, 2001). Power also is defined as the potential to achieve goals.

It is also important to understand why power is used. The most common reasons are to gain a competitive advantage, acquire information, motivate, communicate, improve performance, and improve processes. By developing a power base, you gain the potential for maximum influence. The willingness to use power increases a nurse's ability to acquire the resources needed to improve patient care.

Regardless of when, why, and where care takes place, power centers around an individual's ability to influence others or the behavior of others. To acquire power, maintain it effectively, and use it skillfully, nurses must be aware of the sources and types of power that they will use to influence and transform patient care.

Power and Leadership

Real power—principle-centered power—is based on honor, respect, loyalty, and commitment. Principle-centered power is not forced; it is invited (Covey, 1990). It is defined by the capacity to act and to make choices and decisions. How you choose and what you choose is based on deeply held values. If you choose to live up to your own values and potential, you have an infinite amount of power available. By recognizing your power and the capacity to use it, you can influence and lead others in promoting and creating changes in health care and in your community.

Leadership power then becomes the capacity to create order from conflict, contradictions, and chaos. Leadership power comes from the ability to sustain proactive influence because followers trust and respect the leader to do the right thing for the right reason. As leaders in health care, nurses must understand and select behaviors that activate principle-centered leadership:

- *Get to know people.* Understanding what other people want is not always simple.
- *Be open.* Keep others informed. Trust, honor, and respect spread just as equally as fear, suspicion, and deceit.
- *Know your values and visions.* The power to define your goals is the power to choose.
- *Sharpen your interpersonal competence.* Actively listen to others, and learn to express your ideas well.
- *Use your power to enable others.* Be attentive to the dynamics of power, and give attention to ground rules, such as encouraging dissenting voices and respecting disagreement.
- *Enlarge your sphere of influence and connectedness.* Power sometimes grows out of someone else's need.

Power: How Managers and Leaders Get Things Done

Classically, managers in health care institutions relied on authority to rouse employees to perform tasks and accomplish goals. In contemporary health care organizations, managers use persuasion, enticement, and inspiration to mobilize the energy and talent of a work group and to overcome resistance to change.

A leader's use of power alters attitudes and behavior by addressing individual needs and motivations. There are seven generally accepted types of interpersonal power used in organizations to influence others

MEDIALINK Differentiating the Types of Power

KEY TERMS

Power The potential ability to influence in order to achieve goals.

(French & Raven, 1959; Hersey, Blanchard, & Natemeyer, 1979).

1. **Reward power** is based on the inducements the manager can offer group members in exchange for cooperation and contributions that advance the manager's objectives. The degree of compliance depends on how much the follower values the expected benefits. For example, a nurse manager may grant paid educational leave as a way of rewarding staff nurses for implementing a new patient database system. Reward power often is used in relation to a manager's formal job responsibilities.

2. **Punishment,** or coercive, **power** is based on the penalties a manager might impose on an individual or a group. Motivation to comply is based on fear of punishment or withholding of rewards. For example, the nurse manager might make undesirable job assignments, mete out a formal reprimand, or recommend termination for a nurse who engages in disruptive behavior. Punishment or coercion is used in relation to a manager's perceived authority to determine employment status.

3. **Legitimate power** stems from the manager's right to make a request because of the authority associated with job and rank in an organizational hierarchy. Followers comply because they accept a manager's prerogative to impose requirements, sanctions, and rewards in keeping with the organization's mission and aims. For instance, staff nurses will comply with a nurse manager's directive to take time off without pay when the workload has dropped below projected levels because they know that the manager is charged with maintaining unit expenses within budget limitations.

4. **Expert power** is based on possession of unique skills, knowledge, and competence. Nurse managers, by virtue of experience and advanced education, often are the best qualified to determine what to do in a given situation. Employees are motivated to comply because they respect the manager's expertise. Expert power relates to the development of personal abilities through education and experience. Newly graduated nurses might ask the nurse manager for advice in learning clinical procedures or how to resolve conflicts with co-workers or other health professionals.

5. **Referent power** is based on admiration and respect for an individual. Followers comply because they like and identify with the manager. Referent power relates to the manager's likability and success. For

example, a new graduate might ask the advice of a more experienced and admired nurse about career planning.

6. **Information power** is based on access to valued data. Followers comply because they are motivated by a desire for information that will meet personal needs and facilitate decision making. Information power depends on a manager's organizational position, connections, and communication skills. For example, the nurse manager is frequently privy to information obtained at meetings with administrators about pending organizational changes that affect employees' work situations. A nurse manager may exercise information power by sharing signifi-

---

KEY TERMS

Reward power Power based on inducements offered by the manager in exchange for contributions that advance the manager's objectives.

Punishment (coercive) power Power based on penalties a manager might impose if the individual or group does not comply with authority.

Legitimate power A manager's right to make requests because of authority within an organizational hierarchy.

Expert power Power based on the manager's possession of unique skills, knowledge, and competence.

Referent power Power based on admiration and respect for an individual.

Information power Power based on an individual's access to valued data.

Connection power Power based on an individual's formal and informal links to influential or prestigious persons within and outside an organization.

Position power Power of an individual that is determined by the job description, assigned responsibilities, recognition, advancement, authority, the ability to withhold money, and decision making.

Personal power Power based on an individual's credibility, reputation, expertise, experience, control of resources or information, and ability to build trust.

cant information at staff meetings, thereby improving attendance.

7. **Connection power** is based on an individual's formal and informal links to influential or prestigious persons within and outside an area or organization. Followers comply because they want to be linked to influential individuals. Connection power also relates to the status and visibility of the individual as well as the position. In some cases, nurse managers have personal relationships with an organization's board members that followers believe will protect or advance their work situation.

These power bases are available to managers and may be classified more simply as personal or position power. **Position power** is determined by the job description, assigned responsibilities, recognition, advancement, authority, the ability to withhold money, and decision making. Legitimate, coercive, and reward power are positional because they relate to the "right" to influence others based on rank or role. The extent to which managers mete out rewards and punishment usually is dictated by organizational policy. Information and legitimate power are directly related to the manager's role in the organizational structure.

Expert, referent, information, and connection power are based, for the most part, on personal traits. **Personal power** refers to one's credibility, reputation, expertise, experience, control of resources or information, and ability to build trust. The extent to which one may exercise expert, referent, information, and connection power relates to personal skills and positive interpersonal relationships, as well as employees' needs and motivations.

Leaders and managers often exercise power differently. Leaders tend to rely primarily on personal power sources to provoke interest, inspire commitment, and instill confidence. Managers tend to use position power to ensure adherence to policies and standards and to complete work assignments. Managers also use position power to ensure orderly operation of their areas of responsibility. On the other hand, managers may use personal power to resolve conflicts among members of the work group, to develop an innovative approach to care delivery, or to improve working relationships with other professionals, clients, or organizational decision makers. Managers also rely on personal power to sustain commitment and interest in highly routinized jobs, as well as to maintain an esprit de corps among co-workers.

"Power is interdependent and a balancing act between managers and employees," say King and Koliner (1999,

p. 39). A manager must exercise power judiciously, which is effective because of the dependency that is inherent in a power relationship. The dependency relationship between manager and employee can result in vulnerability and exploitation, as well as benefit.

A manager usually uses both positional and personal power, and both must be used appropriately. The most effective combination depends on the manager's personality, the situation, the needs of followers, and balance in the power–dependency relationship. Box 6-1 provides guidelines for use of power in organizations.

Nurse managers in contemporary health care organizations must recognize that power helps them influence actions and decisions that will benefit staff as well as patients, families, and communities. Nurse managers should view power as a valuable resource that they must acquire, conserve, and invest carefully. Power is used best to support organizational priorities, to facilitate important activities and decisions, and to manage differences among interdependent organization members. Interpersonal skills and technical and managerial competence are far more likely to generate genuine commitment than the use of rewards and punishment.

Managers use power to motivate others, to strengthen their abilities, and to create alliances among diverse parties. Through the effective use of legitimate and expert power, a manager might require staff to improve skills and change personal behavior in anticipation of new technology or services. A manager also may use connection and referent power to bring conflicting parties together to solve problems or develop new programs. When the manager seeks power only to enhance his or her status, however, failures in performance, standoffs, or breakdowns in working relationships result. On the other hand, power used in the service of others—clients, employees, the community, the organization—increases the status and confidence of both the manager and employees. In fast-paced, contemporary organizations, power flows to individuals who have the ability to help the organization deal with complex, difficult tasks. Nurse managers should consider how to demonstrate these principles and further develop their power bases.

Using Power

Despite an increase in pride and self-esteem that comes with using power and influence, some nurses still consider power unattractive. The association of power

Box 6-1 Guidelines for the Use of Power in Organizations

Guidelines for Using Legitimate Authority

- Make polite, clear requests.
- Explain the reasons for a request.
- Don't exceed your scope of authority.
- Verify authority if necessary.
- Follow proper channels.
- Follow up to verify compliance.
- Insist on compliance if appropriate.

Guidelines for Using Reward Power

- Offer the type of rewards that people desire.
- Offer rewards that are fair and ethical.
- Don't promise more than you can deliver.
- Explain the criteria for giving rewards and keep it simple.
- Provide rewards as promised if requirements are met.
- Use rewards symbolically (not in a manipulative way).

Guidelines for Using Coercive Power

- Explain rules and requirements, and ensure that people understand the serious consequences of violations.
- Respond to infractions promptly and consistently without showing any favoritism to particular individuals.
- Investigate to get the facts before using reprimands or punishment, and avoid jumping to conclusions or making hasty accusations.
- Except for the most serious infractions, provide sufficient oral and written warnings before resorting to punishment.

- Administer warnings and reprimands in private, and avoid making rash threats.
- Stay calm and avoid the appearance of hostility or personal rejection.
- Express a sincere desire to help the person comply with role expectations and thereby avoid punishment.
- Invite the person to suggest ways to correct the problem, and seek agreement on a concrete plan.
- Maintain credibility by administering punishment if noncompliance continues after threats and warnings have been made.

Guidelines for Using Expert Power

- Explain the reasons for a request or proposal and why it is important.
- Provide evidence that a proposal will be successful.
- Don't make rash, careless, or inconsistent statements.
- Don't exaggerate or misrepresent the facts.
- Listen seriously to the person's concerns and suggestions.
- Act confidently and decisively in a crisis.

Ways to Acquire and Maintain Referent Power

- Show acceptance and positive regard.
- Act supportive and helpful.
- Use sincere forms of ingratiation.
- Defend and back up people when appropriate.
- Do unsolicited favors.
- Make self-sacrifices to show concern.
- Keep promises.

Adapted from *Leadership in Organizations*, 5th ed. (pp. 146–152), by G. Yukl, 2002, Upper Saddle River, NJ: Prentice Hall. Reprinted by permission.

with aggression and coercion remains strong. In a profession that prides itself on care and compassion, power is viewed as alien. How, then, can nurses bridge the disparity between power as good versus power as bad?

Power grabbing, which has been the traditionally accepted means of relating to power for one's own self-interests and use, is how nurses often think of power. Rather, women and nurses tend to be more comfortable with power sharing and empowerment: power "with" rather than power "over" others. Although nurses need power to ensure that patients have access

to cost-effective quality nursing care, nurses can help transform health care organizations by using power that embraces equality and caring.

Image as Power

A major source of power for nurses is an image of power. Even if one does not have actual power from other sources, the perception by others that one is powerful bestows a degree of power. The same is true for the profession as a whole. If the public sees the profession of nursing as powerful, the profession's ability to achieve its goals and agendas is enhanced.

Images emerge from interactions and communications with others. If nurses present themselves as caring and compassionate experts in health care through their interactions and communications with the public, then a strong, favorable image develops for both the individual nurse and the profession. Nurses, as the ambassadors of care, must understand the importance and benefit of positive therapeutic communications and image. Developing a positive image of power is important for both the individual and the profession.

Individual nurses can promote an image of power by a variety of means.

1. Appropriately introducing yourself by saying your name, using eye contact, and shaking hands can immediately establish you as a powerful person. If nurses introduce themselves by first name to the physician, Dr. Smith, they have immediately set forth an unequal power relationship unless the physician also uses his or her first name. Although women are not socialized to initiate handshakes, it is a power strategy in male-dominated circles, including health care organizations. In Western cultures, eye contact conveys a sense of confidence and connection to the individual to whom one is speaking. These seemingly minor behaviors can have a major impact on whether the nurse is perceived as competent and powerful.

2. Appropriate attire can symbolize power and success. Although nurses may believe that they are limited in choice of attire by uniform codes, it is in fact the presentation of the uniform that can hold the key to power. For example, a nurse manager needs a powerful image both with unit staff and with administrators and other professionals who are setting organizational policy. An astute nurse manager might wear a suit rather than a uniform to work on the day of a high-level interdisciplinary committee meeting. Certainly, attention to details of grooming and uniform selection can enhance the power of the staff nurse as well.

3. Conveying a positive and energetic attitude sends the message that you are a "doer" and someone to be sought out for involvement in important issues. Chronic complaining conveys a sense of powerlessness, whereas solving problems and being optimistic promote a "can do" attitude that suggests power and instills confidence in others.

4. Pay attention to how you speak and how you act when you speak. Nonverbal signs and signals say more about you than words. Make sure your words are reflected in your body language. In other words, keep your facial expression consistent with your message. Stand erect and move energetically. Speak with an even pace and enunciate words clearly. Use only body movements and gestures necessary to make your point.

5. Use facts and figures when you need to demonstrate your point. Policy changes usually evolve from data presented in a compelling story. To position yourself as a powerful player requires the ability to collect and analyze data. Data can be obtained to describe nursing care issues, activities, or concerns. These include patient acuity, daily census, length of stay, overtime budgets, or any data that reflect nursing's overall contribution. Remember that power is a matter of perception; therefore, you must use whatever data are available to support your judgment.

6. Knowing when to be at the right place at the right time is crucial to gain access to key personnel in the organization. This means being invited to events, meetings, and parties not necessarily intended for nurses. It means demanding to sit at the policy table when decisions affecting staffing and patient care are made. Influence is more effective when it is based on personal relationships and when people see others in person: "If I don't see you, I can't ask you for needed information, analysis, and alternative recommendations." Become visible. Be available. Offer assistance. You can be invaluable in providing policymakers with information, interpreting data, and teaching them about the nursing side of health care.

7. In dealing with people outside of nursing, it is important to develop powerful partnerships. Be very careful to use "we" instead of "they." Learn how to share both credit and blame. When working on collaborative projects, be clear about what is needed. If something isn't working well, say so. Never accept another's opinion as fact. Facts can be easily manipulated to fit one's personal agenda. Learn how to probe and obtain additional information. Don't assume you have all the information. Beware of unsolicited commentary. Don't be fearful of giving strong criticism, but always put criticisms in context. Before giving any criticism, give a compliment, if appropriate. Also, make sure your partners are ready to hear all sides of the issue. It's never superfluous to ask, "Do you want to talk about such and such right now?" Once an issue is decided—really decided—don't raise it again.

8. Make it a point to get to know the people who matter in your sphere of influence. Become a part of the power network so that when people are discussing issues or seeking people for important appointments of leadership, your name comes to mind. Be sure to deal with senior people. The more contact you have with the "power brokers," the more support you can generate in the future should the need arise. The more power you use, the more you get.

9. Know who holds the power. Identify the key power brokers. Develop a strategy for gaining access to power brokers through joining alliances and coalitions. Learn how to question others and how to become part of the organizational infrastructure. There is an art to determining when, what, and how much information is exchanged and communicated at any one time and to determining who does so. Powerful people have a keen sense of timing. Be sure to position yourself to be at the right place at the right time. Any strategy will involve a good deal of energy and effort. Direct influence and efforts toward issues of highest priority or when greatest benefits are likely to result.

10. Use power appropriately to promote consensus in organizational goals, develop common means to achieve these goals, and enhance a common culture to bind organizational members together. As the health care providers closest to the patient, nurses best understand patients' needs and wants. In the hospital, nurses are present on the first patient contact and thereafter for 24 hours a day, 7 days a week. In the clinic, the nurse may be the person the patient sees first and most frequently. By capitalizing on the special relationship that they have with patients, nurses can use marketing principles to enhance their position and image as professional caregivers.

Nursing as a profession must market its professional expertise and ability to achieve the objectives of health care organizations. From a marketing perspective, nursing's goal is to ensure that identified markets (e.g., patients, physicians, other health professionals, community members) have a clear understanding of what nursing is, what it does, and what it is going to do. In doing so, nursing is seen as a profession that gives expert care with a scientific knowledge base.

Nursing care often is seen as an indicator of an organization's overall quality. Regardless of the setting, quality nursing care is something that is desired and valued. Through understanding patients' needs and preferences for programs that promote wellness and maintain and restore health, nurses become the organization's competitive edge to enhancing revenues. Marketing an image of expertise linked with quality and cost can position nursing powerfully and competitively in the health care marketplace.

Using Power Appropriately

Using power not only affects what happens at the time, but also has a lasting effect on your relationships. Therefore, it is best to use the least amount of power necessary to accomplish your goals. Also, use power appropriate to the situation (Sullivan, 2004). Table 6-1 lists rules for using power.

Improper use of power can destroy a manager's effectiveness. Power can be overused or underused. Overusing power occurs when you use excessive power relative to the situation. If you fail to use power when it is needed, you are underusing your power. In addition to the immediate loss of influence, you may lose credibility for the future.

Power plays are another way that power is used inappropriately. **Power plays** are attempts by others to diminish or demolish their opponents. Table 6-2 describes several common power plays and their consequences. It is essential that nurses not accept these statements at face value. Often, restating one's initial point in a firm manner is a useful strategy. It is not necessary to respond directly to statements such as those shown in Table 6-2.

Nursing must perceive power for what it really is—the ability to mobilize and focus energy and resources.

Table 6-1 Rules for Using Power
1. Use the least amount of power you can to be effective in your interactions with others.
2. Use power appropriate to the situation.
3. Learn when not to use power.
4. Focus on the problem, not the person.
5. Make polite requests, never arrogant demands.
6. Use coercion only when other methods don't work.
7. Keep informed to retain your credibility when using your expert power.
8. Understand you may owe a return favor when you use your connection power.

From *Becoming influential: A guide for nurses* (p. 35), by E. J. Sullivan, 2004, Upper Saddle River, NJ: Prentice Hall. Reprinted by permission.

Table 6-2   Power Plays

Power Play	Recipient's Response
"Let's be fair."	Feelings of insecurity; insecure about choices because power game is played by someone else's rules.
"Can you prove that?"	Embarrassed by inability to defend self.
"Be specific."	Feelings of incompetence if facts and figures cannot be generated to support position.
"It's either this or that; which is it? Take your pick."	Angered at being forced to choose between limited options.
"But you said . . . and now you say . . . "	Confused about what was meant; believe your position is illogical.

What better position can nurses be in but to assume power to face new problems and responsibilities in reshaping nursing practice to adapt to environmental changes? Power is the means, not the end, to seek new ways for doing things in this uncertain and unsettling time in health care.

Power plus Vision

The key to understanding and gaining power is to identify what you and other people really desire. Once you have decided what you want, look at the total situation or encounter. Take into account, for example, the whole organization, not just your workplace or unit. Rank your wants or needs in order of importance. Determine who controls what you want and who or what stands in your way of achieving it. Identify the resources you control and the individuals who might desire those resources. Power resides not in aggressiveness or assertiveness but in the ability to make a conscious choice. Focus on the choice, not the action.

By making choices about what you want, you develop a strong sense of self-confidence and are aware of and feel good about your true capabilities. Your self-respect depends not on maintaining your role or position of power, but rather on your sense of purpose and direction. A clear vision pulls it all together by building consensus and support; identifying present capabilities; determining success factors; and identifying resources of people, time, and money.

Once you understand how power influences what choices are made and how these choices affect behaviors and feelings, you can appreciate its usefulness. In a constantly dynamic universe, power is a fundamental ingredient. You must ask yourself: Are you willing to use your power to know yourself, set goals, ignite the imagination, direct nursing care, build teams, and reach beyond the unknown into what could be? To use power to change and improve patient care is to recognize that power is natural and desirable.

Politics: The Art of Influencing

Politics is the art of influencing the allocation of scarce resources, which includes money, time, personnel, and materials (Mason, Leavitt, & Chaffee, 2002). Politics is a means to an end, a means for influencing events and the decisions of others. Nurses who renounce politics are essentially saying they do not want to influence events in their everyday work.

Politics

- Is an interpersonal endeavor,
- Is a collective activity,
- Requires analysis and planning, and
- Involves image.

As an *interpersonal endeavor,* politics uses the skills of communication and persuasion. Nurses' communication skills make them particularly effective in political activities. Nurses understand the importance of rapport and how to create meaningful connections with people. They understand the importance of time in developing these connections. They also understand the need to appeal to the other person's needs and interests if the goal is going to be reached. At a "Nurses Night" telephone bank to solicit support for a congressional candidate, the candidate's manager told the nurse organizer of the event, "You nurses are wonderful at this! I was listening to one nurse talking on the phone with a man who I thought must be her uncle or

MEDIALINK Legal and Political Issues in Nursing

KEY TERM

Power plays Power plays are attempts by others to diminish or demolish their opponents.

Politics A means of influencing the allocation of scarce resources, events, and the decisions of others.

someone she knew well—it was a stranger, but they were talking as if they were old friends!"

As a *collective activity,* politics often requires the support and action of many people to bring effective politics to bear on a situation or issue. Furthermore, working with others for political action can be invigorating, more creative, and simply more effective because there are more people to do the work and provide the emotional support that may be needed to sustain long-term political action.

The politically astute nurse develops and carefully uses a support base that crosses the hierarchical lines of each sphere. In the workplace, this means developing connections to other nurses, the maintenance people, top administrators, the social work department, physicians, and other workers at all levels of the organization. Certainly, this takes time, but it can and should be a part of the nurse's everyday work. For example, greet and speak to the person who is cleaning the floor every morning, sit with different people at lunch, and invite the new chief of the medical staff for a cup of coffee. It involves going to professional nursing meetings and exchanging business cards with those you meet. It involves providing support for others' agendas, knowing that they may be able to support you on an issue in the future. And it involves being able to organize and mobilize groups of nurses and coalitions of diverse groups.

It is helpful to have a target list of people with whom you would like to connect to build your support base, remembering that the secretary to the chief officer in the organization may be one of the most powerful persons in the organization by virtue of his or her ability to control access to the top administrator.

Politics is also about *analysis and planning.* Just as the nursing process requires a thorough assessment, good politics arises from a careful and insightful political analysis of the situation, issue, or problem. A political analysis includes assessing the structure and functioning of the sphere in which you are operating. What is the organizational structure? What are the formal and informal lines of communication? Who holds legitimate power? Who holds informal power? What are the stated and unstated missions and agendas of the organization? What individuals are involved in the issue or situation? From a systems perspective, one change on the system can have far-reaching effects on the rest of the system. What are the values, interests, beliefs, priorities, and agendas of these players? What connections and power bases do they have? What is the current context of the situation or issue? What is the climate for change? What outside forces might be influencing the situation or potential solutions or changes? What recent events might influence how others view the situation and their openness to change?

A good political analysis also includes a thorough assessment of the issue or problem itself. Why does the issue exist? What are the contributing factors? Who is affected by the issue? Do efforts need to be devoted to creating an audience interested in the issue? What beliefs and feelings do people hold about the issue? Are more data needed?

Effective political action involves planning. Based on the analysis just described, a group trying to influence an issue or situation would brainstorm about alternative solutions and evaluate their risks and benefits. But the group also would develop a plan for introducing its alternative and persuading others to support its position. Political analysis tells you who can be counted on to play what role in this process. For example, who should introduce the alternative to the person with the formal authority to make the decision to adopt it? Sometimes, the most politically astute approach is not to have the originator of the alternative introduce it, but rather the individual who is most likely to be accepted by the decision maker(s). Is collective action needed? What coalitions need to be formed? The political analysis also will suggest strategies related to timing. Should the alternative be proposed now or in 2 months? Should it be proposed as a pilot project or demonstration project? Should it be gradually phased in or implemented fully at one time? Should group pressure be brought to bear now or later? Timing is often crucial to the effectiveness of political action. People usually are more willing to accept something as a trial or test. Pilot projects also enable those affected to adjust to the change gradually.

Politics is also about *images.* Do people think you can make the change? Do people think the change will be harmful to them? Do people trust you? Do people identify positively with the coalition involved? Your future ability to be politically effective may hinge on the image that others have of you or the group. For example, it is well known that when a workers' contract is settled in a collective-bargaining dispute, both the union and management sides try to come out of the negotiations with the appearance of having won the most. Even losses can be seen as victories, particularly if the effort resulted in the mobilization and empowerment of nurses so that the whole group's power and likelihood of future success are enhanced. Defining the message you want others to receive and effectively marketing that message can create the image needed to further your political agenda.

Some of these guidelines for effective political action stem from long-standing political tenets based on how people (men, in particular) have operated in politics. Machiavelli's *The Prince* is the classic work advocating the use of cutthroat strategies for getting what one wants. Some nursing literature has addressed how to "swim with the sharks," and certainly nurses need to be aware of how the game of politics traditionally is played. However, work by feminist scholars is suggesting that many women may be uncomfortable with cutthroat, Machiavellian politics. It is important for nurses to think about the ethics of their politics. According to Mason (1999) a new ethic is evolving in nursing based on women's ways of knowing and working together. This is particularly relevant to understanding what power is, how to get it, and how it can be used and abused.

Policy and Political Action

Policy can be defined as the decisions that govern action. Policies determine an organization's relationships, activities, and goals. Policies result from political action.

Although most people associate the word *politics* with government, it pertains to every aspect of life that involves competition for allocating scarce resources or influencing decision making. As such, it is relevant to what nurses do in their daily practice, whether as a nurse in a home health agency, a nurse practitioner in a clinic, or a nurse manager in a hospital. What nurses do in their everyday practice is influenced by, and in turn influences, what governments do, what professional organizations do, and what communities do. What nurses do or do not do in one of these areas can have an effect on other areas and on their overall political power.

The steps in political action are shown in Table 6-3. You must first decide what you want to accomplish. Is it realistic? Will you have supporters? Who will be the detractors?

Try to find out what other people involved want. Maybe you could piggyback on their ideas. Congress does this all the time by adding amendments to proposed bills in an attempt to satisfy their opponents.

Start telling your supporters about your idea and see if they will join with you in a coalition. This is not necessarily a formal group but intended for you to know who you can count on in the discussions.

Find out exactly what objections your opponents have and try to figure out a way to alter your plan accordingly or help them understand how your proposal might help them. Political action is never easy, but the most politically astute people accomplish goals far more often than those who don't even try.

Political Action in the Organization

Once a patient gets into a hospital bed, the kind and quality of nursing care he or she receives also can be influenced by politics. For example, the nurse may not find the time to sit with the elderly patient who needs to be fed but will unquestioningly take the time to give the tube feeding that the physician has now ordered (and which will be reimbursed) for a patient who is not eating. The politics of this situation involves what values and policies the organization and third-party payers have embraced. In this case, nursing care requiring a physician's order—and particularly care that involves a technical procedure—is valued, expected, and reimbursed before humanistic, low-technology, personal care.

Politics in the workplace is often regarded with disdain, as reflected in the remark, "She plays politics." This statement is used to imply that the individual got what he or she wanted because of personal connections rather than on merit. And yet, would that same person want a chief nurse administrator who did not understand or use politics in advocating for nursing within the organization? Health care involves multiple special-interest groups all competing for their piece of a limited pool of resources. A group's failure to recognize this fact ensures that the group's ability to influence decision making within the organization will be limited.

Table 6-3	Steps in Political Action

1. Determine what you want.
2. Learn about the players and what they want.
3. Gather supporters and form coalitions.
4. Be prepared to answer opponents.
5. Explain how what you want can help them.

From *Becoming influential: A guide for nurses* (p. 35), by E. J. Sullivan, 2004, Upper Saddle River, NJ: Prentice Hall.

KEY TERM

Policy Decisions that govern action and determine an organization's relationships, activities, and goals.

MEDIALINK   Online Journal of Issues in Nursing

Are nurses involved in defining the mission and philosophy of the organization or third-party payers? They should be. Are nurses participating as equals in committees that set organizational policy? They should be. This is political action.

Something as mundane as which health care providers have reserved parking spaces, a reserved dining room, or the largest offices (or any office!) becomes an important symbol of the power and influence of particular groups. The resources available for nurses to provide safe, effective patient care also reflect the power of nursing within the organization. For example, staff nurses in a medical clinic may waste precious time trying to locate one of the clinic's two tympanic thermometers. Why does the clinic have only two tympanic thermometers available? Most organizations do not purchase the thermometers—the manufacturers often provide them free because the company makes its profit from the sheaths made specifically for the company's thermometer, which must be replaced with each use. Why will the organization spend money on expensive diagnostic equipment such as a nuclear magnetic imager but not on relatively inexpensive equipment that would facilitate cost-effective use of the nurses' time? In organizations where nurses have a high degree of power and influence, the nurse manager controls a budget and is able to negotiate for necessary time-saving equipment.

The delivery of nursing services occurs at many levels in health care organizations. The effectiveness of care delivery is linked to the application of power, politics, and marketing. For the staff nurse, the politics of bedside care involves influencing the allocation of scarce resources (e.g., equipment, supplies, time, or personnel) for the delivery of nursing care. To maintain access to the resources needed for patient care, nurses must connect to the whole organization and beyond, not just their own nursing unit.

Staff nurses need to understand that they belong to a complex organization that is continually confronted with limited resources and is in competition for those resources. With this understanding in mind, staff nurses can use their power when the limitations interfere with and place restrictions on patient care. Whether the restrictions come in the form of limited supplies, money, or time, nurses can use their power and the political skills of artful negotiation, collaboration, and networking to obtain the necessary resources to provide care. Speaking on behalf of patient care, access, and quality are what drives the politics of nursing care.

The politics of nursing care calls for an action plan, not just a care plan. It is time to force those who seek to establish policy without nursing's input to listen to what nurses have to say. Using power often means moving from being a passive observer to an active player. It means responding in politically astute ways by influencing and drafting policies rather than solely abiding by them. Mason (1999) suggests that there are two ways to lose power: by allowing others to take away your power and to become fragmented and self destruct. Unfortunately, both have occurred in nursing.

To respond effectively to the limits placed on clinical nursing practice, nurses must be visible and speak out about the "things nurses do": physical assessment, patient education, primary care, home and hospice care, and other health-related activities. How can nursing become a powerful force in the workplace and the community? How can nurses change the way power, politics, and policy are developed and used? One strategy is to write letters to the editor of your local newspaper or to contact television or radio talk shows explaining what nurses do and how their work improves care and individual lives.

In addition to becoming directly involved with policymakers, nurses can hold grassroots organizational meetings to prepare new policy initiatives or changes. Other strategies include identifying a group of nurses to write letters to the hospital paper explaining the impact the new policy will have on nursing and educating doctors about the public good that can be gained by working together.

What happens in the workplace both depends on and influences what is happening in the larger community, professional organizations, and government. The effective nurse manager understands the connections among these groups and uses them to the advantage of nursing, patients, and the health care organization. Developing influence in each of these three groups takes time and a long-range plan of action. Although the nurse's first priority should be to establish influence in the workplace, the nurse can gradually increase connections and influence with other groups and, later on, make these other groups a priority.

Political Action in the Community

The workplace, government, and organizations all interact with the community, whether local, regional, national, or international. One nurse found that her leadership in a community effort to eliminate improper garbage dumping in her town enabled her to develop important connections to government officials on both state and local levels. It also brought her to the attention of her hospital administrator in a positive and powerful way. The administrator knew that she had developed a positive reputation in the community and made significant connections to other persons of influence as a result of her actions. For many nurses who have children, an important forum for developing their political skills and power is the school's PTA or school board. An identity as a nurse in these groups can and should be made known. The connections developed can be used to further other purposes in the future.

This framework suggests that nurses need to understand the connections between what they do in their everyday work and what takes place in the rest of the community, nation, and world. Such a macroscopic view is particularly needed for the nurse manager. Although the nurse manager is rightfully concerned about how the work group is functioning, she or he must recognize that it does not function in a vacuum. Understanding and considering the broader context in which the unit is functioning makes the difference in whether the nurse manager is seen as visionary, whether the unit is on the cutting edge of nursing practice, and whether the unit sets the standard for excellence in the organization.

Using Power and Politics for Nursing's Future

How can nursing apply the principles of power and politics in the health care environment? Health care is in a state of constant change. Acute care hospitals are downsizing and reorganizing while, at the same time, community sites to deliver nursing care are expanding.

Nurses know the problems and have many of the solutions. Making a case for nursing input into health care policy is no longer an option for nurses. Nurses must be prepared to demand a seat at the policy table, whether that seat is in the board room; at federal, state, or local levels of government; or in any other setting where nurses remain a strong, vital component in health care delivery.

Nurses can have a tremendous impact on health care policy. The best impact is often made with a bit of luck and timing, but never without knowledge of the whole system. This includes knowledge of the policy agenda, the policymakers, and the politics that are involved. Once you gain this knowledge, you are ready to move forward with a political base to promote nursing.

To convert your policy ideas into political realities, consider the following power points:

- Use persuasion over coercion. Persuasion is the ability to share reasons and rationale when making a strong case for your position while maintaining a genuine respect for another's perspective.
- Use patience over impatience. Despite the inconveniences and failings caused by health care restructuring, impatience in the nursing community can be detrimental. Patience, along with a long-term perspective on the health care system, is needed.
- Be open-minded rather than closed-minded. Acquiring accurate information is essential if you want to influence others effectively.
- Use compassion over confrontation. In times of change, errors and mistakes are easy to pinpoint. It takes genuine care and concern to change course and make corrections.
- Use integrity over dishonesty. Honest discourse must be matched with kind thoughts and actions. Control, manipulations, and malice must be pushed aside for change to occur.

To manage nursing care in the future, nurses must come to realize that nursing expertise and clinical judgment are the best combination to effectively influence nursing practice and policy changes. By applying power and politics to the workplace, nurses increase their professional influence. Using influence, knowledge, and expertise can make the health care delivery system work.

What You Know Now

- Power enables nurses and nurse managers to accomplish their goals.
- Exercise of power is an essential aspect of leadership. Power is positional or personal and is based on several different sources, including control over rewards, punishment, information, institutional authority, expertise, personal likability, or connections.
- Nurses must perceive power for what it really is—the ability to mobilize and focus energy and resources.
- Effective use of power is using it appropriately.
- Image is a source of power.
- Politics is the ability to influence the allocation of scarce resources and events in our everyday world.
- Nurses can use political action to influence policies in a variety of areas, including affecting nursing's future.

CASE STUDY 6-1: Using Organizational Politics for Personal Advantage

Karen Keller has been nurse manager of medical and surgical ICUs in a large, urban, for-profit hospital for the past 7 years. Two years ago, Karen completed her master's degree in nursing administration. Her thesis research centered on the acceptance of standardized and computerized documentation methods for critical care units. Karen is well respected in her current role and is a member of several key committees addressing the need for a replacement health information system (HIS) for the hospital. She reports directly to the director of critical care services.

Although Karen enjoys her work as nurse manager, she believes she is ready to assume additional responsibilities on a director level. Through her work on the hospital's HIS selection team and as the nursing representative to the physician's technology committee, Karen identifies the need for a clinical informatics director role. One of Karen's responsibilities on the HIS selection team is to identify talent from clinical areas who could support the HIS implementation. Karen has also agreed to chair several working committees that will assist in determining required clinical functionality for the HIS.

During her tenure at the hospital, Karen has cultivated solid working relationships with several key decision makers within the organization. The human resources director, Ken Harding, has worked with Karen on several large projects over the past 2 years, including implementation of multidisciplinary teams in the ICUs. Karen schedules a lunch with Ken to discuss growth opportunities in the information technology department, the process for creating new roles, and in particular, who will determine the need for and approval of new information technology positions. Using this knowledge and her experience on the HIS selection team and the physicians' technology committee, Karen develops a proposal for the clinical informatics director position.

As the HIS selection team draws closer to selecting a final vendor and an implementation time line is established by the information technology department, Karen approaches her supervisor, Sherrie Wright, with her proposal. Karen also provides Sherrie with an overview of the clinical support that will be necessary for successful implementation of the HIS product. Since the critical care units are targeted for the initial phase of implementation, Sherrie is aware that Karen's high interest in technology and her clinical expertise in the ICU would be invaluable for successful implementation. As a strong manager, Karen can build acceptance among the nurses, physicians, and other members of the health care team.

Sherrie agrees to take Karen's proposal to the chief nursing officer for formal consideration.

Manager's Checklist

The nurse manager is responsible for

- Knowing and understanding the formal lines of authority within the organization,
- Identifying key decision makers and understanding their priorities and how those priorities affect any new initiatives,
- Understanding the importance of timing when initiating change,
- Being in the right place at the right time to take advantage of new opportunities,
- Building strong and credible working relationships with decision makers, and
- Exhibiting a willingness to take on new and challenging tasks that may lead to more responsibility.

Tools for Using Power and Politics

1. Learn the rules for using power and put them into practice.
2. Prepare to combat power plays (Table 6-2) by role-playing better responses.
3. Follow the steps for political action shown in Table 6-3 and in Case Study 6-1.
4. Pay attention to people who are influential and adopt their strategies if appropriate.

Questions to Challenge You

1. Consider a person you believe to have power. What are the bases of that person's power?
2. Evaluate how the person you named uses his or her power. Is it positive or negative?
3. Have you observed people using power inappropriately? Describe what they did and what happened as a result.
4. Assess your own power using the seven types of power discussed in the chapter. Name three ways you could increase your power.

5. Have you been involved in developing policies or political activities? Explain.

Explore 🌐 MediaLink

NCLEX review questions, essay activities, group activities, and other interactive resources for this chapter can be found on the Web site at http://www.prenhall.com/sullivan-decker. Click on "Chapter 6" to select activities for this chapter.

References

Covey, S. (1990). *Principle-centered leadership*. New York: Simon & Schuster.

French, J. R. P., & Raven, B. (1959). The bases of social power. In C. Cartwright & A. Zander (Eds.), *Studies of social power*. Ann Arbor, MI: Institute for Social Research.

Hersey, P., Blanchard, K. H., & Johnson, D. E. (2001). *Management of organizational behavior*. Upper Saddle River, NJ: Prentice Hall.

Hersey, P., Blanchard, K., & Natemeyer, W. E. (1979). Situational leadership perception and the impact of power. *Group and Organizational Studies, 4*(4), 418–428.

King, C., & Koliner, A. (1999). Understanding the impact of power in organizations. *Seminars for Nursing Managers, 7*(1), 39–46.

Mason, D. J. (1999). Nurses dancing with wolves. *American Journal of Nursing, 99*(8), 7.

Mason, D. J., Leavitt, J. K., & Chaffee, M. W. (2002). *Policy and politics in nursing and health care* (4th ed.). St. Louis, MO: Saunders.

Sullivan, E. J. (2004). *Becoming influential: A guide for nurses*. Upper Saddle River, NJ: Prentice Hall.

Key Skills in Nursing Management

CHAPTER 7

Thinking Critically, Making Decisions, Solving Problems

Looking Ahead

Nurses constantly face numerous decisions to make and problems to solve; problem solving and decision making are the very core of nursing, but they are not easy tasks. Developing critical-thinking, decision-making, and problem-solving skills allows nurses to see all sides of an issue, look for creative alternatives and approaches to problems, and make well-thought-out decisions. The effect is a stronger organization and more competent leader. This chapter introduces you to the ways you can become a more critical thinker.

Objectives

In this chapter, you will learn

- Why critical-thinking skills are essential to nurse managers.
- How to use creativity in management.
- How you can enhance your decision-making and problem-solving skills.
- How to make decisions in various situations.
- How to use a problem-solving method.
- How to help groups solve problems.

MediaLink www.prenhall.com/ sullivan-decker

Additional resources for this chapter can be found on the Companion Website at www.prenhall.com/ sullivan-decker. Click on "Chapter 7" to select the activities for this chapter.

- NCLEX Review
- Critical Thinking Activities
- Current Events
- MediaLinks
- *Nursing Leadership & Management in Action:* Developing Critical Thinking Skills

Nurse managers are expected to use knowledge from various disciplines to solve problems with patients, staff, and the organization, as well as problems in their own personal and professional lives. They also must make decisions in dynamic situations, such as

- Do the advantages of the primary nursing care delivery system outweigh proposed advantages of expanded use of unlicensed personnel?
- Would a new model of differentiated practice be more useful?
- Is the present policy requiring 12-hour shifts adequate for both patients and nurses?
- Which is the best staffing pattern to prevent turnover and ensure quality patient care?

Critical thinking helps nurse managers examine all aspects of an issue and look for different and exciting ways to solve new and old problems. This chapter explains and differentiates critical thinking, problem solving, and decision making and describes processes and techniques for using each.

Critical Thinking

Critical thinking is the process of examining underlying assumptions, interpreting and evaluating arguments, imagining and exploring alternatives, and developing a reflective criticism for the purpose of reaching a reasoned conclusion that can be justified. Critical thinking is not the same thing as criticism, though it does require inquiring attitudes, knowledge about evidence and analysis, and skills to combine them.

Critical-thinking skills can be used to resolve problems rationally. Identifying, analyzing, and questioning the evidence and implications of each problem stimulate and illuminate critical thought processes. Critical thinking is also an essential component of decision making. However, compared to problem solving and decision making, which involve seeking a single solution, critical thinking is broader and involves considering a range of alternatives and selecting the best one for the situation (Ignatavicius, 2001). Critical thinking is a higher-level cognitive process that includes creativity, problem solving, and decision making (Figure 7-1).

Using Critical Thinking

The critical-thinking process seems abstract unless it can be related to practical experiences. One way to develop this process is to consider a series of questions when examining a specific problem or making a decision. The following questions are suggested.

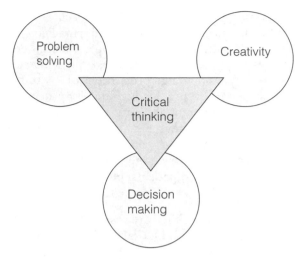

Figure 7-1   Critical-thinking model.

1. *What are the underlying assumptions?* Underlying assumptions are unquestioned beliefs that influence an individual's reasoning. They are perceptions that may or may not be grounded in reality. For example, some people believe the AIDS epidemic is punishment for homosexual behavior. This attitude toward people with AIDS could alter one's approach to care for an AIDS patient.
2. *How is evidence interpreted?* What is the context? Interpretation of information also can be value-laden. Is the evidence presented completely and clearly? Can the facts be substantiated? Are the people presenting the evidence using emotional or biased information? Are there any errors in reasoning?
3. *How are the arguments to be evaluated?* Is there objective evidence to support the arguments? Have all value preferences been determined? Is there a good chance that the arguments will be accepted? Are there enough people to support decisions? For example, many health care institutions changed to a smoke-free environment when it was found that passive smoking was harmful to people's health. At the same time societal values favored nonsmokers, and a strong majority supported the movement.

KEY TERMS

Critical thinking   A process of examining underlying assumptions, interpreting and evaluating arguments, imagining and exploring alternatives, and developing reflective criticism for the purpose of reaching a reasoned, justifiable conclusion.

4. *What are possible alternative perspectives?* Using different basic assumptions and paradigms can help the critical thinker develop several different views of an issue. For instance, a nurse manager who assumes that high proportions of RN staffing are necessary to provide high-quality patient care will have a different alternative solution to a mandated budget cut than a manager who is committed to using assistive personnel. What ideas are reported in the nursing literature? What solutions do staff members, patients, physicians, and others propose? What would be the ideal alternative?

Critical-thinking skills are used throughout the nursing process (see Table 7-1). Managers need to build on the knowledge base they began acquiring in school to make the critical-thinking process a conscious one in daily activities. Learning to be a critical thinker requires a commitment over time, but the skills can be learned. Ignatavicius (2001) describes the characteristics of an expert critical thinker in Box 7-1.

Creativity

Creativity is an essential part of the critical-thinking process. Creativity is the ability to develop and implement new and better solutions. Maintaining a certain level of creativity is the only way to keep an organization alive. One that functions by the rule stifles creativity, is inflexible, and is on the way to oblivion.

Creativity has four stages: preparation, incubation, insight, and verification. Even people who think they are not naturally creative can learn this process (Figure 7-2). First, the individual must acquire information necessary to understand the situation. Anyone can do this through hard work and observation.

Table 7-1	Overview of Critical Thinking Throughout the Nursing Process

The Nursing Process	Critical-Thinking Skills
Assessment	Observing
	Distinguishing relevant from irrelevant data
	Distinguishing important from unimportant data
	Validating data
	Organizing data
	Categorizing data
Diagnosis	Finding patterns and relationships
	Making inferences
	Stating the problem
	Suspending judgment
Planning	Generalizing
	Transferring knowledge from one situation to another
	Developing evaluative criteria
	Hypothesizing
Implementation	Applying knowledge
	Testing hypotheses
Evaluation	Deciding whether hypotheses are correct
	Making criterion-based evaluations

From *Nursing Process in Action: A Critical Thinking Approach* (p. 29), by J. Wilkinson, 1992, Redwood City, CA: Addison-Wesley Nursing.

Creative people are unlikely to view authority as absolute, make few black-and-white distinctions, have a less dogmatic view of life, show more independence of judgment and less conformity, are more willing to

Box 7-1   Characteristics of an Expert Critical Thinker

- Outcome-directed
- Open to new ideas
- Flexible
- Willing to change
- Innovative
- Creative
- Analytical
- Communicator
- Assertive

- Persistent
- Caring
- Energetic
- Risk-taker
- Knowledgeable
- Resourceful
- Observant
- Intuitive
- "Out of the box" thinker

From "Six critical thinking skills for at-the-bedside success," by D. D. Ignatavicius, 2001, *Nursing Management, 32*(1), pp. 37–39.

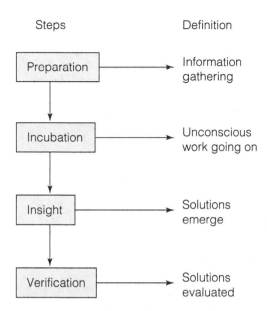

Steps   Definition

Preparation → Information
                gathering

Incubation → Unconscious
               work going on

Insight → Solutions
            emerge

Verification → Solutions
                 evaluated

Figure 7-2 The creative process.

give consideration to their own impulses, have a sense of humor, and are less rigid and freer though less effectively controlled.

For creativity to be of value to the nurse manager, it must be useful to solve problems and make decisions. Using the four stages of creativity, the following steps can help stimulate the generation of new ideas.

1. *Preparation.* A carefully designed planning program is essential. The nurse manager could plan creativity conferences, for example, at which participants will question all work methods. A method of work simplification, built on the premise that most people can increase productivity not by working harder but by eliminating certain steps and creating new services or solutions, could be the goal of these conferences. Some organizations have instituted such conferences on a monthly or bimonthly basis, involving all employees. The focus is on problems any member of the group chooses to bring up that are creating difficulties for the unit or individual. This is not a gripe session, but a setting where problem solving is done in a creative manner. A skillful group leader is important to facilitate progress at these conferences.

   The process follows this sequence:
   • Pick a specific task to improve.
   • Gather relevant facts.

   • Challenge every detail.
   • Develop preferred solutions.
   • Implement improvements.

2. *Incubation.* The nurse manager also needs to meet with new employees routinely as part of the orientation process, at which time everyone seeks information about solutions to problems. New employees are not encumbered with details of accepted practices and can offer suggestions based on their prior experiences or insights before they get set in their ways or have their innovative ideas "turned off." The advantages offered by new employees should be explored because all staff gain from such use of valuable human resources.

3. *Insight.* Most nurse managers are employed in bureaucratic settings that do not foster creativity. Control is exercised over staff, and rigid adherence to formal channels of communication jeopardizes innovation. In addition, there is little room for failure, and when failures do occur they are not tolerated very well. When staff are afraid of the consequences of failure, their creativity is inhibited and innovation does not take place.

   If risk cannot be accepted, special ground rules need to be established that permit innovative managers and staff to function without fear of reprisals or termination if they fail. In addition, nurse managers must realize, as people in other organizations do, that innovative people may not fit the organizational mold. Innovative people generally avoid highly structured and controlled situations and at times may appear disorganized or lackadaisical. The challenge for nurse managers is to know when, for whom, and to what extent control is appropriate. If creativity does have a priority in the health care setting, then the reward system should be geared to and commensurate with that priority.

4. *Verification.* Creativity demands a certain amount of exposure to outside contacts, receptiveness to new and seemingly strange ideas, proper research assistance, a certain amount of freedom, and some permissive management. The climate must promote the survival of potentially useful ideas. Many good new ideas go unused because they arise in an environment grown cold to creativity. A new idea is extremely perishable, and its creator is likely to be its sole supporter, after which it may have none, because the usual reaction is either to ignore it or to look for defects in the new idea. The nurse manager can build an attitude favorable to giving new ideas a fair and proper hearing and thereby reduce

CASE STUDY 7-1: Creative Problem Solving

Jeffrey was just promoted to manager of an acute care clinic, which recently expanded its hours from 6 A.M. until 10 P.M. Jeffrey has realized that staff nurses are reluctant to sign up and do quality chart audits. He gathers information about quality improvement, reviews the literature on motivation and incentives, and discusses the issue with other nurse managers (preparation). He continues to manage the clinic, thinking about the information he has gathered but does not consciously make a decision or reject new ideas (incubation). When working on a new problem, self-scheduling for the change in hours, he realizes a connection between the two problems. Many nurses complain that by the time they receive the schedule the day shifts are filled. Jeffrey states that he will review the chart audits and that those nurses who regularly participate in quality improvement projects will receive a "perk." They will be allowed, on a rotating basis, first choice at selecting the schedule they want to work (this is the insight stage). He discusses the plan with the staff and proposes a 2-month trial period to determine whether the solution is effective (verification).

Manager's Checklist

The nurse manager is responsible for

- Identifying problem areas,
- Generating ideas that might serve as possible solutions,
- Checking with others for advice,
- Selecting motivators,
- Implementing a solution, and
- Evaluating the results.

---

the tendency to destroy the creative process in individuals and within groups.

The major limitation on creativity stems from the initial cost. The greater the creativity sought and the greater the departure from present practice, the greater the investment will be. In the long run, however, creative ideas may turn out to be highly cost-effective. The challenge is to determine if and when they are important, to decide how important they are, and to encourage the creative exchange of such ideas broadly so there is a visible effect of the nurse manager's leadership, measurable in enhanced vitality and productivity.

Case Study 7-1 describes how one nurse manager used creativity to solve a problem.

Decision Making

Considering all the practice individuals get in making decisions, it would seem they might become very good at it. However, the number of decisions a person makes does not correspond to the person's skill at making them. The assumption is that decision making comes naturally, like breathing. It does not.

The decision-making process described in this chapter provides nurses with a system for making decisions that is applicable to any decision. It is a useful procedure for making practical choices. A decision not to solve a problem is also a decision.

The label *decision making* is used inconsistently and often interchangeably with *problem solving*. Although the two processes appear similar and may in some instances depend on one another, they are not synonymous. The main distinctions between the two are that **decision making** may or may not involve a problem, but it always involves selecting one of several alternatives, each of which may be appropriate under certain circumstances, whereas **problem solving** involves diagnosing a problem and solving it, which may or may not entail deciding on one correct solution.

Most of the time, decision making is a subset of problem solving. However, some decisions are not of a problem-solving nature, such as decisions about scheduling, equipment, in-services, or other matters that do not involve problem solving as a deliberate process. Also, habit and tradition may be modes of decision making, such as holding onto the wall when walking down a wet hospital corridor or scheduling patient care activities in traditional ways (e.g., giving every patient a bath every morning).

Research has discredited the early belief that all decisions are choices people make after extensive evaluation of all options in order to find an optimal solution. Simon (1955) and others recognized that evaluation is seldom extensive and virtually never exhaustive. In the 1970s it was recognized that decision makers have a variety of strategies for making choices and a variety of aims in addition to utility. Most often, past experiences provide ways of dealing with problems. Making a deliberate choice is relatively rare and usually is done by screening out the unacceptable options and choosing the best option from the remainders.

Types of Decisions

The types of problems nurse managers encounter and decisions they must make vary widely and determine the problem-solving or decision-making methods they should use. Relatively well defined, common problems can usually be solved with routine decisions, often using established rules, policies, and procedures. For instance, when a nurse makes a medication error, the manager's actions are guided by policy and the report form. **Routine decisions** are more often made by first-level managers than by top administrators.

Adaptive decisions are necessary when both problems and alternative solutions are somewhat unusual and only partially understood. Often they are modifications of other well-known problems and solutions. Managers must make **innovative decisions** when problems are unusual and unclear and when creative, novel solutions are necessary.

Decision-Making Conditions

Managers make decisions both as individuals and in groups that occur in an organizational context. The conditions surrounding decision making can vary and change dramatically. It is essential for the manager to consider the total system, realizing that whatever solutions are created will succeed only if they are compatible with other parts of the system. Within the organization, decisions are made under conditions of certainty, risk, or uncertainty.

Decision Making under Certainty   When nurse managers know the alternatives and the conditions surrounding each alternative, a state of certainty is said to exist. Suppose a nurse manager on a unit with acutely ill patients wants to decrease the number of venipunctures a patient experiences when an IV is started, as well as reduce costs resulting from failed venipunctures. Three alternatives exist:

- Establish an IV team on all shifts to minimize IV attempts and reduce costs.
- Establish a reciprocal relationship with the anesthesia department to start IVs when nurses experience difficulty.

- Set a standard of two insertion attempts per nurse per patient although this does not substantially lower equipment costs.

The manager knows the alternatives (IV team, anesthesia department, standards) and the conditions associated with each (reduced costs, assistance with starting IVs, minimum attempts and some cost reduction). A condition of strong certainty is said to exist and the decision can be made with full knowledge of what the payoff probably will be.

Decision Making under Uncertainty and Risk   Seldom do decision makers have perfect information that McConnell (2000) explains as knowing everything there is to know about a subject or situation. If everything was known, the decision would be obvious for all to realize.

Most critical decision making in organizations is done, therefore, under conditions of *uncertainty* and *risk*. The individual or group making the decision does not know all the alternatives, attendant risks, or likely consequences of each option. Uncertainty and risk are inevitable because of the complex and dynamic nature of health care organizations. Successful decisions, McConnell (2000) asserts, are dependent on human judgment.

Here is an example: If the weather forecaster predicts a 40 percent chance of snow, the nurse manager is operating in a situation of risk when trying to decide how to staff the unit for the next 24 hours.

KEY TERMS

Decision making   A process whereby appropriate alternatives are weighed and one is ultimately selected.

Problem solving   A process whereby a dilemma is identified and corrected.

Routine decisions   The type of decisions made when problems are relatively well defined and common and when established rules, policies, and procedures can be used to solve them.

Adaptive decisions   The type of decisions made when problems and alternative solutions are somewhat unusual and only partially understood.

Innovative decisions   The type of decisions made when problems are unusual and unclear and creative solutions are necessary.

In a risk situation, availability of each alternative, potential successes, and costs are all associated with probability estimates. **Probability** is the likelihood, expressed as a percentage, that an event will or will not occur. If something is certain to happen, its probability is 100 percent. If it is certain not to happen, its probability is 0 percent. If there is a 50–50 chance, its probability is 50 percent.

Suppose a nurse manager decides to use agency nurses to staff a unit during heavy vacation periods. Two agencies look attractive, and the manager must decide between them. Agency A has had modest growth over the past 10 years and offers the manager a 3-month contract, freezing wages during that time. In addition, the unit will have first choice of available nurses. Agency B is much more dynamic and charges more but explains that the reason they have had a high rate of growth is that their nurses are the best and the highest paid in the area. The nurse manager can choose Agency A, which will provide a safe, constant supply of nursing personnel, or B, which promises better care but at a higher cost.

The key element in decision making under conditions of risk is to determine the probabilities of each alternative accurately. The nurse manager can use a **probability analysis,** whereby expected risk is calculated or estimated. Using the probability analysis shown in Table 7-2, it appears as though Agency A offers the best outcome. However, if the second agency had a 90 percent chance of filling shifts and a 50 percent chance of fixing costs, a completely different situation would exist.

The nurse manager might decide that the potential for increased costs was a small tradeoff for having more highly qualified nurses and the best probability of having the unit fully staffed during vacation periods. **Objective probability** is the likelihood that an event will or will not occur based on facts and reliable information. **Subjective probability** is the likelihood that an event will or will not occur based on a manager's personal judgment and beliefs (Figure 7-3).

Janeen, a nurse manager of a specialized cardiac intensive care unit, faces the task of recruiting scarce and highly skilled nurses to care for coronary bypass patients. The obvious alternative is to offer a salary and benefit package that rivals that of all other institutions in the area. However, this means Janeen will have costly specialized nursing personnel in her budget who are not easily absorbed by other units in the organization. The probability that coronary bypass procedures will become obsolete in the future is unknown. In addition, other factors (e.g., increased competition, government regulations regarding reimbursement) may contribute to conditions of uncertainty.

The Decision-Making Process

The management literature describes decisions as discrete events made by an individual manager or a group using an orderly, rational process. This process, the **rational,** or **normative, decision-making model,** is a series of steps that managers take in an effort to make logical, well-grounded rational choices that maximize the achievement of objectives (Figure 7-4). The rationality of the decision made depends on the manager's ability to use information and analysis and on his or her values, beliefs, and objectives. The decision-making process is a sequence of the basic steps, however, not every step is used in every decision. In making adaptive and innovative decisions, managers rarely use these steps in sequence.

An application of the normative decision-making method is the optimizing strategy. The decision maker first identifies all possible outcomes, examines the probability of each alternative, and then takes the action that yields the highest probability of achieving the most desirable outcome. The rational or normative

Table 7-2

	Probability Analysis
Agency A	60% Filling shifts
	100% Fixed wages
Agency B	50% Filling shifts
	70% Fixed wage

Figure 7-3 **Conditions under which decisions are made. From** *Management: A Competency-based Approach,* **9th ed. (p. 221), by Hellriegel, D., Jackson, S. E. & Slocum, J. W., Jr., 2002, Cincinnati, OH: South-Western.**

decision-making model is thought of as the ideal but often cannot be fully used.

Individuals seldom make major decisions at a single point in time and often are unable to recall when a decision was finally reached. Some major decisions are the result of many small actions or incremental choices the person makes without regarding larger strategic issues. In addition, decision processes are likely to be characterized more by confusion, disorder, and emotionality than by rationality. For these reasons, it is essential that the nurse manager develop appropriate technical skills and the capacity to find a good balance between lengthy processes and quick, decisive action.

The **descriptive,** or **bounded, rationality model,** developed by Simon in 1955 and supported by research in the 1990s (Simon, 1993), emphasizes the limitations of the rationality of the decision maker and the situation. It recognizes three ways in which decision makers depart from the rational decision-making model:

- The decision maker's search for possible objectives or alternative solutions is limited because of time, energy, and money.
- Managers frequently lack adequate information about problems and cannot control the conditions under which they operate.
- Managers often use a satisficing strategy.

Satisficing is not a misspelled word; it is a decision-making strategy whereby the individual chooses an alternative that is not ideal but either is good enough (suffices) under existing circumstances to meet minimum standards of acceptance or is the first acceptable alternative.

KEY TERMS

Probability The likelihood that an event will or will not occur.

Probability analysis A calculation of the expected risk made to accurately determine the probabilities of each alternative.

Objective probability The likelihood that an event will or will not occur based on facts and reliable information.

Subjective probability The likelihood that an event will or will not occur based on a manager's personal judgment and beliefs.

Rational (normative) decision-making model A decision-making process based on logical, well-grounded rational choices that maximize the achievement of objectives.

Descriptive (bounded) rationality model A decision-making process that emphasizes the limitations of the rationality of the decision maker and the situation.

Satisficing A decision-making strategy whereby the individual chooses a less than ideal alternative that meets minimum standards of acceptance.

Figure 7-4 **Rational decision-making model. From *Management: A Competency-based Approach,* 9th ed. (p. 229), by Hellriegel, D., Jackson, S. E. & Slocum, J. W., Jr., 2002, Cincinnati, OH: South-Western.**

Nursing management situations present a multitude of problems that are ineffectively solved with satisficing strategies. *Elena, a nurse manager in charge of a busy neurosurgical floor with high turnover rates and high patient acuity levels, uses a satisficing alternative when hiring replacement staff. She hires all nurse applicants in order of application until no positions are open. A better approach would be for Elena to replace staff only with nurse applicants who possess the skills and experiences required to care for neurosurgical patients, regardless of the number of applicants or desire for immediate action. Elena also should develop a plan to promote job satisfaction, the lack of which is the real reason for the vacancies.*

Nurse managers who solve problems using satisficing may lack specific training in problem solving and decision making. They may view their units or floors as drastically simplified models of the real world and be content with this simplification because it allows them to make decisions with relatively simple rules of thumb or from force of habit. However, *optimizing techniques,* where the best of all possible alternatives is chosen, make demands on managers' willingness and ability to collect information, analyze it, and choose the best alternative.

The **political decision-making model** describes the process in terms of the particular interests and objectives of powerful stakeholders, such as hospital boards, medical staffs, corporate officers, and regulatory bodies. Power is the ability to influence or control how

problems and objectives are defined, what alternative solutions are considered and selected, what information flows, and, ultimately, what decisions are made (see Chapter 6).

The decision-making process begins when the nurse manager perceives a gap between what is actually happening and what should be happening, and it ends with action that will narrow or close this gap. The simplest way to learn decision-making skills is to integrate a model into one's thinking by breaking the components down into individual steps. The seven steps of the decision-making process (Box 7-2) are as applicable to personal problems as they are to nursing management problems. Each step is elaborated by pertinent questions clarifying the statements, and they should be followed in the order in which they are presented.

Decision-Making Techniques

Decision-making techniques vary according to the nature of the problem or topic, the decision maker, the context or situation, and the decision-making method or process. For routine decisions, choices that are tried and true can be made for well-defined, known situations or problems. Well-designed policies, rules, and standard operating procedures can produce satisfactory results with a minimum of the manager's time. **Artificial intelligence,** including programmed computer systems such as **expert systems** that can store,

---

Box 7-2   Steps in Decision Making

1. Identify the purpose:	Why is a decision necessary? What needs to be determined? State the issue in the broadest possible terms.
2. Set the criteria:	What needs to be achieved, preserved, and avoided by whatever decision is made? The answers to these questions are the standards by which solutions will be evaluated.
3. Weight the criteria:	Rank each criterion on a scale of values from 1 (totally unimportant) to 10 (extremely important).
4. Seek alternatives:	List all possible courses of action. Is one alternative more significant than another? Does one alternative have weaknesses in some areas? Can these be overcome? Can two alternatives or features of many alternatives be combined?
5. Test alternatives:	First, using the same methodology as in step 3, rank each alternative on a scale of 1 to 10. Second, multiply the weight of each criterion by the rating of each alternative. Third, add the scores and compare the results.
6. Troubleshoot:	What could go wrong? How can you plan? Can the choice be improved?
7. Evaluate the action:	Is the solution being implemented? Is it effective? Is it costly?

retrieve, and manipulate data, can diagnose problems and make limited decisions.

For adaptive decisions involving moderately ambiguous problems and modification of known and well-defined alternative solutions, there are a variety of techniques. Many types of decision grids or tables can be used to compare outcomes of alternative solutions. Decisions about units or services can be facilitated, with analyses comparing output, revenue, and costs over time or under different conditions. Analyzing the costs and revenues of a proposed new service is an example.

Making innovative decisions requires both discovering and diagnosing unfamiliar and ambiguous problems and developing unique and creative solutions. These decisions involve considerable uncertainty and, often, risk. Adding home care to the services offered by a hospital maternity nursing unit is an example of a situation requiring innovative decisions.

Regardless of the decision-making model or strategy chosen, data collection and analysis are essential. In many health care organizations, quality teams are using a variety of tools to gather, organize, and analyze data about their work. Based on the work of Deming (Walton, 1988), nurses are using tools such as cause-and-effect diagrams, flow charts, Pareto charts, run charts, histograms, control charts, and scatter diagrams to help understand facts and relationships in processes they are examining. Figure 7-5 illustrates a cause-and-effect diagram that a team of nurses created to help them improve the documentation process for their ambulatory oncology unit.

Group Decision Making

The widespread use of participative management, quality improvement teams, and shared governance in health care organizations requires every nurse manager to determine when group, rather than individual, decisions are desirable and how to use groups effectively. A number of studies have shown that professional people do not function well under micromanagement. As an alternative, group problem solving of substantial issues casts the manager in the role of facilitator and consultant. Compared to individual decision making, groups can provide more input, often produce better decisions, and generate more commitment. The nurse manager must understand the group decision-making process, troubleshoot, and be a positive role model. Several group decision-making techniques can be used.

Nominal Group Technique The **nominal group technique (NGT),** developed by Delbecq, VandeVen, and Gustafson (1975), is a structured and precise method of eliciting written questions, ideas, and reactions from group members. NGT is a group process in name only because no direct exchange occurs among members. NGT consists of

- Silently generating ideas in writing,
- Round-robin presentation by group members of their individual ideas in a terse phrase on a flip chart,
- Discussion of each recorded idea for clarification and evaluation, and
- Voting individually on priority ideas, with the group solution being derived mathematically through rank ordering or rating using the group's decision rule.

Delphi Technique In the **Delphi technique,** judgments on a particular topic are systematically gathered from participants who do not meet face to face. Ideas are collected through a carefully designed sequence of questionnaires interspersed with summaries of information and opinions derived from previous questionnaires. The process may involve many iterations but normally does not exceed three. This technique can rely on the input of experts widely dispersed geographically. It can be used to evaluate the quality of research proposals or to

KEY TERMS

Political decision-making model A decision-making process in which the particular interests and objectives of powerful stakeholders influence how problems and objectives are defined.

Artificial intelligence Computer technology that can diagnose problems and make limited decisions.

Expert systems Computer programs that provide complex data processing, reasoning, and decision making.

Nominal group technique (NGT) A decision-making technique that elicits written questions, ideas, and reactions from group members.

Delphi technique A decision-making technique in which judgments on a particular topic are systematically gathered from participants who do not meet face to face.

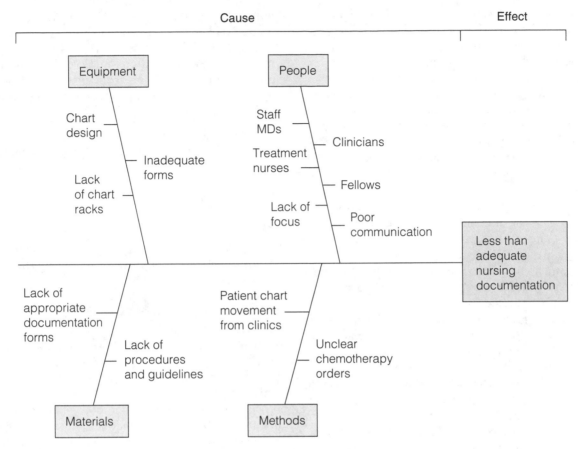

Figure 7-5   **Brainstorming session of a nursing quality focus team.**

make predictions about the future based on current scientific knowledge. This technique is useful when expert opinions are needed and expense would prohibit bringing them together.

For fact-finding problems with no known solution, the NGT and the Delphi technique are superior to other group techniques. Both NGT and the Delphi technique minimize the chances of more vocal members dominating discussion and allow independent consideration of ideas.

Statistical Aggregation   Like the Delphi technique, **statistical aggregation** does not require a group meeting. Individuals are polled regarding a specific problem, and their responses are tallied. It is a very efficient technique, but it is limited to problems for which a quantifiable answer can be obtained. One disadvantage of both statistical aggregation and the Delphi technique is that no opportunity exists for group members to strengthen their interpersonal ties or for the generative effect of group interaction.

Brainstorming   In **brainstorming**, group members meet together and generate many diverse ideas about the nature, cause, definition, or solution to a problem without consideration of their relative value. A premium is placed on generating lots of ideas as quickly as possible and on coming up with unusual ideas. (The wilder the idea, the better.) Most importantly, members do not critique ideas as they are proposed. Evaluation takes place after all the ideas have been generated.

KEY TERMS

Statistical aggregation   A decision-making technique in which individuals are polled regarding a specific problem and their responses are tallied.

Brainstorming   A decision-making method in which group members meet and generate diverse ideas about the nature, cause, definition, or solution to a problem.

Members are encouraged to improve on each other's ideas. These sessions are very enjoyable but are often unsuccessful because members inevitably begin to critique ideas, and as a result, meetings shift to the ordinary interacting group format. Criticisms of this approach are the high cost factor, the time consumed, and the superficiality of many solutions.

Stumbling Blocks

Nurse managers' personality traits, inexperience, lack of adaptability, and preconceived ideas are several obstacles to problem solving and decision making.

Personality   The nurse manager's personality can and often does affect how and why certain decisions are made. Many nurse managers are selected because of their expert clinical, not management, skills. Inexperienced in management, they may resort to various unproductive activities. On the one hand, a nurse manager who is insecure may base decisions primarily on approval seeking. When a truly difficult situation arises, the manager, rather than face rejection from the staff, makes a decision that will placate people rather than one that will achieve the larger goals of the unit and organization. On the other hand, a nurse manager who demonstrates an authoritative type of personality might make unreasonable demands on the staff, fail to reward staff for long hours because he or she has a "workaholic" attitude, or give the staff no control over patient care activities. Similarly, an inexperienced manager may cause a unit to flounder because the manager is not inclined to act on new ideas or solutions to problems. Managerial traits of optimism, humor, and a positive approach are crucial to energizing staff and promoting creativity.

Rigidity   Rigidity, an inflexible management style, is another obstacle to problem solving. It may result from ineffective trial-and-error solutions, fear of risk taking, or inherent personality traits. The nurse manager can avoid ineffective trial-and-error problem solving by gathering sufficient information and determining a means for early correction of wrong or inadequate decisions. Also, to minimize risk in problem solving, the manager should know and understand alternative risks and expectations.

The nurse manager who uses a rigid style in problem solving easily develops tunnel vision—the tendency to look at new things in old ways and from established frames of reference. It then becomes very difficult to see things from another perspective, and problem solving becomes a process whereby one person makes all of the

decisions with little information or data from other sources. In the current changing health care setting, rigidity can at times be a nurse manager's greatest barrier to effective problem solving.

Preconceived Ideas   Effective nurse managers do not start out with the preconceived idea that one proposed course of action is right and all others wrong. Nor do they assume that only one opinion can be voiced and others will be silent. They start out with a commitment to find out why staff members or others disagree. If the staff, other professionals, or patients see a different reality or even a different problem, nurse managers need to integrate this information into a database to develop additional problem-solving alternatives.

Most people have preconceived ideas about problems and their solutions. Those who are certain that only their perception is accurate may never accept the final decision. Nurse managers, however, have formal responsibility for problem solving and decision making and must put personal ideas on hold until they have gathered enough information to view the situation objectively and in the widest possible perspective.

Pederson (1993) identified qualities that staff nurses most consistently attributed to excellent head nurses. Excellent head nurses are characterized as positive, happy, energetic, authentic, sincere, honest, and open. They develop relationships that are supportive, caring, sensitive, and appreciative. Effective head nurses also are forward-thinking, courageous, creative, and willing to take risks. They advocate for others and support professional standards and growth. They do not avoid conflict but are skilled in resolving it and solving problems. In a nationwide survey of nurse administrators and managers in academic health centers, human management skill was ranked as the most important criterion of nurse manager effectiveness; the characteristics of flexibility, negotiation, and compromise were second (Patz, Biordi, & Holm, 1991).

Problem Solving

People use problem solving when they perceive a gap between an existing state (what is going on) and a desired state (what should be going on). How one perceives the situation influences how the problem is identified or solved. Therefore, perceptions need to be clarified before problem solving can occur.

Questioning also is central to problem solving. Questioning identifies central issues, examines reasoning, clarifies ambiguities in defining the problem, explores value conflicts, and challenges assumptions (Boychuk, 1999). This type of reflection allows problems to become opportunities to enhance professional growth and organizational efficiency and effectiveness. The scientific problem-solving process requires searching for information to clarify the problem and to discover a variety of solutions. These solutions are carefully evaluated and the best one is chosen for implementation. The implemented solution is maintained over time to ensure its immediate and continued effectiveness. If difficulties are encountered, some or all of the process is repeated. One problem-solving method is the nursing process shown in Table 7-1.

Problem-Solving Methods

A variety of methods can be used to solve problems. People with little management experience tend to use the **trial-and-error method,** applying one solution after another until the problem is solved or appears to be improving. These managers often cite lack of experience and of time and resources to search for alternative solutions.

In a step-down unit with an increasing incidence of medication errors, Max, the nurse manager, uses various strategies to decrease errors, such as asking nurses to use calculators, having the charge nurse check medications, and posting dosage and medication charts in the unit. After a few months, by which time none of the methods has worked, it occurs to Max that perhaps making nurses responsible for their actions would be more effective. Max develops a point system for medication errors: When nurses accumulate a certain amount of points, they are required to take a medication test; repeated failure of the test may eventually lead to termination. Max's solution is effective, and a low level of medication errors is restored.

As the above example shows, a trial-and-error process can be time consuming and may even be detrimental. Although some learning can occur during the process, the nurse manager risks being perceived as a poor problem solver who has wasted time and money on ineffective solutions.

Experimentation, another type of problem solving, is more rigorous than trial and error. Pilot projects or limited trials are examples of experimentation. Experimentation involves testing a theory (hypothesis) or hunch to enhance knowledge, understanding, or prediction. A project or study is carried out in either a controlled setting (e.g., in a laboratory) or an uncontrolled setting (e.g., in a natural setting such as an outpatient clinic). Data are collected and analyzed and results interpreted to determine whether the solution tried has been effective.

Lin, a nurse manager of a pediatric floor, has received many complaints from mothers of children who think the nurses are short-tempered. Lin has a hunch that 12-hour shifts, which have been recently implemented on her floor, are contributing to the problem; she believes that nurses who must interact frequently with families would perform better on 8-hour shifts. She can test her theory by setting up a small study comparing the two staffing patterns with patient satisfaction.

Experimentation may be creative and effective or uninspired and ineffective, depending on how it is used. As a major method of problem solving, experimentation may be inefficient because of the amount of time and control involved. However, a well-designed experiment can be persuasive in situations in which an idea or activity, such as a new staffing system or care procedure, can be tried in one of two similar groups and results objectively compared.

Still other problem-solving techniques rely on *past experience* and *intuition.* Everyone has various and countless experiences. Individuals build a repertoire of these experiences and base future actions on what they considered successful solutions in the past. If a particular course of action consistently resulted in positive outcomes, the person will try it again when similar circumstances occur. In some instances, an individual's past experience can determine how much risk he or she will take in present circumstances. The nature and frequency of the experience also contribute significantly to the effectiveness of this problem-solving method. How much the person has learned from these experiences, positive or negative, can affect the current viewpoint and can result in either subjective and narrow judgments or very wise ones. This is especially true in human relations problems. A nurse manager who has an unfortunate experience with a nurse recovering from chemical dependency may, in the future, judge negatively the performance of all nurses with acknowledged chemical dependency problems. Intuition relies heavily on past experience and trial and error. The extent to which past experience is related to intuition is difficult to determine, but nurses' wisdom, sensitivity, and intuition are known to be valuable in solving problems.

Some problems are self-solving: If permitted to run a natural course, they are solved by those personally involved. This is not to say that a uniform laissez-faire management style solves all problems. The nurse manager must not ignore managerial responsibilities, but often difficult situations become more manageable when participants are given time, resources, and support to discover their own solutions. This typically happens, for example, when a newly graduated nurse joins a unit where most of the staff are associate degree RNs who resent the new nurse's level of education as well as the nurse's lack of experience. If the nurse manager intervenes, a problem that the staff might have worked out on their own becomes an ongoing source of conflict. The important skill required here is knowing when to do nothing. Chapter 9 discusses this issue further.

The Problem-Solving Process

Many nursing problems require immediate action. Nurses don't have time for formalized processes of research and analysis specified by the scientific method. Therefore, learning an organized method for problem solving is invaluable. One practical method for problem solving is to follow this seven-step process, which is also outlined in Box 7-3.

1. *Define the problem.* The most important part of problem solving is defining the problem. How problems are perceived determines the solutions or identifies needed changes. The nurse manager identifies a problem as a departure from what he or she perceives to be a desirable state of affairs. The nurse manager is responsible not only for dealing with the situation, but also for dealing with it with foresight.

   Suppose a nurse manager reluctantly implements a self-scheduling process and finds that each time the schedule is posted, evenings and some weekend shifts are not adequately covered. The manager might identify the problem as the immaturity of the staff and their inability to function under democratic leadership. The causes may be lack of interest in group decision making, minimal concern over providing adequate patient coverage, or, perhaps more correctly, a few nurses' lack of understanding of the process.

The definition of a problem should be a descriptive statement of the state of affairs, not a judgment or conclusion. If one begins the statement of a problem with a judgment, the solution may be equally judgmental, and critical descriptive elements could be overlooked. If the nurse manager defines the above problem as immaturity and reverts to making out the schedules without further fact-finding, a minor problem could develop into a full-blown crisis.

Sometimes the problem is not easily identified. In this case, tools may be helpful. One such tool is the **affinity map.** Lepley (1998) describes six steps to the process (see Figure 7-6 for an example).

- A problem is acknowledged and a thoughtful question is raised to stimulate ideas.
- Without talking among the group, ideas about the problem are generated and recorded on individual slips of paper or cards.
- Then, again without talking, the group is asked to organize similar ideas into no more than six categories.
- The group facilitator names the categories, explains the rationale used for the naming process, and ensures agreement on category names.
- The group is allowed an opportunity to explain their thinking. In doing so, perceptions about the problem are discovered and consensus is built. One rule during this

---

KEY TERMS

Trial-and-error method   A method whereby one solution after another is tried until the problem is solved or appears to be improving.

Experimentation   A type of problem solving in which a theory is tested to enhance knowledge, understanding, or prediction.

Affinity map   A tool used to identify problems.

Box 7-3   Steps in Problem Solving

1. Define the problem.
2. Gather information.
3. Analyze the information.
4. Develop solutions.

5. Make a decision.
6. Implement the decision.
7. Evaluate the solution.

Affinity map

Barriers to staff nurse performance

Staffing policies	Interpersonal skills	Resources	Technical skills	Miscellaneous
Scheduling	Use of proper communication channels	Time	Need for in-servicing on new equipment	Paperwork
RN:patient ratios		Supplies		Meetings
Patient acuity	Conflict management	Functioning equipment	Need for in-servicing on new policies and procedures	In-services
Use of PRN staff	Inadequate delegation skills	Assistive personnel		
Floating	Customer service		Computer technology	
	Inadequate leadership skills			

Cause-and-effect diagram

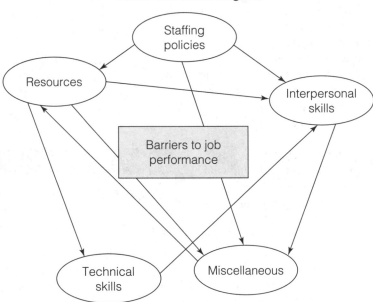

Figure 7-6 **The affinity map and cause-and-effect diagram. From "Problem-Solving Tool for Analyzing System Problems," by C. J. Lepley, 1998, *Journal of Nursing Administration, 28*(2), pp. 44–50.**

step is that there are no right or wrong answers; therefore, none of the ideas should be criticized.

- Finally, the affinity map can be used to determine cause-and-effect relationships. The name of each category is written down in a circular format to create a diagram. The relationships between categories are identified and directional arrows used. The category with the most number of outgoing arrows is considered the root cause of the problem. The category with the most incoming arrows is the effect.

Premature interpretation can alter one's ability to deal with facts objectively. For example, are there other explanations for the apparent behavior that do not entail negative assumptions about the maturity of the staff? Premature interpretations can be avoided by using reflective inquiry.

Schmieding (1999) describes four characteristics of *reflective inquiry:*

- Objective data are tested against one's thoughts and feelings.
- Past experiences and knowledge are used to evaluate the situation.
- Ideas about the problem are validated or refuted based on empirical evidence through a serial rather than a linear process.
- The facts and ideas generated are verified through deliberate investigation.

Accurate assessment of the scope of the problem also determines whether the manager needs to seek a lasting solution or just a stopgap measure. Is this just a situational problem requiring only intervention with a simple explanation, or is it more complex, involving the leadership style of the manager? The manager must define and classify problems in order to take action.

In defining a problem, the nurse manager should determine the area it covers and ask:

- Do I have the authority to do anything about this myself?
- Do I have all the information? The time?
- Who else has important information and can contribute?
- What benefits could be expected? A list of potential benefits provides the basis for comparison and choice of solutions. The list also serves as a means for evaluating the solution.

2. *Gather information.* Problem solving begins with collecting facts. This information gathering initiates a search for additional facts that provides clues to the scope and solution of the problem. A careful, systematic, complete search facilitates the accomplishment of goals and evaluates the possible effects of the solution. Information gathered will probably be a combination of facts and feelings. The manager should obtain relevant, valid, accurate, and detailed descriptions from appropriate people or sources and put the information in writing.

This step encourages people to report facts accurately. The nurse manager or team may choose to have everyone involved provide information. Although this may not always provide objective information, it reduces misinformation and allows everyone an opportunity to tell what he or she thinks is wrong with a situation. Lack of time, of course, may prevent gathering written data.

Experience is another source of information—one's own experience as well as the experience of other nurse managers and staff. Everyone involved usually has ideas about what should be done about a problem, and many of these ideas provide good information and valuable suggestions. Yet information gathered may never be complete. Some data will be useless, some inaccurate, but some will be useful to develop innovative ideas worth pursuing.

3. *Analyze the information.* The manager should analyze the information only when all of it has been sorted into some orderly arrangement. The following is suggested:

- Categorize information in order of reliability.
- List information from most important to least important.
- Set information into a time sequence. What happened first? Next? What came before what? What were the concurrent circumstances?
- Set up information in terms of cause and effect. Is A causing B, or vice versa?
- Classify information into categories: human factors, such as personality, maturity, education, age, relationships among people, and problems outside the organization; technical factors, such as nursing skills or the type of unit; temporal factors, such as length of service, overtime, type of shift, and double shifts; and policy factors, such as organizational procedures or rules applying to the problem, legal issues, and ethical issues.
- Consider how long the situation has been going on.

Because no amount of information is ever complete or comprehensive enough, critical-thinking skills are important to the manager's ability to examine the assumptions, evidence, and potential value conflicts.

4. *Develop solutions.* As the nurse manager or group analyzes information, numerous possible solutions will suggest themselves. These should be written down and plans made to immediately start developing the best of them. It is not wise to limit consideration only to simple solutions, because doing so may constrain creative thinking and cause overconcentration on detail. Developing alternative solutions makes it possible to combine the best parts of several solutions into a superior one. Also,

alternatives are valuable in case the first-order solutions prove impossible to implement.

When exploring a variety of solutions, the nurse manager should maintain an uncritical attitude toward the way the problem has been handled in the past. Some problems have had a long-standing history by the time they reach the nurse manager, and attempts may have been made to resolve them over a long period of time. "We tried this before and it didn't work," is often said and may apply—or more likely, may not apply—in a changed situation.

Past experience may not always supply an answer, but it can aid the critical-thinking process and help prepare for future problem solving. Nurse managers and others can review the literature, attend relevant seminars, and brainstorm ideas. Sometimes others have solved similar problems and those methods can be applied to a comparable problem.

5. *Make a decision.* After reviewing the list of potential solutions, the nurse manager should select the one that is most feasible and satisfactory and has the fewest undesirable consequences. Some solutions have to be put into effect quickly; matters of discipline or compromises in patient safety, for example, need immediate intervention. Nurse managers should have, in advance, the authority to act in an emergency and know the penalties to be imposed for various infractions.

If the problem is a technical one and its solution brings about a change in the method of doing work (or using new equipment), there may be resistance. All people become disturbed by changes that reorder their habit patterns and threaten personal security or status. Many solutions fail because the manager does not recognize the change process that must be initiated before solutions can be implemented. If the solution involves change, the manager should fully involve those who will be affected by it, if possible, or at least inform them of the process. (See Chapter 16 for discussion of the change process.)

6. *Implement the decision.* The manager implements the decision after selecting the best course of action. If unforeseen new problems emerge after implementation, the manager must evaluate these impediments as carefully as any other problem. Nurse managers must be careful, however, not to abandon a workable solution just because a few people object. A minority always will. If the previous steps in the problem-solving process have been followed, the solution has been carefully thought out, and potential problems have been addressed, implementation should move forward. Nurses must remember that no solution is perfect and that regardless of the benefits, all change is stressful.

Most employees cooperate only with solutions that fit into their "zone of acceptance." Some solutions are clearly unacceptable, some are neutral, others are barely acceptable, and some are fully acceptable. This last group lies within the zone of acceptance. Thus, if the nurse manager chooses a solution that he or she knows may not be accepted, the manager must take steps to educate or motivate the staff to comply with it.

The nurse manager may decide that when the census is low, nurses will "float" to other units. The unit's own staff, however, has negative ideas about floating and do not wish to cooperate. If the nurse manager cannot educate or motivate staff to see floating as an acceptable solution to fluctuating census problems, the solution, no matter how good, will fail because it is not within the staff's zone of acceptance. Participative management techniques, which are discussed throughout this book, help identify acceptable solutions to problems.

7. *Evaluate the solution.* After the solution has been implemented, nurses should review the plan instituted and compare the actual results and benefits to those of the idealized solution. People tend to fall back into old patterns of habit, only giving lip service to change and carrying out the same old behavior. The nurses must ask, Is the solution being implemented? If so, are the results better or worse than expected? If they are better, what changes have contributed to its success? How can we ensure that the solution continues to be used and to work? Such a periodic checkup gives the nurse manager valuable insight and experience to use in other situations and keeps the problem-solving process on course.

The nurse manager should study outcomes of the solution somewhat as a football coach studies videotapes of a football game. Where were mistakes made? How can they be avoided in the future? What decisions were successes? Why? Many ineffective solutions are never challenged once they are implemented. If the nurse manager evaluates the outcome to ensure that the problem has indeed been solved and builds on that experience, problem solving becomes an expert skill that the nurse can use throughout a management career.

See Case Study 7-2 to learn how one nurse manager used critical thinking to solve a problem.

CASE STUDY 7-2: Critical Thinking and Problem Solving

Latonia Wilson is nurse manager for a busy 20-bed telemetry unit. In addition to providing postsurgical care for cardiac patients, nurses also prepare patients for cardiac lab procedures. Latonia's staff includes 8 graduate nurses, almost half of her nursing staff. The new nurses have attended most of the required nursing orientation for the hospital.

Three times in one month, telemetry unit patients who had orders for heparin drips were instead administered heparin flush. Premixed IV bags for heparin drips as well as heparin flush for indwelling arterial catheters are stocked on the IV solutions cart in the medication room. While no adverse patient outcomes had been reported, procedures have been delayed.

Geena Donati is a graduate nurse on the telemetry unit. Recently, she took a bag of heparin drip from the IV cart and started to attach it to the IV tubing. She noticed that the label stated heparin flush instead of heparin. Upon returning to the med room, she checked the heparin drip bin and found heparin flush bags mixed in with the heparin drip. The pharmacy technician came into the med room and began stocking the IV cart. Geena noticed that the pharmacy technician put extra heparin drip bags in the heparin flush bin. She questioned the pharmacy technician and he told Geena that since the unit used a lot of heparin solution, he had started bringing extra to decrease his trips to the unit.

Geena met with Latonia later during her shift. She told her manager about the extra heparin bags being mixed into the wrong bins. Latonia asked Geena if she would be interested in working with two other RNs on the unit to develop new procedures to decrease heparin medication errors. Geena and the task force worked with the pharmacy department to change the label color for heparin drip and heparin flush solutions, physically separated the bins on the IV cart onto different shelves, and provided a short educational segment at the monthly staff meeting. Since the new procedures were developed, no further heparin errors have occurred on the telemetry unit.

Manager's Checklist

The nurse manager is responsible for

- Tracking and identifying reoccurring negative performance issues on the unit,
- Analyzing adverse outcomes to determine what factors contributed to the outcome,
- Empowering staff to improve work processes on the unit,
- Understanding the organizational structure and assisting staff in working with other departments within the organization, and
- Including a "lessons learned" agenda at staff meetings, as needed, to review with staff how problems have been resolved within the unit.

Group Problem Solving

Traditionally, managers solved most problems in isolation. This practice, however, is outdated. Both the complexity of problems and the staff's desire for meaningful involvement at work create the impetus for using group approaches to problem solving. Today consensus-based problem solving is more often the norm.

Advantages of Group Problem Solving Groups collectively possess greater knowledge and information than any single member and may access more strategies to solve a problem. Under the right circumstances and with appropriate leadership, groups can deal with more complex problems than a single individual, especially if there is no one right or wrong solution to the problem. Individuals tend to rely on a small number of familiar strategies; a group is more likely to try several approaches.

Group members may have a greater variety of training and experiences and approach problems from more diverse points of view. Together, a group may generate more complete, accurate, and less biased information than one person. Groups may deal more effectively with problems that cross organizational boundaries or involve change that requires support from all departments affected. Participative problem solving has additional advantages: It increases the likelihood of acceptance and understanding of the decision, and it enhances cooperation in implementation.

Disadvantages of Group Problem Solving Group problem solving also has disadvantages: It takes time and resources and may involve conflict. Group problem solving also can lead to the emergence of benign tyranny within the group. Members who are less informed or less confident may allow stronger members to control group discussion and problem solving. A disparity in participation may contribute to a power struggle between the nurse manager and a few assertive group members.

Group problem solving also can be affected by **groupthink.** Groupthink is a negative phenomenon that occurs in highly cohesive groups that become isolated. Through prolonged close association, group members come to think alike and have similar prejudices and blind spots, such as stereotypical views of outsiders. They exhibit a strong tendency to seek concurrence, which interferes with critical thinking about important decisions. In addition, the leadership of such groups suppresses open, free-wheeling discussion and controls what ideas will be discussed and how much dissent will be tolerated. Groupthink seriously impairs critical thinking and can result in erroneous and damaging decisions.

The phenomenon of groupthink was studied in depth by Janis (1982), who cited the problem-solving process of the Kennedy administration's ad hoc committee on the Bay of Pigs invasion as a classic illustration.

Two phenomena are associated with groupthink (Forsyth, 1983): premature concurrence seeking, and illusions and misperceptions. **Premature concurrence seeking** is evidenced in several features of groupthink, such as

- High pressure to conform and taboos against expressing dissent or criticizing ideas presented by the majority, a leader, or some other powerful member,
- Self-censorship of dissenting opinions, in which members with questions or concerns remain silent,
- **Mindguards,** who use "gate keeping" to protect the group from controversial information and discourage dissent by diverting doubts about the group's decisions or beliefs, and
- Apparent unanimity, reflected in the illusion that the group is in concurrence despite objections and concerns.

Misperceptions and illusions are also characteristic of groupthink. They may include

- A belief that the group is morally correct, which encourages members to ignore the ethical and moral consequences of their decisions,
- Rationalization of warnings and other forms of negative feedback,
- Biased perceptions of the out-group, and
- Collective rationalization of contradictory information (Janis, 1982).

Leaders and group members may use the following tactics to prevent groupthink in cohesive groups (Janis, 1982):

1. Promote open inquiry by assigning the crucial evaluator role to each member. Encourage the group to give high priority to airing objections and doubts. Reinforce by accepting criticism.
2. The leader initially should delay stating his or her preferences and expectations until others' views have been fully disclosed.
3. The leader may set up several independent work groups to tackle the same issue. The groups then reconvene to explore a variety of approaches to problem solving and to hammer out differences.
4. Each member of the decision-making group should discuss periodically the group's deliberations with trusted associates in his or her own unit of the organization and report back nonmembers' views and reactions.
5. One or more outside experts within the organization who are not core members of the problem-solving group should be invited to each meeting on a rotating basis to challenge the views of the core members.
6. At every problem-solving meeting, at least one group member should be assigned the role of devil's advocate by attempting to find fault with any argument that might be considered valid.
7. Whenever problem solving involves relations with a rival, all warning signals from the rival should be analyzed and possible interpretations of the rival's intentions examined.
8. After reaching a preliminary consensus (agreement that everyone can support, arrived at without formal voting) about the best alternative, the problem-solving group should hold a second chance meeting at which every member is expected to express as vividly as possible all residual doubts and to rethink the entire issue before making a final choice.

Managers must recognize that although managing dissent may be complicated, time consuming, and at times unpleasant, conflict is not always dysfunctional, and it is often necessary for quality decision making.

Dialectical inquiry is another technique to minimize groupthink. In dialectical inquiry, advocates of a plan and a counterplan undertake a formal debate. This technique formalizes conflict by allowing disagreement, encourages the exploration of alternative solutions, and reduces the emotional aspects of conflict. This approach can be used regardless of a manager's feelings. The benefits from this method come from the presentation and debate of the basic assumptions underlying proposed courses of action. Any false or misleading assumptions become apparent, and the process promotes better understanding of problems and leads to higher levels of confidence in a decision. Some potential drawbacks to this method are that it can lead to an emphasis on who won the debate rather than what the best decision is or it can lead to inappropriate compromise.

Risky Shift Groups tend to make riskier decisions than individuals. Groups are more likely to support unusual or unpopular positions (e.g., public demonstrations). Groups tend to be less conservative than individual decision makers and frequently display more courage and support for unusual or creative solutions to problems. This phenomenon is referred to as **risky shift** (Napier & Gershenfeld, 1981).

Several factors contribute to this phenomenon. Individuals who lack information about alternatives may make a safe choice, but after group discussion they acquire additional information and become more comfortable with a less secure alternative. The group setting also allows for the diffusion of responsibility. If something goes wrong, others also can be assigned the blame or risk. In addition, leaders may be greater risk takers than individuals, and group members may attach a social value to risk taking because they identify it with leadership. Risky shift may be less of a problem in health care organizations because society discourages risk about health matters. However, nurse managers should be aware of this phenomenon, especially in relation to organizational decisions (e.g., starting or terminating a service).

When to Use Groups for Problem Solving Vroom and Jago (1974, 1988) developed a model for determining when to use a group for problem solving. In practice, several factors determine the degree of participation in group problem solving:

- Who initiates ideas
- How much support from subordinates is required to implement a solution
- How completely an employee is involved in each phase of problem solving (identifying the problem,

analyzing the problem, finding alternatives, estimating consequences, and making choices)
- How much weight the nurse manager attaches to the ideas received
- How much the nurse manager knows about the issue

Generally, groups should be used for problem solving when time and deadlines allow for a group decision; the problem is complex or unstructured; the group members share the organization's goals; there is need for acceptance, or at least understanding, of the decision if it is to be implemented properly; and the process will not lead to unacceptable conflict.

What You Know Now

- Critical thinking requires examining underlying assumptions about current evidence, interpreting information, and evaluating the arguments presented to reach a new and exciting conclusion.
- The creative process involves preparation, incubation, insight, and verification, which can be learned by individuals and used in groups.
- Problem-solving and decision-making processes use critical-thinking skills.
- The decision-making process may employ several models: rational or normative, descriptive or bounded rationality, satisficing, and political.
- Decision-making techniques vary according to the problem and the degree of risk and uncertainty in the situation.

KEY TERMS

Groupthink A negative phenomenon occurring in highly cohesive, isolated groups in which group members come to think alike, which interferes with critical thinking.

Premature concurrence seeking A result of groupthink caused by pressure to conform, self-censorship, mindguards, and apparent unanimity.

Mindguards A feature of groupthink in which the group is "protected" from controversial information.

Dialectical inquiry A technique used to minimize groupthink through the use of a formal debate format.

Risky shift A phenomenon seen in groups in which riskier, more controversial decisions are made.

- Methods of problem solving include trial and error, intuition, experimentation, past experience, tradition, and recognizing problems that are self-solving.
- The problem-solving process involves defining the problem, gathering information, analyzing information, developing solutions, making a decision, implementing the decision, and evaluating the solution.

Tools for Making Decisions and Solving Problems

1. Ask questions, interpret data, and consider alternatives to make decisions and solve problems.
2. Recognize when decisions are made under certainty, uncertainty, and risk, and evaluate the alternatives appropriately.
3. Identify opportunities to use groups appropriately to make decisions and solve problems.
4. Follow the problem-solving process described in the chapter.
5. Realize that you cannot solve all problems.

Questions to Challenge You

1. Identify someone you believe has critical-thinking skills. What are they?
2. Describe a situation when you made an important decision. What content in the chapter applied to that situation? What was the outcome?
3. Have you been involved in group decision making at school or work? What techniques were used? Were they effective?
4. From the models discussed in the chapter, describe fictional or real situations using these models.
5. A number of ways that problem solving might fail were discussed in the chapter. Name three more.

Explore 🌐 MediaLink

NCLEX review questions, essay activities, group activities, and other interactive resources for this chapter can be found on the Web site at http://www.prenhall.com/sullivan-decker. Click on "Chapter 7" to select activities for this chapter.

References

Boychuk, J. E. D. (1999). Catching the wave: Understanding the concept of critical thinking. *Journal of Advanced Nursing, 29*(3), 577–583.

Delbecq, A. L., VandeVen, A. H., & Gustafson, D. H. (1975). *Group techniques for program planning.* Glenview, IL: Foresman.

Forsyth, D. R. (1983). *An introduction to group dynamics.* Monterey, CA: Brooks/Cole.

Ignatavicius, D. D. (2001). Six critical thinking skills for at-the-bedside success. *Nursing Management, 32*(1), 37–39.

Janis, I. L. (1982). *Groupthink: Psychological studies of policy decisions and fiascoes*, 2nd ed. Boston: Houghton Mifflin.

Lepley, C. (1998). Problem-solving tools for analyzing system problems: The affinity map and the relationship diagram. *Journal of Nursing Administration, 28*(12), 44–50.

McConnell, C. R. (2000). The anatomy of a decision. *Health Care Manager, 18*(4), 63–74.

Napier, R. W., & Gershenfeld, M. K. (1981). *Groups: Theory and experience.* Boston: Houghton Mifflin.

Patz, J., Biordi, D., & Holm, K. (1991). Middle nurse manager effectiveness. *Journal of Nursing Administration, 21*(1), 15–24.

Pederson, A. (1993). Qualities of the excellent head nurse. *Nursing Administration Quarterly, 18*(1), 40–50.

Schmieding, N. J. (1999). Reflective inquiry framework for nurse administrators. *Journal of Advanced Nursing, 30*(3), 631–639.

Simon, H. A. (1955). A behavioral model of rational choice. *Quarterly Journal of Economics, 69*, 99–118.

Simon, H. A. (1993). Decision making: Rational, nonrational, and irrational. *Education Administration Quarterly, 29*(3), 392–411.

Vroom, V. H., & Jago, A. G. (1974). Decision making as a social process: Normative and descriptive models of leader behavior. *Decision Sciences, 5*, 743–769.

Vroom, V. H., & Jago, A. G. (1988). *The new leadership.* Englewood Cliffs, NJ: Prentice Hall.

Walton, M. (1988). *The Deming management method.* Northbrook, IL: Dodd, Mead.

Communicating Effectively

Looking Ahead

As one of the most fundamental components of society and one of the most basic tools of management, communication encompasses so much that it nearly defies definition. We communicate to relay information, and the methods, implications, and results vary immensely. This chapter provides an overview of communication skills and techniques that you can use to be more effective within your organization.

Successful and effective management and leadership depend on well-developed interpersonal skills. Communicating clearly and effectively is critical because managers spend the majority of the day communicating. Communication skills are needed to facilitate team building, manage conflict, and demonstrate insight, empathy, caring, and trustworthiness. This chapter discusses communication in management and leadership.

Objectives

In this chapter, you will learn

- Why communication skills are essential for leadership.
- What factors influence communication.
- How communication can be distorted and misunderstood.
- Which communication mode to use depending on the message and the relationship.
- How communication strategies vary according to the situation and those involved.
- How to communicate with difficult people.

MediaLink ● www.prenhall.com/
sullivan-decker

Additional resources for this chapter can be found on the Companion Website at www.prenhall.com/sullivan-decker. Click on "Chapter 8" to select the activities for this chapter.

- NCLEX Review
- Critical Thinking Activities
- Current Events
- MediaLinks
- *Nursing Leadership & Management in Action:* Evaluating Personal Communication Techniques; Communicating Effectively through Writing; Developing Assertiveness

Communication

Communication is a complex, ongoing, dynamic process in which the participants simultaneously create shared meaning in an interaction. The goal of communication is to approach, as closely as possible, a common understanding of the message sent and the one received. At times, this can be difficult because both participants are influenced by past conditioning, the present situation, each person's purpose in the current communication, and each person's attitudes toward self, the topic, and each other. It is important that participants construct messages as clearly as possible, listen carefully, monitor each other's response, and provide feedback.

Modes of Communication

Messages may be written (handwritten, typed, electronically mailed, faxed), oral (face-to-face, one-on-one, or in groups; by telephone; on voice mail), or interactive video. The purpose of the message is one characteristic that helps determine the best mode to use. In general, the more important or delicate the issue, the more intimate the mode should be. Any difficult issue should be communicated face-to-face, such as terminating an individual's employment. Conflict or confrontation also is usually best handled in person so that the individual's response can be seen and answered appropriately.

Levels of personal intimacy in communication are influenced, in descending order:

- in person
- on the telephone
- voice mail messages
- electronic mail
- memos, faxes, and written mail

The telephone is slightly less intimate than in-person communication. Tone of voice, for instance, can be conveyed and may facilitate cooperation. Voice mail is the next level of communication. Voice mail is useful to convey information that is not necessarily sensitive and may or may not require a reply. The time and place of an upcoming meeting, for example, can be communicated by voice mail, which has the added advantage of avoiding "phone tag." Electronic mail (e-mail) is useful for information similar to that conveyed by voice mail and has the added advantage of being able to broadcast messages to large groups via a listserv. The dates and times for a blood drive are a good example of a broadcast e-mail message. Conveying complicated information that may require thought before the receiver replies is another value of using e-mail.

The level of formality of the communication also affects the mode used. Applying for a position requires a written letter, usually mailed, although some organizations accept faxed applications today. Also, the relationship between the sender and receiver also affects the mode. If a staff nurse, for example, wants to nominate a co-worker for an award given by the hospital board of directors, a written letter is required. Memos are less formal than written letters; they can be sent by fax or through the mail.

Distorted Communication

Nonverbal communication can distort the meaning of the words spoken. Oral messages are accompanied by a number of nonverbal messages known as **metacommunications.** These behaviors include head or facial agreement or disagreement; eye contact; tone, volume, and inflection of the voice; gestures of the shoulders, arms, hands, or fingers; body posture and position; dress and appearance; timing; and environment.

Nonverbal communication is more powerful than the words one speaks. When a verbal message is incongruent with the nonverbal message, the recipient has difficulty interpreting the intended meaning; this results in **intrasender conflict.** For example, a manager who states, "Come talk to me anytime," but keeps the office door closed at all times, sends a conflicting message to the staff. **Intersender conflict** occurs when a person receives two conflicting messages from differing sources. For example, the risk manager may encourage a nurse to report medication errors, whereas the nurse manager follows up with discipline over the error. The nurse is caught between conflicting messages from the two.

Other common causes of distorted communication are

- Using inadequate reasoning,
- Using strong, judgmental words,
- Speaking too fast or too slowly,
- Using unfamiliar words, and
- Spending too much time on details.

Distortion also occurs when the recipient is busy or distracted, bases understanding on previous experiences with the sender, or has a biased perception of the meaning of the message or the messenger. Consider the example of distortion of written communication provided in Box 8-1.

KEY TERMS

Communication A complex, ongoing, dynamic process in which the participants simultaneously create shared meaning in an interaction.

Metacommunications Nonverbal messages in communication, including body language and environmental factors.

Intrasender conflict Difficulty in interpreting the intended meaning of a message due to incongruity between verbal and nonverbal communication.

Intersender conflict Difficulty in interpreting the intended meaning of a message due to two conflicting messages received from differing sources.

Box 8-1 Distortion in Written Communication

There is ample opportunity for distortion in the complicated process of sending, receiving, and responding to messages, as demonstrated by the following correspondence between a plumber and an official of the National Bureau of Standards (Donaldson & Scannell, 1979).

Bureau of Standards
Washington, D.C.
Gentlemen:
I have been in the plumbing business for over 11 years and have found that hydrochloric acid works real fine for cleaning drains. Could you tell me if it's harmless?

Sincerely,
Tom Brown, Plumber

Mr. Tom Brown, Plumber
Yourtown, U.S.A.
Dear Mr. Brown:
The efficacy of hydrochloric acid is indisputable, but the chlorine residue is incompatible with metallic permanence!

Sincerely,
Bureau of Standards

Bureau of Standards
Washington, D.C.
Gentlemen:
I have your letter of last week and am mightily glad you agree with me on the use of hydrochloric acid.

Sincerely,
Tom Brown, Plumber

Mr. Tom Brown, Plumber
Yourtown, U.S.A.
Dear Mr. Brown:
We wish to inform you we have your letter of last week and advise that we cannot assume responsibility for the production of toxic and noxious residues with hydrochloric acid and further suggest you use an alternate procedure.

Sincerely,
Bureau of Standards

Bureau of Standards
Washington, D.C.
Gentlemen:
I have your most recent letter and am happy to find you still agree with me.

Sincerely,
Tom Brown, Plumber

Mr. Tom Brown, Plumber
Yourtown, U.S.A.
Dear Mr. Brown:
Don't use hydrochloric acid, it eats the hell out of pipes!

Sincerely,
Bureau of Standards

For communication among more than two people, the chance of distortion increases proportionally.

Directions of Communication

Formal or informal communication may be downward, upward, lateral, or diagonal. **Downward communication** (manager to staff) is often directive. The staff is told what needs to be done or given information to facilitate the job to be done. **Upward communication** occurs from staff to management or from lower management to middle or upper management. Upward communication often involves reporting pertinent information to facilitate problem solving and decision making. **Lateral communication** occurs between individuals or departments at the same hierarchical level (e.g., nurse managers, department heads). **Diagonal communication** involves individuals or departments at different hierarchical levels (e.g., staff nurse to chief of the medical staff). Both lateral and diagonal communication involve information sharing, discussion, and negotiation.

An informal channel commonly seen in organizations is the grapevine (i.e., rumors and gossip). Grapevine communication is usually rapid, haphazard, and prone to distortion. It is also useful. Sometimes the only way you learn about a pending change is through the grapevine. One problem with grapevine communication is that no one is accountable for the misinformation relayed. Keep in mind also that information gathered this way has undergone subtle changes as the message has passed from person to person. It is a slightly altered version of the truth.

Gender Differences in Communication

Men and women communicate differently, according to linguist Deborah Tannen (1994). They have become socialized through communication patterns that reflect their societal roles. Men tend to talk more, longer, and faster, whereas women are more descriptive, attentive, and perceptive. Women tend to use tag questions (e.g., "I can take off this weekend, can't I?") and tend to

self-disclose more than men (Donaldson & Donaldson, 1996). Women tend to ask more questions and solicit more input than their male counterparts. Men tend to be more aggressive, express their opinion, and disagree more than women managers (Davidhizar & Cramer, 2000). In unpleasant situations, men talk more whereas women withdraw. Table 8-1 lists some of the differences in the ways that men and women communicate.

Using gender-neutral language in communication helps bridge the gap between men's and women's ways of communicating. Jurma and Powell (1994) found subordinates rated managers who used both male and female communication strategies as better handlers of conflict. Recommendations for gender-neutral communication are listed in Table 8-2.

Cultural Differences in Communication

Cultural attitudes, beliefs, and behaviors all affect communication. Such elements as body movement, gestures, tone, and spatial orientation are culturally defined. A great deal of misunderstanding results from

---

KEY TERMS

Downward communication Communication, generally directive, given from an authority figure or manager to staff.

Upward communication Communication that occurs from staff to management.

Lateral communication Communication that occurs between individuals at the same hierarchical level.

Diagonal communication Communication involving individuals at different hierarchical levels.

Table 8-1 Gender Differences in Communication

Men tend to	Women tend to
Interrupt more frequently	Wait to be noticed
Talk more, longer, louder, and faster	Use qualifiers (prefacing and tagging)
Disagree more	Use questions in place of statements
Focus on the issue more than the person	Relate personal experiences
Boast about accomplishments	Promote consensus
Use banter to avoid a one-down position	Withdraw from conflict

From *Becoming Influential: A Guide for Nurses* (p. 52), by E. J. Sullivan, 2004, Upper Saddle River, NJ: Prentice Hall. Reprinted by permission.

Table 8-2	Recommendations for Gender-Neutral Communication

Men may need to	Women may need to
Listen to objections and suggestions	State your message clearly and concisely
Listen without feeling responsible	Solve problems without personalizing them
Suspend judgment until information is in	Say what you want without hinting
Explain your reasons	Eliminate unsure words ("sort of") and nonwords ("truly")
Not yell	Not cry

From *Becoming Influential: A Guide for Nurses* (p. 52), by E. J. Sullivan, 2004, Upper Saddle River, NJ: Prentice Hall. Reprinted by permission.

people's lack of understanding of each other's cultural expectations. For example, people of Asian descent take great care in exchanges with superiors so that there is no conflict or "loss of face" for either person.

Understanding the cultural heritage of employees and learning to interpret cultural messages is essential for the nurse manager to communicate effectively with staff from diverse backgrounds. Personal and professional cultural enrichment training is recommended. This includes reading the literature and history of the culture; participating in open, honest, respectful communication; and exploring the meaning of behavior. It is important to recognize, however, that subcultures exist within all cultures; therefore, what applies to one individual will not be true for everyone else in that culture.

Differences in Organizational Culture

As discussed in Chapter 2, the customs, norms, and expectations within an organization are powerful forces that shape behavior. Focusing on relevant issues regarding the organizational culture can identify failures in communication. Communication is a frequent source of job dissatisfaction as well as a powerful determinant of an organization's effectiveness. Just as violation of other norms within the organization results in repercussions, so does violation of communication rules.

To discover what rules affect communication in your organization, ask yourself:

- Who has access to what information? Is information withheld? Shared widely?
- What modes of communication are used for which messages? Are they used appropriately?
- How clear are the messages? Or are they often distorted?
- Does everyone receive the same information?

- Do you receive too much information? Not enough?
- How effective is the message?

The Role of Communication in Leadership

Although communication is inherent in the manager's role, the manager's ability to communicate often determines his or her success as a leader. Leaders who engage in frank, open, two-way communication and whose nonverbal communication reinforces the verbal communication are seen as informative. Communication is enhanced when the manager listens carefully and is sensitive to others. The major underlying factor, however, is an ongoing relationship with the manager's employees.

Successful leaders are able to persuade others and enlist their support. The most effective means of persuasion is the leader's personal characteristics. Competence, emotional control, assertiveness, consideration, and respect promote trustworthiness and credibility. A participative leader is seen as a careful listener who is open, frank, trustworthy, and informative.

Communicating with Different Populations

Subordinates

Depending on the organization's policies, the nurse manager's responsibilities may include selecting, interviewing, evaluating, counseling, and disciplining employees; handling their complaints; and settling conflicts. The principles of effective communication are especially pertinent in these activities because good communication is the adhesive that builds and maintains an effective work group.

Giving direction is not, in itself, communication. If the manager receives an appropriate response from the

MEDIALINK Interpersonal Communication

subordinate, however, communication has occurred. To give directions and achieve the desired results, the nurse manager needs to develop a message strategy. The techniques that follow can help improve effective responses from others.

- *Know the context of the instruction.* Be certain you know exactly what you want done, by whom, within what time frame, and what steps should be followed to do it. Be clear in your own mind what information a person needs to carry out your instruction, what the outcome will be if the instruction is carried out, and how that outcome can or will be evaluated. When you have thought through these questions, you are ready to give the proper instruction.
- *Get positive attention.* Avoid factors that interfere with effective listening. Informing the person that the instructions will be given is one simple way to try to get positive attention. Highlighting the background, giving a justification, or indicating the importance of the instructions also may be appropriate.
- *Give clear, concise instructions.* Use an inoffensive and nondefensive style and tone of voice. Be precise, and give all the information receivers need to carry out your expectations. Follow a step-by-step procedure if several actions are needed.
- *Verify through feedback.* Make sure the receiver has understood your specific request for action. Ask for a repeat of the instructions.
- *Give follow-up communication.* Understanding does not guarantee performance. Follow up to determine the outcome of your instruction and give feedback to the receiver.

The nurse manager is responsible both for the quality of the work life of individual employees and for the quality of patient care in the entire unit. To carry out this job, the nurse manager should acknowledge the needs of individual employees, especially if the needs of one conflict with needs of the department; the manager should speak directly with those involved and state clearly and accurately the rationale for the decisions made.

Superiors

The manager's interaction with higher administration is comparable to the interaction between the manager and a subordinate, except that the manager is now the subordinate. The nurse manager must recognize that higher administration is responsible for the consequences of decisions made for a larger area, such as all of nursing service or the entire organization. The principles used in communicating with subordinates are equally appropriate. Managers must be organized and prepared to state their needs clearly, explain the rationale for requests, suggest benefits for the larger organization, and use appropriate channels. They also must be prepared to listen objectively to their supervisor's response and be willing to consider reasons for possible conflict with needs of other areas.

Working effectively with a supervisor is important because a supervisor directly influences personal success in a career and within the organization. Managing a supervisor, or managing upward, is a crucial skill for nurses. To manage upward, remember that the relationship requires participation from both parties. Managing upward is successful when power and influence move in both directions. Rules for managing your supervisor are found in Box 8-2.

One aspect of managing upward is to understand the supervisor's position from her or his frame of reference. This will make it easier to propose solutions and ideas that the supervisor will accept. Understand

---

Box 8-2   Rules for Managing Your Supervisor

- Give immediate positive feedback for good things that the supervisor does; positive feedback is a welcome change.
- Never let your supervisor be surprised; keep her or him informed.
- Always tell the truth.
- Find ways to compensate for weaknesses of your supervisor. Fill in weak areas tactfully. Volunteer to do something the supervisor dislikes doing.

- Be your own publicist. Don't brag, but keep your supervisor informed of what you achieve.
- Keep aware of your supervisor's achievements and acknowledge them.
- If your supervisor asks you to do something, do it well and ahead of the deadline if possible. If appropriate, add some of your own suggestions.
- Establish a positive relationship with the supervisor's assistant.

that a supervisor is a person with even more responsibility and pressure. Learn about the supervisor from a personal perspective: What pressures, both personal and professional, does the supervisor face? How does the supervisor respond to stress? What previous experiences are liable to affect today's issues? This assessment will allow you to identify ways to help your supervisor with his or her job and for your supervisor to help you with yours.

Influencing Your Supervisor Nurse managers need to approach their supervisor to exert their influence on a variety of issues and problems. Support for the purchase of capital equipment, for changes in staffing, or for a new policy or procedure all require communicating with your supervisor. Timing, rationale, choice of form or format, and possible objections all are important factors to consider as you prepare to make such a request. Timing is critical; choose an opportunity when the supervisor has time and appears receptive. Also, consider the impact of your ideas on other events occurring at that time.

Should ideas be presented in spoken or written form? Usually some combination is used. Even if you have a brief meeting about a relatively small request, it is a good idea to follow up with a memorandum detailing your ideas and the plans to which you both agreed. Sometimes the procedure works in reverse. If you provide the supervisor a written proposal prior to a meeting, both of you will be familiar with the idea at the start. In the latter case, careful preparation of the written material is essential.

What can be done if, in spite of careful preparation, your supervisor says no? First, make sure you have understood the objections and associated feelings. **Negative inquiry** (e.g., "I don't understand") is a helpful technique to use. Do not interrupt or become defensive or distraught; remain diplomatic. **Fogging,** agreeing with part of what was said, or **negative assertion,** accepting some blame, are two additional techniques that you can use.

The next step is confrontation. Keep your voice low and measured; use "I" language; and avoid absolutes, why questions, put-downs, inflammatory statements, and threatening gestures. Finally, if you feel you have lost and compromise is unlikely, table the issue by saying, "Could we continue discussing this at another time?" Then, think through your supervisor's reasoning and evaluate it.

Afterward ask yourself: "What new information did I get from the supervisor?" "What are ways I can renegotiate?" "What do I need to know or do to overcome objections?" Once you can answer these questions,

approach your supervisor again with the new information. This behavior shows that the proposal is a high priority, and the new information may cause him or her to reevaluate.

Managers often succeed in influencing superiors through persistence and repetition, especially if supporting data and documentation are supplied. If the issue is important enough, you may want to take it to a higher authority. If so, tell your supervisor you would like an administrator at a higher level to hear the proposal. Keep an open mind, listen, and try to meet objections with suggestions of how to solve problems. Be prepared to compromise, which is better than no movement at all, or to be turned down.

Taking a Problem to Your Supervisor No one wants to hear about a problem, and your boss is no different. Nonetheless work involves problems, and the manager's job is to solve them. Go to your supervisor with a goal to problem solve together. Have some ideas about solving the problem in hand if you can but do not be so wedded to them that you are unable to listen to your supervisor's ideas. Keep an open mind. Use the following steps to take a problem to your supervisor:

- Find an appropriate time to discuss a problem, scheduling an appointment if necessary.
- State the problem succinctly and explain why it is interfering with work.
- Listen to your supervisor's response and provide more information if needed.
- If you agree on a solution, offer to do your part to solve it. If you cannot discover an agreeable solution, schedule a follow-up meeting or decide to gather more information.
- Schedule a follow-up appointment.

By solving the problem together and, if necessary, by taking active steps together, you and your supervisor are more likely to accept the decision and be committed to

---

KEY TERMS

Negative inquiry A communication technique used to clarify objections and feelings (e.g., I don't understand . . .).

Fogging A communication technique in which one agrees with part of what was said.

Negative assertion A communication technique in which one accepts some blame for what was said.

it. Setting a specific follow-up date can prevent a solution from being delayed or forgotten.

If All Else Fails . . . Sometimes no matter what you do, working with your supervisor seems nearly impossible. Kimura (2003) calls such supervisors "toxic." Toxic managers foster a negative work environment, and employees become dissatisfied, angry, and depressed. High absenteeism and turnover result. As a manager you are charged with supporting your superior. If working with that superior is too difficult for you to manage your work satisfactorily, you may have to transfer elsewhere or leave. (Consult *Becoming Influential: A Guide for Nurses* by E. J. Sullivan for more on this topic.)

Peers

Relationships with peers can vary from comfortable and easy to challenging and complex. Because peers often have much in common with respect to authority and power, they can share similar concerns. Camaraderie may be present; peers can exchange ideas and address problems creatively. Peers can provide support, and the strengths of one can be developed in the other. Conversely, there may also be competition or conflicts (e.g., battles over territory, personality clashes, differences of opinion). Interactions with peers are inevitable. Even when there are conflicts, peers should interact on a professional level; tactics for communicating with difficult people and negotiating may be helpful. Both topics are discussed later in this chapter.

Medical Staff

Communication with the medical staff may be difficult for the nurse manager because the relationship of physicians and nurses has been that of superior and subordinate. Gender-based differences in nursing (although less so in medicine today) may add to the difficulty. Furthermore, physician training in communication skills has often been absent (Cegala & Lenzmeier-Broz, 2002).

Complicating physician–nurse relationships is the employee status of the medical staff. They may not be employees of the organization but still have considerable power in the health care setting because of their ability to attract patients to the organization, and, finally, the medical staff is in itself diverse, consisting of physicians who are organizational employees, residents, physicians in private practice, and consulting physicians. Obviously, principles of effective communication are very important in interactions with the medical staff.

Today's nurse managers are role models and leaders for establishing nurse–physician relationships on their units. Nurse–physician communication has been shown to affect patient outcomes in two landmark studies. Lower-than-expected death rates in intensive care units were related to excellent coordination and communication among the nurse–physician staff in one study (Knaus, Draper, Wagner, & Zimmerman, 1986), and lack of communication and coordination among health care providers was related to unnecessarily high-cost stays for patients in another (Gavett, Drucker, McCrum, & Dickenson, 1985). Nurse managers have important reasons, then, for setting a positive tone that fosters mutual respect among nurses and physicians on their units.

In today's competitive health care marketplace, it also is necessary to view the physician as a nursing service customer. Organizations are competing for patients, and physicians (as well as insurers) are sources of patients. The product of nursing service is patient care; physicians help provide the patients.

What do physicians want? Physicians first want quality staff—nurses, health care workers, and other physicians. They want up-to-date facilities and equipment, quality care, and adequately trained nursing personnel. Physicians also want respect (as do nurses and others who work in health care) and regard patient care as their primary concern. These are many of the same goals that nurses have.

To support greater collaboration between nurses and physicians and to improve the product of nursing service—patient care—keep these principles in mind:

- Respect physicians as persons, and expect them to respect you.
- Consider yourself and your staff equal partners with physicians in health care.
- Build your staff's clinical competence and credibility. Ensure that your staff has the clinical preparation necessary to meet required standards of care.
- Actively listen and respond to physician complaints as customer complaints. Create a problem-solving structure. Stop blaming physicians exclusively for communication problems.
- Use every opportunity to increase your staff's contact with physicians and to include your staff in meetings that include physicians. Remember that limited interactions contribute to poor communication.
- Establish a collaborative practice committee on your unit whose membership is composed equally of nurses and physicians. In the meetings, identify problems, develop mutually satisfactory solutions,

and learn more about each other. Emphasize similarities and quality care. Begin with those physicians who have a positive attitude toward collaboration.

- Serve as a role model to your staff in nurse–physician communication.
- Support your staff in participating in collaborative efforts by words and by your actions.

But if you are confronted with power plays or intimidation, what is the best way to respond? Intimidation results from vulnerability and a threat to self-worth. Intimidation can be counteracted by increasing self-confidence and personal feelings of power. Umiker (1990) describes four ways to generate power.

1. With words:
   - Use the other person's name frequently.
   - Use strong statements.
   - Avoid discounters, such as "I'm sorry, but. . . . "
   - Avoid clichés.
   - Avoid fillers (such as "ah," "uh," and "um").
2. Through delivery:
   - Be enthusiastic.
   - Speak clearly and forcefully.
   - Make one point at a time.
   - Do not tolerate interruptions.
3. By listening:
   - For facts.
   - For feelings.
   - For what is not being said (e.g., body language, mixed messages, hidden messages).
4. Through body posture and body language:
   - Sit next to your antagonist; turn 30 degrees toward the person when you address that person.
   - Lean forward.
   - Expand your personal space.
   - Use gestures.
   - Stand when you talk.
   - Smile when you are pleased, not in order to please.
   - Maintain eye contact, but do not stare.

One nurse manager handled a problem with a physician as shown in Case Study 8-1. Additional techniques to counteract intimidation and threat are included in Chapter 9.

CASE STUDY 8-1: Communication

Josie Randolph is nurse manager of a perioperative unit, including responsibility for the preoperative testing unit, 18 OR suites, preop holding, and sterile processing. The OR department supports the hospital's Level I trauma service as well as all other surgical services.

Dr. Jonas Welborne is a plastic surgeon with a history of aggressive behavior. He has several cases on today's OR schedule. While he is in his first surgery, a trauma case is brought to the OR. Susan Richardson, the OR charge nurse, decides to bump Dr. Welborne's second case out of OR #3 to make room for the trauma case. When Dr. Welborne has finished his first case, he is informed of the delay in his second case. Dr. Welborne storms into the OR scheduling office and begins yelling at Susan. The situation quickly escalates to the point where Dr. Welborne uses obscenities and throws several charts on the floor. Loretta Donnelly, an OR tech, runs to Josie's office and asks her to come immediately to the OR scheduling office.

Susan and Dr. Welborne continue to yell at one another, in full view of patients in the preop area. Josie immediately steps between Dr. Welborne and Susan and firmly asks both of them to lower their voices. She instructs Susan to wait in the Staff Lounge while she speaks with Dr. Welborne. Josie asks Dr. Welborne to step into her office so they can calmly discuss the situation. Dr. Welborne is still visibly agitated but agrees to discuss the problem. After hearing his side of the story, Josie apologizes for the inconvenience, but reminds him of the OR policies. Emergent cases take precedence over elective cases, and no other elective cases were on the schedule at that time. She asks Dr. Welborne if there are alternatives to scheduling his cases that would minimize delays or bumps. As they talk, Dr. Welborne becomes calmer. Josie informs Dr. Welborne that his earlier behavior is unacceptable. Within a few minutes, he apologizes to Josie and asks to speak with Susan. He also apologizes to Susan. Josie and Susan discuss the incident and ways Susan can help diffuse similar situations in the future. As with Dr. Welborne, Josie indicates that Susan's behavior was unprofessional.

Manager's Checklist
The nurse manager is responsible for

- Mediating conflict in a timely manner,
- Knowing organizational policies and procedures that support staff decisions,
- Allowing open and complete discussion of the problem,
- Actively listening to both participants, and
- Using assertive communication to facilitate problem solving.

Other Health Care Personnel

The nurse manager has the overwhelming task of coordinating the activities of a number of personnel with varied levels and types of preparation and different kinds of tasks. The patient may receive regular care from a registered nurse, unlicensed assistive personnel, a respiratory therapist, a physical therapist, and a dietitian, among others. The nurse manager must use considerable skill to communicate effectively with the diverse personnel and managers involved in health care. In interacting with personnel from other departments, the nurse manager must recognize and respond to differences between the goals of their departments and the nursing unit. Recognizing this helps both parties to identify their commonalities and to deal with their differences.

Patients and Families

Nurse managers deal with many difficult issues. Patient or family complaints about the delivery of care (e.g., complaints about a staff member, violations of policy) are one example. When dealing with patient or family complaints, keep the following principles in mind:

- *The patient (and family) are the principal customers of the organization.* Treat patients and families with respect; keep communication open and honest. Dissatisfied customers fail to continue to use a service and also inform their friends and families about their negative experiences. Handle complaints or concerns tactfully and expeditiously. Many times, even lawsuits can be avoided if the patient or family feels that someone has taken the time to listen to their complaints. (See the section on risk management in Chapter 13.)
- *Most individuals are unfamiliar with medical jargon.* Use words that are appropriate to the recipient's level of understanding. However, take care not to be condescending or intimidating. It is just as important to assess the person's knowledge base and level of understanding as it is to know his or her vital signs or liver status.
- *Maintain privacy and identify a neutral location for dealing with difficult interactions.*
- *Make special efforts to find interpreters if a patient or family does not speak English.* Have readily available a list of individuals who are able to communicate in a variety of languages. The list also should include individuals experienced in sign language and Braille. Another resource is AT&T's language line

service (1-800-752-6096), which provides interpreters for over 140 languages 24 hours a day.
- *Recognize cultural differences in communicating with patients and their families.* People in some cultures do not ask questions for fear of imposing on others. Some cultures prefer interpreters from their own culture; others do not. Cultural education for the staff can help identify some of these differences and teach them appropriate, culturally sensitive responses.

Communicating with Difficult People

Difficult personalities exist in all groups of people—subordinates, superiors, physicians, other health care team members, patients, and family members alike. Strategies for coping with difficult people follow (Nations, 1990a, 1990b, 1990c).

1. *Put physical distance between you and the difficult person.* A common method to achieve physical distance is to limit the time you spend with the individual. Match the person's energy level in speed, pitch, and volume; this conveys awareness and empathy. This technique is particularly effective with hostile, aggressive individuals. However, negative behavior, such as yelling and tantrums, should not be mirrored; instead, remain calm but assertive.
2. *Psychologically distance yourself from the individual.* View the person from a different perspective; try "putting on his shoes." Also "lose the shoulds" (for example, "Who does he think he is? He shouldn't be allowed to talk to us like that.") Ask: What does this person's behavior accomplish? What type of personality trait is being exhibited?
3. *Identify the individual's feelings and information level.* Then validate those feelings and information as well as your relationship, but don't patronize. This technique is particularly successful with a "know-it-all" who may be under the illusion that only he or she is right.
4. *Ask extensional questions.* Questions that begin with "how" or "what" often help the person to focus on his or her concerns and rethink what has just been said. Focusing on holes in the individual's argument provides an opportunity for a graceful retreat.
5. *Use physical movement.* Lead an upset individual to your office or another neutral location, or suggest that the two of you go for a cup of coffee. Physical activity often diminishes stress and hostility.

6. *Try humor.* If the situation is not too serious, humor is an excellent method to defuse anger and frustration; however, be careful to avoid sarcasm or putdowns.

The effort to develop excellent communication skills is well worth the manager's effort. As Porter-O'Grady (2003) reminded us, today's relationship-oriented environments require superb interpersonal skills. A facilitative leadership style encourages others, empowers them to do their best work, and supports them when problems and conflict inevitably emerge.

What You Know Now

- Communication is a complex, ongoing, dynamic process in which participants simultaneously create meaning in an interaction.
- Expert communication skills are essential for a nurse manager's success.
- Gender, cultural background, and the organizational culture influence communication and its outcome.
- Messages can be distorted or misconstrued. Your job is to be as clear as possible and ensure that you have been understood.
- Communication strategies vary according to the situation and the roles of people involved.

Tools for Communicating Effectively

1. Identify and use the appropriate method (in person, phone, voice mail, e-mail, letter) for your communications.
2. Evaluate your communication skills in various situations. Think of ways to improve.
3. Practice using the skills described in specific situations, such as with your supervisor, with the medical staff, or with difficult people.
4. Become sensitive to others' responses, both verbal and nonverbal, and craft your messages appropriately.
5. Gather feedback and continue to assess the effectiveness of your communications.
6. Strive to improve your communication skills.

Questions to Challenge You

1. What are the communication channels in your workplace or clinical site? Are they congruent with the published organizational chart? How well does communication flow both upward and downward?

2. Are messages received in a timely fashion?
3. Is the medium (in person, phone, e-mail, etc.) appropriate to the message?
4. Are messages worded appropriately? For example, bad news is suitably serious; good news more positive.
5. Are messages negative in tone? For example, "Everyone *must*. . . . " rather than "The requirements are. . . . " (The difference is subtle, but important.)

Explore MediaLink

NCLEX review questions, essay activities, group activities, and other interactive resources for this chapter can be found on the Web site at http://www.prenhall.com/sullivan-decker. Click on "Chapter 8" to select activities for this chapter.

References

Cegala, D. J., & Lenzmeier-Broz, S. (2002). Physician communication skills training: A review of theoretical backgrounds, objectives and skills. *Medical Education, 36*(1), 1004–1017.

Davidhizar, R., & Cramer, C. (2000). Gender differences in leadership in the health professions. *Health Care Manager, 18*(3), 18–24.

Donaldson, L., & Scannell, E. (1979). *Human response development: The new trainer's guide.* Reading, MA: Addison-Wesley.

Donaldson, M. C., & Donaldson, M. (1996). *Negotiating for dummies.* Foster City, CA: IDG Books Worldwide.

Gavett, J. W., Drucker, W. R., McCrum, M. S., & Dickenson, J. C. (1985). *A study of high cost inpatients in Strong Memorial Hospital.* Rochester, NY: Rochester Area Hospital Corporation and University of Rochester.

Jurma & Powell (1994). Perceived gender roles of managers and effective conflict management. *Psychological Reports, 74*(1), 104–106.

Kimura, H. (2003). Overcome toxic management. *Nursing Management, 34*(1), 26–29.

Knaus, W. A., Draper, E. A., Wagner, D. P., & Zimmerman, J. E. (1986). An evaluation of outcome from intensive care in major medical centers. *Annals of Internal Medicine, 104,* 410–418.

Nations, K. H. (1990a). Coping with difficult people. Part 1. *Medical Laboratory Observer, 22*(9), 22–25.

Nations, K. H. (1990b). Coping with difficult people. Part 2: Dealing with know-it-alls even if you are one yourself. *Medical Laboratory Observer, 22*(10) 29–30, 32.

Nations, K. H. (1990c). Coping with difficult people. Part 3: Effective ways to deflect hostility. *Medical Laboratory Observer, 22*(11), 40–42.

Porter-O'Grady, T. (2003). A different age for leadership, Part 1: New context, new content. *Journal of Nursing Administration, 32*(2), 105–110.

Sullivan, E. J. (2004). *Becoming influential: A guide for nurses.* Upper Saddle River, NJ: Prentice Hall.

Tannen, D. (1994). *Talking from 9 to 5: How women's and men's conversational styles affect who gets heard, who gets credit, and what gets done at work.* New York: Morrow.

Umiker, W. (1990). How to generate power in meetings. *Health Care Supervisor, 9*(1), 33–38.

CHAPTER 9

Handling Conflict

Conflict

Conflict Process Model

> Antecedent Conditions
> Perceived and Felt Conflict
> Outcomes

Conflict Management

> Managing Conflict
> Other Conflict Management
> Strategies

Looking Ahead

Conflict is one of the most difficult problems managers face, and learning how to deal with conflict is essential for nurse managers to be successful. Conflicts occur between staff members, with patients and their families, between nurses and other health care professionals, and with the manager's own supervisor. Conflict management skills can be learned. This chapter shows you how.

Objectives

In this chapter, you will learn

- Why conflict can be positive or negative.
- How conflict can help generate change.
- What the components of conflict are.
- What different types of conflict exist.
- How to manage conflict.

MediaLink 🌐 **www.prenhall.com/ sullivan-decker**

Additional resources for this chapter can be found on the Companion Website at www.prenhall.com/sullivan-decker. Click on "Chapter 9" to select the activities for this chapter.

- NCLEX Review
- Critical Thinking Activities
- Current Events
- MediaLinks
- *Nursing Leadership & Management in Action:* Recognizing Role Conflicts; Strategies for Resolving Conflict

Conflict

A manager's communication often centers around conflict. A study by the American Management Association (McElhaney, 1996) reports that nurse managers spend approximately 20 percent of their time dealing with conflict. Conflict is a natural, inevitable condition in organizations, and it is often a prerequisite to change in people and organizations.

Conflict is defined as the consequence of real or perceived differences in mutually exclusive goals, values, ideas, attitudes, beliefs, feelings, or actions (a) within one individual (*intrapersonal conflict*), (b) between two or more individuals (*interpersonal conflict*), (c) within one group (*intragroup conflict*), or (d) between two or more groups (*intergroup conflict*). Conflict is dynamic. It can be positive or negative, healthy or dysfunctional.

A certain amount of conflict is beneficial to an organization. It can provide heightened sensitivity to an issue, further piquing the interest and curiosity of others. Conflict also can increase creativity by acting as a stimulus for developing new ideas or identifying methods for solving problems. Disagreements can help all parties become more aware of the tradeoffs, especially costs versus benefits, of a particular service or technique.

Conflict also helps people recognize legitimate differences within the organization or profession and serves as a powerful motivator to improve performance and effectiveness, as well as satisfaction. For example, during intergroup conflict, individual groups become more cohesive and task oriented, whereas communication between groups diminishes.

Aggressive behavior can occur. Groups placed in "win–lose" competition have the tendency to increase the in-group versus out-group bias between them. Scapegoating may occur, with each group viewing the other as an enemy. This may make it difficult for the groups to work together in the future.

Conflict may be covert and inappropriate. Anger may be displaced to innocent bystanders. Others may repress their frustration or anger, which may surface later in behavior (e.g., increased errors, accidents, or illness). Other inappropriate responses to conflict are retaliation, projection, rationalization, attention-seeking behaviors, repression, or escape tactics, such as resignation or flight into fantasy.

Competition, such as that which occurs between health care organizations, also is a frequent source of conflict. Competition occurs when two or more groups attempt the same goals and only one group can attain those goals. Filley (1975) defines **competitive conflict** as a victory for one side and a loss for the other side. The process by which the conflict is resolved is determined by a set of rules. The goals of each side are mutually incompatible, but the emphasis is on winning, not the defeat or reduction of the opponent. When one side has clearly won, competition is terminated.

Disruptive conflict, in contrast, does not follow any mutually acceptable set of rules and does not emphasize winning. The parties involved are engaged in activities to reduce, defeat, or eliminate the opponent. This type of conflict takes place in an environment charged with fear, anger, and stress. For example, a resident on night call may contribute to disruptive behavior by refusing to answer pages, turning off the beeper, or belittling nurses for calling with "minor" problems. Nurses often react to this type of behavior with their own disruptive behavior: frequent, "by the book," middle-of-the-night phone calls to get back at the offending resident. An example of a more subtle disruptive behavior would be the failure to extend minor work-saving courtesies to an unpopular resident. Disruptive conflict can, in unusual circumstances, result in irrational, upsetting, or even violent behavior.

Conflict Process Model

Filley's model of conflict resolution provides a generalized format for examining conflict behavior in relation to the nurse manager's job. This model provides a framework that helps explain how and why conflict occurs and, ultimately, how one can minimize conflict or resolve it with the least amount of negative aftermath.

KEY TERMS

Conflict The consequence of real or perceived differences in mutually exclusive goals, values, ideas, attitudes, beliefs, feelings, or actions.

Competitive conflict A type of conflict that is resolved through competition, in which victory for one side and loss for the other side is determined by a set of rules.

Disruptive conflict A type of conflict in which winning is not emphasized and there is no mutually acceptable set of rules; parties involved are engaged in activities to reduce, defeat, or eliminate the opponent.

Filley suggests that conflict and its resolution develop according to a specific process. This process begins with certain preexisting conditions (antecedent conditions). The parties are influenced by their feelings or perceptions about the situation (perceived or felt conflict), which initiates behavior (manifest behavior). The conflict is either resolved or suppressed (conflict resolution or suppression), and in the aftermath (resolution aftermath), new attitudes and feelings between the parties evolve.

Antecedent Conditions

Antecedent conditions are associated with increases in conflict. Antecedent conditions propel a situation toward conflict; they may or may not be the cause. In nursing, antecedent conditions include incompatible goals, differences in values and beliefs, task interdependencies (especially asymmetric dependencies, in which one party is dependent on the other but not vice versa), unclear or ambiguous roles, competition for scarce resources, differentiation or distancing mechanisms, and unifying mechanisms.

Incompatible Goals   The most important antecedent condition to conflict is incompatible goals. As discussed in Chapter 3, goals are desired results toward which behavior is directed. Even though the common goal in health care organizations is to give quality patient care in a cost-effective manner, conflict in achieving these goals is inevitable because individuals often view this from different perspectives. In addition, individuals and organizations have multiple goals that change over time. A health care organization may have specific goals to achieve the best possible care for patients and control costs to stay within budget and, at the same time, to provide intrinsically satisfying jobs for its employees. These multiple goals will frequently conflict with each other, so they will have to be prioritized. Priority setting can be one of the most difficult but important activities a health care manager must face. Goals are important because they become the basis for allocating resources and thus become an important source (antecedent) of conflict in the organization.

Similarly, individuals themselves have multiple goals, and those goals may also conflict. Individuals allocate scarce resources, such as their time, on the basis of priority and, therefore, might achieve one goal at the expense of others. The inability to attain multiple (and mutually incompatible) goals—whether those goals are personal or organizational—can cause conflict.

An example of goal conflict in nursing is the dichotomy between health care providers and third-party payers. This issue can best be described as a conflict between groups with differing goals. Health care providers want to maximize the quality of care, whereas payers are concerned with minimizing health care costs.

Role Conflicts   Roles are defined as other people's expectations regarding behavior and attitudes. Roles become unclear when one or more parties have related responsibilities that are ambiguous or overlapping. The nurse manager might experience conflict between his or her responsibilities as an administrator and responsibilities as a staff member. Similarly, unclear or overlapping job descriptions or assignments may lead to conflict. For example, there could be conflict over such mundane issues as who has responsibility to deliver a patient to the radiology department—the nurse or the transport staff?

Task interdependence is another potential source of conflict. Nursing and housekeeping, for example, are interdependent. Housekeeping cannot completely clean a room until nursing has discharged the patient. Other examples of interdependence are the relationships among shifts and those between physicians and nurses. Interdependent relationships have the potential to initiate conflict.

Structural Conflict   One conflict commonly seen in the health care environment is structural conflict. Structured relationships (superior to subordinate, peer to peer) provoke conflict because of poor communication, competition for resources, opposing interests, or a lack of shared perceptions or attitudes. A nurse manager (superior) stimulates conflict with a staff member (subordinate) by reprimanding the staff member for some inappropriate act. If the nurse manager is unable to communicate to the staff member why the act was unacceptable, opposing interests develop, and the conflict is sustained. In this situation, positional power is often imposed. Positional power is the authority inherent in a certain position—for example, the nurse administrator has greater positional power than a nurse manager.

Competitions for Resources   Competition for scarce resources can be internal (among different units in the organization) or external (among different organizations). Internally, competition for resources may involve assigning staff from one unit to another or purchasing high-technology equipment when another unit is desperate for staff.

Externally, health care organizations compete for finite external resources (e.g., managed-care contracts).

Organizations are using a variety of means, such as developing new services and advertising, to try to capture the market in health care. With increased numbers of nurse practitioners, competition between nurses and physicians for patients also has increased.

Values and Beliefs   Differences in values and beliefs frequently contribute to conflict in health care organizations. Values and beliefs result from the individual's socialization experience. Conflicts between physicians and nurses, between nurses and administrators, or even between nurses with associate degrees versus those with baccalaureate degrees, often occur because of differences in values, beliefs, and experiences.

Distancing mechanisms or differentiation serve to divide a group's members into small, distinct groups, thus increasing the chance for conflict. This tends to lead to a "we–they" distinction. One of the more frequently seen examples is distancing between physicians and nurses. Opposition between intensive care nurses and nurses on medical floors, night versus day shifts, and unlicensed versus licensed personnel also are examples. Differentiation among subunits also occurs and is due to differences in structure. The administrative unit may be bureaucratic, the nursing unit structured on a more professional basis, and staff physicians on an even different structure. Nonstaff physicians may be relatively independent of the health care organization.

Unifying mechanisms occur when greater intimacy develops or when unity is sought. All nurse managers might be expected to reach consensus over an issue, but they might experience internal conflict if they are forced to accept a group position even though individually they may not be wholly committed to the decision. A classic example of a unifying mechanism is the relationship between husband and wife. As intimacy increases, issues arise that would not normally cause conflict in a casual relationship but do affect closer relationships. A nurse manager's friendship with a staff member also may lead to this type of conflict.

Perceived and Felt Conflict

Perceived and felt conflict account for the conflict that may occur when the parties involved view situations or issues from differing perspectives, when they misunderstand each other's position, or when positions are based on limited knowledge. **Perceived conflict** refers to each party's perception of the other's position. **Felt conflict** refers to the feelings of opposition within the relationship of two or more parties. It is characterized by mistrust, hostility, and fear.

To demonstrate how this process works, consider this situation. A nurse manager and a surgeon have worked together for years. They have mutual respect for each other's ability and skills, and they communicate frequently. When their subordinates clash, they are left with conflicting accounts of a situation, in which the only agreed-upon fact is that a patient received less-than-appropriate care. Now consider the same scenario if the nurse and doctor have never dealt with each other or if one feels that the other will not approach the problem constructively.

In the first situation (perceived conflict), their positive regard for each other's abilities makes the nurse and physician believe they can constructively solve the conflict. The nurse does not feel the physician will try to dominate, and the physician respects the nurse manager's managerial ability. With these preexisting attitudes, the physician and nurse can remain neutral while helping their subordinates solve the conflict. If the nurse and physician were experiencing felt conflict, they might approach the situation differently. Each might assume the other will defend her or his subordinates at all costs and communication will be inhibited. The conflict is resolved by domination of the stronger person, either in personality or position. One wins; the other loses.

Outcomes

Manifest behavior is the first outcome of conflict. Behaviors may be overt or covert. Overt behavior may take the form of aggression, competition, debate, or problem solving. Covert behavior may be expressed by a variety of indirect tactics, such as scapegoating, avoidance, or apathy.

The final stages of the conflict process are **suppression** or **resolution** and the resulting aftermath. Suppression occurs when one person or group defeats the other. Only the dominant side is committed to the agreement, and the loser may or may not carry out the agreement. Resolution occurs when a mutually agreed-upon solution is arrived at and both parties commit themselves to carrying out the agreement.

The optimal solution is to manage the issues in a way that will lead to a solution wherein both parties see themselves as winners and the problem is solved. This leaves a positive aftermath that will affect future relations and influence feelings and attitudes. In the example of conflict between the nurse manager and the physician, consider the difference in the aftermath and how future issues would be approached if both parties felt positive about the outcome, as compared to future interactions if one or both parties felt they had lost.

Conflict Management

Managing conflict is an important part of the nurse manager's job. Nurse managers often are involved in conflict management on several different levels. They may be participants in the conflict as individuals, supervisors, or representatives of a unit. In fact, they must often initiate conflict by confronting staff, individually or collectively, when a problem develops. They also may serve as mediators or judges to conflicting parties. There could be a conflict within the unit, between parties from different units, or between internal and external parties (for example, a nursing instructor from the university may have a conflict with staff on a particular unit).

The nurse manager and other participants in conflict management must be realistic regarding the outcome. Often those inexperienced in conflict negotiation expect unrealistic outcomes. When two or more parties hold mutually exclusive ideas, attitudes, feelings, or goals, it is extremely difficult, without the commitment and willingness of all concerned, to arrive at an agreeable solution that meets the needs of both.

Conflict management begins with a decision regarding if and when to intervene. Failure to intervene can allow the conflict to get out of hand, whereas early intervention may be detrimental to those involved, causing them to lose confidence in themselves and reduce risk-taking behavior in the future. Some conflicts are so minor, particularly if they are between only two people, that they do not require intervention and would be better handled by the two people involved. Allowing them to resolve their conflict might provide a developmental experience and improve their abilities to resolve conflict in the future. When the conflict might result in considerable harm, however, the nurse manager must intervene.

Sometimes the nurse manager may postpone intervention purposely to allow the conflict to escalate, because increased intensity can motivate participants to seek resolution. The manager can escalate the conflict even further by exposing participants to each other more frequently without the presence of others and without an easy means of escape. Participants are then forced to face the conflict between them. Giving participants a shared task or shared goals not directly related to the conflict may help them understand each other better and increase their chances to resolve their conflicts by themselves. Using such a method is useful only if the conflict is not of high intensity, if the participants are not highly anxious about it, and if the

KEY TERMS

Perceived conflict   One's perception of the other's position in a conflict.

Felt conflict   The feelings of opposition within the relationship of two or more parties.

Suppression   The stage of conflict that occurs when one person or group defeats the other and only the dominant side is committed to the agreement; the loser may or may not carry out the agreement.

Resolution   The stage of conflict that occurs when a mutually agreed-upon solution is arrived at and both parties commit themselves to carry out the agreement.

manager believes that the conflict will not decrease the efficiency of the department in the meantime.

If a nurse manager decides to intervene in a conflict between two or more parties, he or she can apply mediation techniques, deciding when, where, and how the intervention should take place. Routine problems can be handled in either the superior's or subordinate's office, but serious confrontations should take place in a neutral location unless the parties involved are of unequal power. In this case, the setting should favor the disadvantaged participant, thereby equalizing their power.

The place should be one where distractions will not interfere and adequate time is available. Because conflict management takes time, the manager must be prepared to allow sufficient time for all parties to explain their points of view and arrive at a mutually agreeable solution. A quick solution that inexperienced managers often resort to is to impose positional power, making a premature decision. This results in a win–lose outcome, which leads to feelings of elation and eventual complacency for the winners and loss of morale for the losers.

The following are basic rules on how to mediate a conflict between two or more parties:

1. Protect each party's self-respect. Deal with a conflict of issues, not personalities.
2. Do not put blame or responsibility for the problem on the participants. The participants are responsible for developing a solution to the problem.
3. Allow open and complete discussion of the problem from each participant.

MEDIALINK Strategies for Resolving Conflict

4. Maintain equity in the frequency and duration of each party's presentation. A person of higher status tends to speak more frequently and longer than a person of lower status. If this occurs, the mediator should intervene and ask the person of lower status for response and opinion.

5. Encourage full expression of positive and negative feelings in an accepting atmosphere. The novice mediator tends to discourage expressions of disagreement.

6. Make sure both parties listen actively to each other's words. One way to do this is to ask one person to summarize the comments of the other prior to stating her or his own.

7. Identify key themes in the discussion, and restate these at frequent intervals.

8. Encourage the parties to provide frequent feedback to each other's comments; each must truly understand the other's position.

9. Help the participants develop alternative solutions, select a mutually agreeable one, and develop a plan to carry it out. All parties must agree to the solution for successful resolution to occur.

10. At an agreed-upon interval, follow up on the progress of the plan.

11. Give positive feedback to participants regarding their cooperation in solving the conflict.

Conflict management is a difficult process, consuming both time and energy. Management and staff must be concerned and committed to resolving conflict by being willing to listen to others' positions and to find agreeable solutions.

Managing Conflict

Filley's Strategies   Filley (1975) identified three basic strategies for dealing with conflict according to the outcome: win–lose, lose–lose, and win–win. In the **win–lose strategy,** one party exerts dominance, usually by power of authority, and the other party submits and loses. Forcing, competing, and negotiation are techniques likely to lead to win–lose competition. Majority rule is another example of the win–lose outcome, especially within groups. It may be a satisfactory method of resolving conflict, however, if various factions vote differently on different issues and the group functions over time so that members win some and lose some. Win–lose outcomes often occur between groups. Frequent losing, however, can lead to the loss of cohesiveness within groups and diminish the authority of the group leader.

In the **lose–lose strategy,** neither side wins. The settlement reached is unsatisfactory to both sides. Avoiding, withdrawing, smoothing, and compromising may lead to lose–lose outcomes. One compromising strategy is to use a bribe to influence another's cooperation in doing something he or she dislikes. For example, the nurse manager may promise a future raise in an attempt to coerce a staff member to work an extra weekend. Using a third party as arbitrator can lead to a lose–lose outcome. Because an outsider may want to give something to each side, neither gets exactly what he or she desires, resulting in a lose–lose outcome. This is a common strategy in arbitration of labor–management disputes. Another strategy that may result in a lose–lose or win–lose outcome is resorting to rules. The outcome is determined by whatever the rules say, and confrontation is avoided.

The win–lose and lose–lose methods share some common characteristics:

1. The conflict is person-centered (we–they) rather than problem-centered. This is likely to occur when two cohesive groups that do not share common values or goals are in conflict.

2. Parties direct their energy toward total victory for themselves and total defeat for the other. This can cause long-term problems for the organization.

3. Each sees the issue from her or his own point of view rather than as a problem in need of a solution.

4. The emphasis is on outcomes rather than definition of goals, values, or objectives.

5. Conflicts are personalized.

6. Conflict-resolving activities are not differentiated from other group processes.

7. There is a short-run view of the conflict; the goal is to settle the immediate problem rather than resolve differences.

Win–win strategies focus on goals and attempt to meet the needs of both parties. Two specific win–win strategies are consensus and integrative decision making. **Consensus** involves attention to the facts and to the position of the other parties and avoidance of trading, voting, or averaging, where everyone loses something. The consensus decision is often superior to even the best individual one. This technique is most useful in a group setting because it is sensitive to the negative characteristics of win–lose and lose–lose outcomes. True consensus occurs when the problem is fully explored, the needs and goals of the involved parties are understood, and a solution that meets these needs is agreed upon.

Integrative decision making focuses on the means of solving a problem rather than the ends. They are most useful when the needs of the parties are polarized. Integrative decision making is a constructive process in which the parties jointly identify the problem and their needs. They explore a number of alternative solutions and come to consensus on a solution. The focus of this group activity is to solve the problem, not to force, dominate, suppress, or compromise. The group works toward a common goal in an atmosphere that encourages the free exchange of ideas and feelings. Using integrative decision-making methods, the parties jointly identify the value needs of each, conduct an exhaustive search for alternatives that could meet the needs of each, and then select the best alternative. Like the consensus methods, integrative decision making focuses on defeating the problem, not each other.

Other Conflict Management Strategies

Several other strategies can be used to manage conflict. Some tend to be more successful than others depending on the situation, those involved, and the organization.

Confrontation is considered the most effective means for resolving conflicts. This is a problem-oriented technique in which the conflict is brought out into the open and attempts are made to resolve it through knowledge and reason. The goal of this technique is to achieve win–win solutions. Facts should be used to identify the problem. The desired outcome should be explicit. "This is the third time this week that you have not been here for report. According to hospital policy, you are expected to be changed, scrubbed, and ready for report in the lounge at 7:00 A.M." is an example.

Confrontation is most effective when delivered in private as soon as possible after the incident occurs. Employee respect and manager credibility are two important considerations when a situation warrants confrontation. A more immediate confrontation also helps both the employee and manager sort out pertinent facts. In an emotionally charged situation, however, it may be best for the parties to wait. Regardless of timing, the message is usually more effective if the manager listens and is empathetic.

Many other techniques besides intervention can be used to resolve conflict and are consistent with the problem-solving approach. Some of these include changing or clarifying goals, making appeals to the hierarchy, providing cooling-off periods, using interme-

> ### KEY TERMS
>
> ***Win–lose strategy*** A strategy used during conflict in which one party exerts dominance and the other submits and loses.
>
> ***Lose–lose strategy*** A conflict strategy in which neither side wins; the settlement reached is unsatisfactory to both sides.
>
> ***Win–win strategy*** A conflict strategy that focuses on goals and attempts to meet the needs of both parties.
>
> ***Consensus*** A conflict strategy in which a solution that meets everyone's needs is agreed upon.
>
> ***Integrative decision making*** A conflict strategy that focuses on the means of solving a problem rather than the ends.
>
> ***Confrontation*** The most effective means of resolving conflict, in which the conflict is brought out in the open and attempts are made to resolve it through knowledge and reason.
>
> ***Negotiation*** A conflict management technique in which the conflicting parties give and take on various issues.

diaries, and dividing the resources so each party can partially achieve its goals.

Negotiation involves give-and-take on various issues among the parties. Its purpose is to achieve agreement even though consensus will never be reached. Therefore, the best solution is not often achieved. Negotiation often becomes a structured, formal procedure, as in collective bargaining (see Chapter 24). However, negotiation skills are important in arriving at an agreeable solution between any two parties. Staff learn to negotiate schedules, advanced practice nurses negotiate with third-party payers for reimbursement, insurance companies negotiate with vendors and hospitals for discounts, and clinic managers negotiate employment contracts with physicians. Although negotiation involves adept communication skills, its usefulness revolves around issues of conflict. Without differences in opinion, there would be no need for negotiation.

Levenstein (1984) lists ten commandments for negotiators:

1. Clarify the common purpose.
2. Keep the discussion relevant.

MediaLink Helping Skills

3. Get agreement on terminology.
4. Avoid abstract principles; concentrate on the facts.
5. Look for potential tradeoffs.
6. Listen.
7. Avoid debating tactics; use persuasive tactics.
8. Keep in mind the personal element.
9. Use logic logically.
10. Look for solutions that satisfy the other person's real interests.

Collaboration implies mutual attention to the problem, in which the talents of all parties are used. In collaboration, the focus is on solving the problem, not defeating the opponent. The goal is to satisfy both parties' concerns. Collaboration is useful in situations in which the goals of both parties are too important to be compromised.

Compromise is used to divide the rewards between both parties. Neither gets what she or he wants. Compromise can serve as a backup to resolve conflict when collaboration is ineffective. It is sometimes the only choice when opponents of equal power are in conflict over two or more mutually exclusive goals. Compromising also is expedient when a solution is needed rapidly.

Competing is an all-out effort to win, regardless of the cost. Competing may be needed in situations involving unpopular or critical decisions. Competing also is used in situations in which time does not allow for more cooperative techniques.

In **avoiding,** the participants never acknowledge that a conflict exists. Avoidance is the conflict resolution technique often used in highly cohesive groups. The group avoids disagreement because they do not want to do anything that may interfere with the good feelings they have for each other.

Accommodating is an unassertive, cooperative tactic used when individuals neglect their own concerns in favor of others' concerns. Accommodating frequently is used to preserve harmony when one person has a vested interest in an issue that is unimportant to the other party.

In situations where conflict is discouraged, suppression is often used. **Suppression** could even include the elimination of one of the conflicting parties through transfer or termination. Other, less effective techniques for managing conflict include withdrawing, smoothing, and forcing, although each mode of response is useful in given situations.

Withdrawal from the conflict simply removes at least one party, thereby making it impossible to resolve the situation. The issue remains unresolved, and feelings about the issue may resurface inappropriately.

Smoothing is accomplished by complimenting one's opponent, downplaying differences, and focusing on minor areas of agreement, as though little disagreement existed. Smoothing may be appropriate in dealing with minor problems, but in response to major problems, it produces the same results as withdrawing.

Forcing is a method that yields an immediate end to the conflict but leaves the cause of the conflict unresolved. A superior can resort to issuing orders, but the subordinate will lack commitment to the demanded action. Forcing may be appropriate in life-or-death situations but is otherwise inappropriate. Negotiation and confrontation are generally more effective modes of responding to conflict.

See how one nurse manager handled a conflict between two members of her staff in Case Study 9-1.

KEY TERMS

Collaboration   All parties work together to solve a problem.

Compromise   A conflict management technique in which the rewards are divided between both parties.

Competing   An all-out effort to win, regardless of the cost.

Avoiding   A conflict management technique in which the participants deny that conflict exists.

Accommodating   An unassertive, cooperative tactic used in conflict management when individuals neglect their own concerns in favor of others' concerns.

Suppression   A technique used to manage conflict in which one party is eliminated through transfer or termination.

Withdrawal   The removal of at least one party from the conflict, making it impossible to resolve the situation.

Smoothing   Managing conflict by complimenting one's opponent, downplaying differences, and focusing on minor areas of agreement.

Forcing   A conflict management technique that forces an immediate end to conflict but leaves the cause unresolved.

CASE STUDY 9-1: Conflict Management

Mai Tran is the nurse manager of a 20-bed medical–surgical unit in a large university hospital. Her nursing staff is diverse in experience and educational background. Working in a teaching hospital, Mai believes that nurses should be open to new methods and work processes, with an emphasis on evidenced-based practice.

Ken Robertson, RN, has worked for 2 years on the unit and is in his final semester of a master's program focusing on geriatric care. Eileen Holcomb, RN, has worked on the same unit for the past 28 years and was a graduate of the hospital's former diploma program. Ken recently completed a clinical rotation in dermatology and has worked with the skin care team at the hospital to develop new protocols for preventing skin breakdown. During a recent staff meeting, Ken presents the new protocols to the staff. Eileen makes several comments during the presentation that simply getting patients out of bed and making sure they have adequate nutrition is easier and less time consuming than the new protocol. "All these new protocols are just a way to justify all those credentials behind a name," Eileen says, gathering a chorus of chuckles from some of the older nurses on the staff. Ken glares at Eileen and responds, "As nurses become educated we need to reflect a professional practice." Mai notices that several staff members are uncomfortable as the meeting ends.

Ken and Eileen continue to exchange sarcastic comments and glares over the next two shifts. The obvious disagreement is affecting their co-workers and gossiping is decreasing productivity on the unit. Mai schedules individual meetings with Ken and Eileen to discuss their perspective. After reviewing the situation and determining that the issue is simply one of personality conflict, Mai brings Ken and Eileen together for a meeting in her office. Mai reviews the facts of the situation with them and shares her opinion that both have acted inappropriately and that their actions have affected not only their work, but that of the unit as a whole. She informs Ken and Eileen that they must act in a professional and respectful manner with each other or disciplinary action will be taken. She encourages to them to work out any future problems in a cooperative manner.

Manager's Checklist

The nurse manager is responsible for

- Understanding how to manage conflict among staff members in a timely manner,
- Understanding generational perceptions and how they impact group dynamics,
- Understanding when disciplinary action is necessary,
- Informing the human resource department of a potential personnel problem and the proposed solution,
- Meeting with staff to assist them in resolving conflict,
- Determining whether all staff should be educated on respect in the workplace, and
- Documenting interventions and outcomes as appropriate.

What You Know Now

- Conflict is a dynamic process, the consequence of real or perceived differences between individuals or groups.
- Conflict can be positive and the first step in initiating change.
- Antecedent conditions include incompatible goals, role conflicts, structural conflict, competition for scarce resources, and differences in values and beliefs.
- A number of strategies exist to handle conflict; choosing the best one to use is based on the situation and the people involved.
- Learning to manage conflict is a requirement for nurse managers.

Tools for Handling Conflict

1. Evaluate conflict situations to decide if and when to intervene.
2. Understand the antecedent conditions for the conflict and the positions of those involved.
3. Enlist others to help solve conflicts.
4. Select a conflict management strategy appropriate to the situation.
5. Practice the conflict management strategies discussed in the chapter and evaluate the outcomes.

Questions to Challenge You

1. How are conflicts handled at work or school? Are leaders good conflict managers? Use an example to explain.

2. Select a situation in which you have been involved in conflict. How did you handle your part in it? How about others involved? Did it turn out well? Explain.

3. What is the most difficult part of handling conflicts for you? Understanding others' positions? Devising a successful solution? Enlisting others' help? Encouraging participants to agree to a solution?

4. Study the chapter for help in improving your areas of weakness. Evaluate your performance.

Explore 🌐 MediaLink

NCLEX review questions, essay activities, group activities, and other interactive resources for this chapter can be found on the Web site at http://www.prenhall.com/sullivan-decker. Click on "Chapter 9" to select activities for this chapter.

References

Filley, A. C. (1975). *Interpersonal conflict resolution.* Glenview, IL: Scott, Foresman.

Levenstein, A. (1984). Negotiation vs. confrontation. *Nursing Management, 15*(1), 52–53.

McElhaney, R. (1996). Conflict management in nursing administration. *Nursing Management, 27*(3), 49–50.

Delegating Successfully

Looking Ahead

Delegation is the act of entrusting and empowering another with responsibility. It is a dynamic process that can often be difficult to learn but is an essential part of the nurse's job. Effective delegation is a tool that benefits both the individual and the organization. Chapter 10 outlines the process of delegation, dealing with both authority and acceptance, and the obstacles faced by those who delegate.

Objectives

In this chapter, you will learn

- How to differentiate delegation from work allocation.
- Why delegation involves responsibility, accountability and authority.
- How effective delegation benefits the patient, the staff and the organization.
- What the process of effective delegation is.
- What obstacles to effective delegation can emerge.

MediaLink 🌐 **www.prenhall.com/ sullivan-decker**

Additional resources for this chapter can be found on the Companion Website at www.prenhall.com/

MEDIALINK · Differentiating Responsibility, Accountability, and Authority

sullivan-decker. Click on "Chapter 10" to select the activities for this chapter.

- NCLEX Review
- Critical Thinking Activities
- Current Events
- MediaLinks
- *Nursing Leadership & Management in Action:* Differentiating Responsibility, Accountability, and Authority

Report is over. Where do you begin? Assessments. Patients to prepare for surgery. Medicines to give. Breakfast trays to deliver and set up. Baths to give. Treatments to do. An admission coming. Charting. Too much to do and so little time. Have you ever felt this way? How can you get it all done, be efficient, provide quality care, and survive the day? Delegate!

It is easy to say delegate, but delegation is a difficult leadership skill for nurses to learn and one that may not have been taught in undergraduate education. With changes in health care delivery, both new graduates and experienced nurses are struggling to develop their delegation skills. Managers also must continually improve their delegation skills to survive. Never before has delegation been as critical a skill for nurses to perfect as it is today, with the emphasis on doing more with less. This chapter describes the delegation process, the benefits and barriers to delegation, and tips on how to avoid ineffective delegation and liability.

Defining Delegation

What is delegation? **Delegation** is the process by which responsibility and authority for performing a task (function, activity, or decision) is transferred to another individual who accepts that authority and responsibility. Although the delegator remains accountable for the task, the delegate is also accountable to the delegator for the responsibilities assumed. Therefore, delegation is a dynamic process that involves responsibility, accountability, and authority. As a process, delegation empowers others and builds trust, enhances communication and leadership skills, and develops teamwork.

Delegation is also a tool. With effective delegation, a manager can accomplish more tasks, and productivity increases. Delegation can also be a tool to develop skills and abilities of others and to promote harmony in the organization.

To delegate efficiently, the nurse manager must realize that delegation is an art and, fortunately, a learnable skill. To perfect this skill, the manager must first appreciate what is and isn't delegation. The place to start is with a clear understanding of the underlying concepts of responsibility, accountability, and authority.

Responsibility and Accountability

Although *responsibility* and *accountability* are often used synonymously, the two words represent different concepts that go hand in hand. **Responsibility** denotes an obligation to accomplish a task, whereas **accountability** is accepting ownership for the results or lack thereof. In delegation, responsibility is transferred whereas accountability is shared.

The first principle to remember about delegation is *you can delegate only those tasks for which you are responsible.* If you have no direct responsibility for the task, then you can't delegate that task. For instance, if a manager is responsible for filling holes in the staffing schedule, the manager can delegate this responsibility to another individual. However, if staffing is the responsibility of a central coordinator, the manager can make suggestions or otherwise assist the staffing coordinator, but cannot delegate the task.

Likewise, if an orderly who is responsible for setting up traction is detained and a nurse asks a physical therapist on the unit to assist with traction, this is not delegation, because setting up traction is not the responsibility of the nurse. However, if the orderly (the person responsible for the task) had asked the physical therapist to help, this could be an act of delegation if the other principles of delegation are met.

To clearly understand who is responsible, it is important to look at practice acts, standards of care, job descriptions, and policy statements. The nurse practice acts in each state define the scope of nursing practice.

The National Council of State Boards of Nursing (1997) provides a decision-making tree shown in Figure 10-1.

These regulations, however, seldom provide a list of tasks that may or may not be delegated because nursing is a knowledge-based, not a task-based, discipline (Lindsay, 2003).

KEY TERMS

Delegation The process by which responsibility and authority are transferred to another individual.

Responsibility An obligation to accomplish a task.

Accountability The act of accepting ownership for the results or lack thereof.

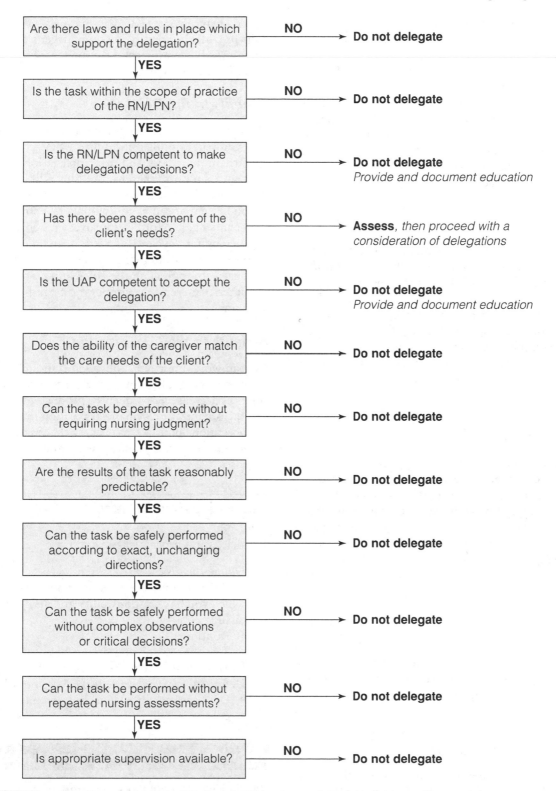

Figure 10-1 Delegation decision-making tree. Authority to delegate varies, so licensed nurses must check the jurisdiction's statutes and regulations. RNs may need to delegate to the LPN the authority to delegate to the UAP. Adapted from the Delegation Decision Tree developed by the Ohio Board of Nursing. *Note:* National Council of State Boards of Nursing (1997). Retrieved September 2003, from www.ncsbn.org.

Also, check professional standards. Several organizations have provided position statements regarding delegation. It is also important to be familiar with job descriptions and policy statements at your organization. What may have been allowed at one organization may not be permitted at another. It is also important to realize that an employer cannot decide what to delegate.

In reporting on a study of delegation in home care, Hirst and Foley (2001) suggest that specific tasks can be delegated but responsibility for the client remains with the case manager.

Authority

The second principle of delegation is that *along with responsibility, you must transfer authority.* **Authority** is the right to act. Therefore, by transferring authority, the delegator is empowering the delegate to accomplish the task. Too often this principle of delegation is neglected. Managers retain authority, crippling the delegate's abilities to accomplish the task, setting the individual up for failure, and minimizing efficiency and productivity. This pitfall is discussed later in the chapter.

Differentiating Delegation from Work Allocation

Delegation is often confused with work allocation. As previously discussed, delegation is a mutual transfer of responsibility and authority that occurs on the basis of competence and trust. In **work allocation,** no transfer of authority occurs. Instead, assignments are a bureaucratic function that reflect job descriptions and requirements.

Benefits of Delegation

Effective delegation benefits both the individual and the organization. Some of these benefits have been previously mentioned. This section describes the benefits to the manager, delegate, organization, and patient.

Benefits to the Manager

Delegation yields a number of personal benefits for the manager. First, the manager will be able to devote more time to those tasks that cannot be delegated. With more time available, the manager can develop new skills and abilities, facilitating the opportunity for career advancement. Having individuals with advanced skills provides continuity in the manager's absence and offers a ready replacement if the manager has an opportunity for advancement.

Benefits to the Delegate

The delegate also benefits from delegation. The delegate gains new skills and abilities that can facilitate upward mobility. In addition, delegation can bring trust and support, thereby building self-esteem and confidence. Subsequently, job satisfaction and motivation are enhanced as individuals feel stimulated by new challenges. Morale improves; a sense of pride and belonging develops as well as greater awareness of responsibility. Individuals feel more appreciated and learn to appreciate the roles and responsibilities of others, increasing cooperation and enhancing teamwork.

Benefits to the Organization

As teamwork improves, the organization benefits by achieving its goals more efficiently. Overtime and absences decrease. Subsequently, productivity increases, and the organization's financial position may improve. As delegation increases efficiency, the quality of care improves. As quality improves, patient satisfaction increases.

The Delegation Process

The delegation process has five steps:

1. *Define the task.*
    Delegate only an aspect of your own work for which you have responsibility and authority. These include:
    - Routine tasks
    - Tasks for which you do not have time
    - Tasks that have moved down in priority
    Define the aspects of the task. Ask yourself:
    - Does the task involve technical skills or cognitive abilities?

KEY TERMS

Authority   The right to act or empower.

Work allocation   The assignment of tasks that reflect job descriptions and requirements.

- Are specific qualifications necessary?
- Is performance restricted by practice acts, standards, or job descriptions?
- How complex is the task?
- Is training or education required?
- Are the steps well defined, or are creativity and problem solving required?
- Would a change in circumstances affect who could perform the task?

While you are trying to define the complexity of the task and its components, it is important not to fall into the trap of thinking no one else is capable of performing this task. Often others can be prepared to perform a task through education and training. The time taken to prepare others can be recouped many times over. Also know well the task to be delegated.

An alternative would be to subdivide the task into component parts and delegate the components congruent with the available delegate's capabilities. For example, developing a budget is a managerial responsibility that cannot be delegated, but someone else could explore the types of tympanic thermometers on the market, their costs, advantages, and so on. A committee of staff nurses could evaluate the options and make a recommendation that you could include in the budget justification.

But how do you know what should not be delegated? Before a task is delegated, two questions must be addressed. First, what areas of authority, or what resources, must the person control to achieve the expected results? Second, what are the limits, boundaries, or parameters for each area of authority or resource to be used? A unit manager who is responsible for maintaining adequate supplies needs budget authority. The authority to spend money on supplies, however, may be limited to a specific amount for specific supplies or may be allocated to supplies in general.

Certain tasks should never be delegated. Discipline should not be delegated nor should a highly technical task. Also any situation that involves confidentiality or controversy should not be delegated to others.

2. *Decide on delegate.*

Match the task to the individual. It is important to analyze individuals' skill levels and abilities to evaluate their capability to perform the various tasks; it is also important to determine characteristics that might prevent them from accepting responsibility for the task. Conversely experience and individual characteristics, such as initiative, intelligence, and enthusiasm, can expand the individual's capabilities. A rule of thumb is to delegate to the lowest person in the hierarchy who has the requisite capabilities and who is allowed to do the task legally and by organizational policy.

Next determine availability. For example, Su Ling might be the best candidate, but she leaves for vacation tomorrow and won't be back before the project is due. Then ask who would be willing to assume responsibility. Delegation is a contractual agreement that is entered into voluntarily.

3. *Determine the task.*

The next step in delegation is clearly defining your expectations for the delegate. Communication should be clear and complete. Plan your meeting with the delegate. Attempting to delegate in the middle of a crisis is not delegation; that is directing. Provide for enough time to describe the task and your expectations and to entertain questions. Also, meet in an environment as devoid of distractions as possible.

Key behaviors in delegating tasks are:

a. Describe the task using "I" statements, such as "I would like . . . " and appropriate nonverbal behaviors—open body language, face-to-face positioning, and eye contact. The delegate needs to know what is expected, when the task should be completed and where and how, if that is appropriate. The more experienced delegates may be able to define for themselves the where and how. Decide whether written reports are necessary or if brief oral reports are sufficient. If written reports are required, indicate whether tables, charts, or other graphics are necessary. Be specific about reporting times. Identify critical events or milestones that might be reached and brought to your attention.

b. Provide the delegate with a reason for the task. Describe the importance to the organization, you, the patient, and the delegate. Provide the delegate with an incentive for accepting both the responsibility and the authority to do the task.

c. Inform the delegate by what standard the task will be evaluated and how often. Clearly describe the expected outcome and the timeline for completion. Establish how closely the assignment will be supervised. Monitoring is important because you remain accountable for the task, but controls should never limit an individual's opportunity to grow.

d. Identify any constraints for completing the task as well as risks. Also identify any situational variables by which authority and responsibility for the task will change. For example, you may ask an assistant to feed a patient for you as long as the patient is coherent and awake, but you would feed the patient if he were confused.

e. Validate understanding of the task and your expectations by eliciting questions and providing feedback.

4. *Reach agreement.*

Once you have outlined your expectations, you must be sure that the delegate agrees to accept responsibility and authority for the task. You need to be prepared to equip the delegate to complete the task successfully. This might mean providing additional information or resources or informing others about the arrangement as needed to empower the delegate. Before meeting with the individual, anticipate areas of negotiation, and identify what you are prepared and able to provide.

5. *Monitor performance and provide feedback.*

Monitoring performance provides a mechanism for feedback and control that ensures that the delegated tasks are carried out as agreed. Give careful thought to monitoring efforts when objectives are established. When defining the task and expectations, clearly establish the where, when, and how. Remain accessible. Support builds confidence and reassures the delegate of your interest in the delegate and negates any concerns about dumping undesirable tasks.

Monitoring the delegate too closely, however, conveys distrust. Analyze performance with respect to the established goal. If problem areas are identified, privately investigate and explain the problem, provide an opportunity for feedback, and inform the individual how to correct the mistake in the future. Provide additional support as needed. Also, be sure to give the praise and recognition due, and don't be afraid to do so publicly.

See how a school nurse handled delegation in Case Study 10-1.

CASE STUDY 10-1: Delegation

Lisa Ford is a school nurse for a suburban school district. She has responsibility for three school buildings, including a middle school, a high school and vocational rehabilitation workshop for mentally and physically handicapped secondary students. Her management responsibilities include providing health services for 1,000 students, 60 faculty members, and 25 staff members and supervising 2 unlicensed school health aides and 3 special education health aides. The logistics of managing multiple school sites results in the delegation of many daily health room tasks, including medication administration, to the school-based health aides.

Nancy Andrews is an unlicensed health aide at the middle school. This is her first year as a health aide and she has a limited background in health care. The nurse practice act in the state allows for the delegation of medication administration in the school setting. Lisa is responsible for training Nancy to safely administer medication to students, documenting the training, evaluating Nancy's performance, and providing ongoing supervision. Part of Nancy's training will also include a discussion of those medication-related decisions that must be made by a registered nurse.

Manager's Checklist

The nurse manger is responsible for

- Understanding the state nurse practice act and its applicability to the school setting,

- Implementing school district policies related to health services and medication administration,

- Developing and implementing an appropriate training program,

- Limiting opportunities for error and decreasing liability by ensuring that unlicensed health aides are appropriately trained to handle delegated tasks,

- Maintaining documentation related to training and observation of medication administration by unlicensed staff,

- Auditing medication administration records to ensure accuracy and completeness,

- Conducting several "drop in" visits during the school year to track competency of health aides, and

- If necessary, reporting any medication errors to administration and following up with focused training and closer supervision.

Accepting Delegation

When you accept delegation, it is important to understand what is being asked of you. First, acknowledge the delegator's confidence in you, but realistically examine whether you have the skills and abilities for the task and the time to do it. If you do not have the requisite skills, it is your responsibility to inform the delegator. However, it does not mean you cannot accept the responsibility. See whether the person is willing to train or otherwise equip you to accomplish the task. If not, then you need to refuse the offer.

Accepting delegation means that you accept full responsibility for the outcome and its benefits or liabilities. Just as the delegator has the option to delegate parts of a task, you also have the option to negotiate for those aspects of a task you feel you can accomplish. Recognize, however, that this may be an opportunity for growth. You may decide to capitalize on it, obtaining new skills or resources in the process.

Once you agree on the role and responsibilities you are to assume, make sure you are clear on the time frame, feedback mechanisms, and other expectations. Don't assume anything. As a minimum, repeat to the delegator what you heard said; better yet, outline the task in writing.

Throughout the project, keep the delegator informed. Explore any concerns you have as they come up. Foremost, complete the task as agreed. Successful completion can open more doors in the future.

In the event you are not qualified or do not have the time, do not be afraid to say no. Thank the delegator for the offer and clearly explain why you must decline at this time. Express your interest in working together in the future.

Obstacles to Delegation

Although delegation can yield many benefits, there are potential barriers. Some barriers are environmental; others are the result of the delegator's or delegate's beliefs or inexperience. Table 10-1 summarizes potential obstacles to delegation.

A Nonsupportive Environment

Environments both within and external to the organization may present obstacles to delegation. As described earlier, state practice acts may limit what can be delegated and to whom. Professional standards, job descriptions, and policy statements also may impose limitations. In a study by Thomas and Hume (1998) new graduates identified support from members of the health care team, especially supervisors, as contributing to successful delegation.

Organizational Culture The culture within the organization may restrict delegation. Hierarchies, management styles, and norms may all preclude delegation. Rigid chains of command and autocratic leadership

Table 10-1 Potential Obstacles to Delegation

Environmental	Delegator	Delegate
Practice acts	Lack of trust and confidence	Inexperience
Standards	Believe others incapable	Fear of failure and reprisal
Job descriptions	Believe self indispensable	Lack of confidence
Policies	Fear of competition	Overdependence on others
Organizational structure	Fear of criticism	Avoidance of responsibility
Management styles	Fear of liability	
Norms	Fear of blame for others' mistakes	
Resources	Fear of loss of control	
	Fear of overburdening	
	Fear of decreased job satisfaction	
	Insecurity	
	Inexperience in delegation	
	Inadequate organizational skills	

Reprinted with permission from "Delegation: How to deliver care through others," R. Hansten and M. Washburn, 1992, *American Journal of Nursing*, 92(3), pp. 87–88.

styles do not facilitate delegation and rarely provide good role models. The norm is to do the work oneself because others are not capable or skilled. An atmosphere of distrust prevails as well as a poor tolerance for mistakes. Additional environmental factors include a norm of crisis management and poorly defined job descriptions or chains of command.

Personal Qualities   Poor communication and interpersonal skills can also be a barrier to delegation. Thomas and Hume (1998) note that in addition to good communication skills and respecting and treating staff fairly, a willingness to work with the other, to be open to suggestions, to provide feedback and acknowledgment for work well done is essential. They also note that delegates must be reliable and willing to follow instructions.

Resources   Another difficulty frequently encountered is a lack of resources. For example, there may be no one to whom you can delegate. Consider the sole registered nurse in a skilled nursing facility. If practice acts define a task as one that only a registered nurse can perform, there is no one else to whom that nurse can delegate that task.

Another limiting factor may be finances. For instance, someone from your department must attend the annual conference in your nursing specialty area. However, the organization will only pay the manager's travel and conference expenses, which precludes anyone else from attending.

Educational resources may be another limiting factor. Perhaps others could learn how to do a task if they could practice with the equipment, but the equipment is not available.

Time can also be a limiting factor. For example, it is Friday and the schedule needs to be posted Monday. No one on your staff has experience developing schedules and you need to go out of town for a family emergency, so there is no one else to do the schedule.

An Insecure Delegator

The majority of the barriers to delegation arise from the delegator. Three conflicts have been identified by del Bueno (1993):

1. Trust versus control
2. Approval versus affiliation
3. Democratic ideal versus the classical hierarchy

Trust is paramount to delegation, but to trust another individual means to give up some control. Everyone has the need for both approval and affiliation, but which is more important—the need to be liked, or the need to belong and be accepted? Which is more valued—teamwork and empowerment, or control and the established hierarchy? These are difficult to address.

Hansten and Washburn (1992) have developed a simple quiz, found in Box 10-1, to help identify your readiness to delegate.

Commonly voiced concerns about delegation are:

- "I can do it better."
- "I can do it faster."
- "I'd rather do it myself."
- "I don't have time to delegate."

Often underlying these statements are erroneous beliefs, fears, and inexperience in delegation. As previously indicated, a delegator should delegate those things that the delegator can do well. Therefore, there is a degree of truth in the first three statements; however, one of the roles of a manager is to develop staff. Hence, by failing to delegate, the manager is shirking this responsibility.

Delegation does take time, but failing to delegate is a time waster. Time invested in developing staff today is later repaid many times over.

Additional problems are inherent in the two statements, "I can do it better" and "I can do it faster." These statements suggest a lack of trust and confidence in the staff. The manager also sends the message that the staff is incapable, whereas the manager is indispensable. Both are erroneous. In the process, the staff is demoralized, and the manager loses respect. More often than not, these statements are smokescreens for the delegator's own fears and weaknesses.

Common fears are:

- *Fear of competition or criticism.* What if someone else can do the job better or faster than I? Will I lose my job? Be demoted? What will others think? Will I lose respect and control? This fear is unfounded if the delegator has selected the right task and matched it with the right individual. In fact, the delegate's success in the task provides evidence of the delegator's leadership and decision-making abilities.
- *Fear of liability.* Some individuals are not risk takers and shy away from delegation for this reason. There are risks associated with delegation, but the delegator can minimize these risks by following the steps of delegation, as previously described. More about risks is discussed in the section on liability later in the chapter. A related concern is a fear of being blamed for the delegate's mistakes. If the delegator used prudence in selecting the task and delegate, then the responsibility for any mistakes made are

Box 10-1 Delegation Assessment

1. Mr. Jones, a bedridden but stable patient, needs a complete bed bath. You
   a. Assign the task to the nurse assistant.
   b. Work together with the nursing assistant to give the bath.
   c. Do the job yourself because Mr. Jones is a VIP and you know you'll do the best job.

2. You are the charge nurse, and one of your team members is a float nurse who has never worked on the unit before. You
   a. Spend 15 minutes with her assessing her abilities and providing a brief orientation to the unit so that she can take the full assignment.
   b. Give her three of the "easiest patients" and pick up the rest of the assignment yourself.
   c. Call the supervisor and tell her that you have no time to orient someone and the float will be more trouble than she's worth.

3. Another new admission is arriving on your unit. You
   a. Assign the patient to the LPN, recognizing that one of the registered nurses will be overseeing and completing the admission assessment.
   b. Ask the nursing assistant to get the vital signs, and you complete the admission before assigning the patient to another RN.
   c. Take the admission yourself because everyone else seems too busy.

4. You and a nursing assistant are assigned to 10 patients on a medical surgical floor. You
   a. Spend 15 minutes making walking rounds with the nursing assistant, then decide how to distribute patient care tasks.
   b. Assign tasks according to the assignment board from yesterday.

   c. Send the nursing assistant to take vital signs without further information or communication.

5. You are uncertain about a nursing assistant's skill in giving a cleansing enema. You
   a. Review the hospital procedure with the nursing assistant and observe him performing the task so that next time he can do it alone.
   b. Give the enema yourself today, promising that the next time you'll teach the nursing assistant.
   c. You never assign him to give an enema.

6. Your manager tells you that the care delivery system on your unit is changing and you'll need to use assistive personnel. You
   a. Welcome the opportunity to free up some of your time to do more of your professional duties.
   b. Keep an open mind and wait to review the job description of the new assistants.
   c. Take a wait-and-see attitude, but if it doesn't work out in the next two weeks, you'll apply to another hospital in town where you can still be a "real nurse."

If you answered mostly "a"s, congratulations! You have overcome many of the typical barriers to delegation. You can be a mentor to your co-workers who are learning the skill.

If you answered mostly "b"s, you are on the way to overcoming your personal barriers to delegation. Keep an open mind and read on.

If you answered mostly "c"s, oops! You have strong objections to sharing your work load with others. Read on. Learning this skill and applying it will enhance your daily work life.

Reprinted with permission from "Delegation: How to deliver care through others," R. Hansten and M. Washburn, 1992, *American Journal of Nursing*, 92(3), pp. 87–88.

solely those of the delegate; it is not necessary to take on guilt for another's mistakes. To help keep this issue in perspective, it is important to recall the benefits of delegation and balance the rewards with the risks while making the delegation decision.

- *Fear of loss of control.* Will I be kept informed? Will the job be done right? How can I be sure? The more one is insecure and inexperienced in delegation, the more this fear is an issue. This is also a predominant concern in individuals who tend

toward autocratic styles of leadership and perfectionism. The key to retaining control is to clearly identify the task and expectations and then to monitor progress and provide feedback.

- *Fear of overburdening others.* They already have so much to do; how can I suggest more? Everyone has work to do. Such a statement belittles the decisional capabilities of others. Recall that delegation is a voluntary, contractual agreement; acceptance of a delegated task indicates the availability and willingness of the delegate to perform the task. Often, the delegate welcomes the diversion and stimulation, and what the delegator perceives as a burden is actually a blessing. The onus is on the delegator to select the right person for the right reason.

- *Fear of decreased personal job satisfaction.* Because the type of tasks recommended to delegate are those that are familiar and routine, the delegator's job satisfaction should actually increase with the opportunity to explore new challenges and obtain other skills and abilities.

Additional hindrances to delegation include inadequate organizational skills, such as poor time management, and inexperience in delegation.

An Unwilling Delegate

Inexperience and fear of failure can motivate a potential delegate to refuse to accept a delegated task. Much reassurance and support are needed. In addition, the delegate should be equipped to handle the task. If proper selection criteria are used and the steps of delegation followed, then the delegate should not fail. The delegator can boost the delegate's lack of confidence by building on simple tasks. The delegate needs to be reminded that everyone was inexperienced at one time. Another common concern is how mistakes will be handled. When describing the task, the delegator should provide clear guidelines for handling problems, guidelines that adhere to organizational policies.

Another barrier is the individual who avoids responsibility or is overdependent on others. Success breeds success; therefore, it is important to use an enticing incentive to engage the individual in a simple task that guarantees success.

Ineffective Delegation

When the steps of delegation are not followed or barriers remain unresolved, delegation is often ineffective. Inefficient delegation can result from unnecessary duplication, underdelegation, reverse delegation, and overdelegation.

Unnecessary Duplication

If staff are duplicating the work of others, the manager may have given related tasks to too many people (Barter, 2002). To avoid unnecessary duplication, try to delegate associated tasks to as few people as possible. This allows the person to complete the assignment without spending time negotiating with others about which task should be done by which person. Also reporting is simplified for both the employee and the manager.

To prevent work duplication, Barter (2002, p. 57) suggests that you ask:

- How often does staff duplicate an activity that someone else has recently performed?
- Why does this duplication occur and is it necessary?
- How could managers delegate to prevent duplication?

Underdelegation

Underdelegation occurs when

- The delegator fails to transfer full authority to the delegate,
- The delegator takes back responsibility for aspects of the task, or
- The delegator fails to equip and direct the delegate.

As a result, the delegate is unable to complete the task, and the delegator must resume responsibility for its completion.

Reverse Delegation

In **reverse delegation,** someone with a lower rank delegates to someone with more authority. Consider Celina, a staff nurse who says to her nurse manager, "I'm really swamped today. Can you hang Mr. Morino's chemo so I can go to lunch?" Though the manager could assist Celina, this is not an efficient use of her time. Instead, the manager could help Celina organize her own time and efficiently delegate some responsibilities.

Overdelegation

Overdelegation occurs when the delegator loses control over a situation by providing the delegate with too much authority or too much responsibility. This places the delegator in a risky position, increasing the potential for liability.

Liability and Delegation

The National Council of State Boards of Nursing (1995) suggests five rights of delegation:

- Right task
- Right circumstances
- Right person

- Right direction and communication
- Right supervision

The nurse is responsible for exercising informed judgment and basing the decision to delegate on the individual's competencies and qualifications, according to the American Nurses Association (2001) Code of Ethics for Nurses. Failure to do so constitutes negligence. Therefore, it is imperative that the right task be given to the right person. This means that the delegator must follow the steps of delegation in defining the task and determining who can and should perform the task.

The delegator needs to be delegating for the right reasons; that is, not to gain personal prestige or dump undesirable tasks, but to accomplish the goals of the organization more efficiently. In addition, the delegator needs to ensure that the task is being completed correctly and that clear guidelines and parameters for the task have been given. If these considerations are included in the steps of delegating, then the risks should be acceptable and liabilities minimal.

Delegation is a skill that can be learned, but not easily (Jones, 2003). Like other skills, delegating successfully requires practice. Sometimes it seems it might be easier to do it yourself. But it is not. Once you learn how to delegate, you will extend your ability to accomplish more by using others' help. No one in health care today can afford to fail to delegate.

What You Know Now

- Delegation is a contractual agreement in which authority and responsibility for a task is transferred by the person accountable for the task to another individual.

- Delegation involves skill in identifying and determining the task and level of responsibility, determining who has the requisite skills and abilities, describing expectations clearly, reaching mutual agreement, and monitoring performance and providing feedback.
- Delegatable tasks are personal, routine tasks that the delegator can perform well; that do not involve discipline, highly technical tasks, or confidential information; and that are not controversial.
- Delegation benefits the manager, delegate, organization, and patients.
- Various organizational, delegator, and delegate barriers can prevent effective delegation.
- Ineffective delegation usually results from inadequate or inappropriate transference of authority or responsibility.
- Adhering to the steps of delegation—in particular, prudently selecting a qualified person as delegate and providing appropriate supervision—minimizes the risk of liability.
- All managers must learn to delegate in order to be successful in their positions.

Tools for Delegating Successfully

1. Delegate only tasks for which you have responsibility.
2. Transfer authority when you delegate responsibility.
3. Be sure you follow state regulations, job descriptions, and agency policies when delegating.
4. Follow the delegation process and key behaviors for delegating described in the chapter.
5. Accept delegation when you are clear about the task, time frame, reporting, and other expectations.
6. Confront your fears about delegation; recognize those that are realistic and those that are not.

Questions to Challenge You

1. Review your state's nurse practice act. How is delegation defined? What tasks can and cannot be delegated? How is supervision defined? Are there any other guidelines for supervision? Are responsibilities regarding advanced practice delineated? How does the scope of practice differ between registered and licensed practical/vocational nurses? What is the scope of practice of other health care providers?
2. What are your agency's policies on delegation?
3. Describe a situation when you delegated a task to someone else. Did you follow the steps of delegation

explained in the chapter? Was the outcome positive? If not, what went wrong?

4. Describe a situation when someone else delegated a task to you. Did your delegator explain what to do? Did you receive too much information? Not enough? Was supervision appropriate to the task and to your abilities? What was the outcome?

5. How did you score on the delegation assessment shown in Box 10-1? What did you learn about how to improve your delegation skills?

Explore ⊕ MediaLink

NCLEX review questions, essay activities, group activities, and other interactive resources for this chapter can be found on the Web site at http://www.prenhall.com/sullivan-decker. Click on "Chapter 10" to select activities for this chapter.

References

American Nurses Association (ANA). (1985). *Code of ethics for nurses.* Washington, DC: Author.

Barter, M. (2002). Follow the team leader. *Nursing Management, 33*(10), 54–57.

del Bueno, D. J. (1993). Delegation and the dilemma of the democratic ideal. *Journal of Nursing Administration, 23*(3), 20–21, 25.

Hansten, R., & Washburn, M. (1992). Delegation: How to deliver care through others. *American Journal of Nursing, 92*(3), 87–90.

Hirst, S. P., & Foley, L. (2001). Delegation: The views of case managers. *Home Health Care Management & Practice, 13*(4), 301–307.

Jones, R. (2003). Perspectives in leadership: The art of delegation. *Nursing Spectrum, 13*(6), 7.

Lindsay, C. (2003). Decoding delegation. *Nursing Spectrum, 4*(1), 20.

National Council of State Boards of Nursing. (1995). Delegation: Concepts and decision-making process. Retrieved July 28, 2003, from www.ncsbn.org

National Council of State Boards of Nursing. (1997). Delegation decision-making tree. Retrieved July 28, 2003, from www.ncsbn.org

Thomas, S., & Hume, G. (1998). Delegation competencies: Beginning practitioners' reflections. Nurse Educator, 23(1), 38–41.

Building and Managing Teams

Looking Ahead

What distinguishes a group from a team? To understand the concept more clearly, think about an orchestra. The very first day the musicians come together, they are a group of people, each with individual skills and knowledge. The conductor, their leader, gives them a framework: the music. To achieve their goal, creating music, the musicians must learn to cooperate and rely on each other as a team. The orchestra analogy is not unlike nursing, a team-oriented profession with many different types of players. This chapter looks at the different types of groups and group dynamics and offers strategies that nurses and nurse managers can employ to develop teams within the work environment.

Objectives

In this chapter, you will learn

- How to differentiate groups from teams.
- What the characteristics of different types of groups are.
- How groups form, function, and end.
- Why the nurse manager is a team leader.
- How to manage groups, task forces, and patient care conferences.

MediaLink 🌐 **www.prenhall.com/sullivan-decker**

Additional resources for this chapter can be found on the Companion Website at www.prenhall.com/sullivan-decker. Click on "Chapter 11" to select the activities for this chapter.

- NCLEX Review
- Critical Thinking Activities
- Current Events
- MediaLinks
- *Nursing Leadership & Management in Action:* Identifying Stages of Group Development; Differentiating Roles People Assume in Groups

Most often, nursing occurs in a team environment. Work groups that share common objectives function in a harmonious, coordinated, purposeful manner as teams. High-performance teams require expert nurse manager leadership skills. In a health care delivery system integrated across settings, a team environment becomes increasingly essential. Nurse managers must skillfully orchestrate the activity and interactions of interdisciplinary teams as well as conventional nursing work groups. Understanding the nature of groups and how groups are transformed into teams is essential to the nurse manager's effectiveness.

Unfortunately, research indicates that many managers experience considerable difficulty in transforming work groups into effective teams. Some managers lack the planning and organizing skills needed to facilitate work group performance. The manager may not know how to work with group members to identify goals, tasks, and practical work plans.

Managers also may lack skills in conflict management. Although conflict within any work group is inevitable, the manner in which conflict is managed depends on the manager's skill in assisting co-workers to sort out personal differences and to improve their understanding and acceptance of differing views and styles.

In addition, some managers have difficulty managing their own interpersonal relationships with group members. They may play favorites, ignore reticent members, give up including the withdrawn individual, or allow animosity to develop with an individual or a subgroup. Achieving balanced relationships with even the most difficult members is part of successful management and is essential to the work group's function. Close teamwork is difficult to achieve when managers lack group planning and organizing skills, do not know how to manage conflict, or cannot maintain healthy interpersonal relationships with group members.

Because staff nurses work in close proximity and frequently depend on each other to perform their work,

the quality of group leadership and interaction is vital. A positive climate is one in which there is mutual high regard and in which group members safely may discuss work-related concerns, critique and offer suggestions about clinical practice, and comfortably experiment with new behaviors. Maintaining a positive work group climate and building a team is a complex and demanding leadership task.

Differentiating Groups from Teams

A **group** is an aggregate of individuals who interact and mutually influence each other. Both formal and informal groups exist in organizations. **Formal groups** are clusters of individuals designated temporarily or permanently by an organization to perform specified organizational tasks. Formal groups may be structured laterally, vertically, or diagonally. Task groups, teams, task forces, and committees may be structured in all of these ways, whereas command groups generally are structured vertically.

Group members include

- Individuals from a single work group or individuals at similar job levels from more than one work group,
- Individuals from different job levels, or
- Individuals from different work groups and different job levels in the organization.

Groups may be permanent or temporary. Command groups, teams, and committees usually are permanent, whereas task groups and task forces are often temporary.

Informal groups evolve naturally from social interactions. Groups are informal in the sense that they are not defined by an organizational structure. Examples of informal groups include individuals who regularly eat lunch together or who convene spontaneously to discuss a clinical dilemma.

Real (command) groups accomplish tasks in organizations and are recognized as a legitimate organizational entity. Its members are interdependent, share a set of norms, generally differentiate roles and duties among themselves, are organized to achieve ongoing organizational goals, and are collectively held responsible for measurable outcomes. The group's manager has line authority in relation to group members individually and collectively. The group's assignments are usually routine and designed to fulfill the specific mission of the agency or organization. The regularly assigned staff who work together under the direction of a single manager constitute a command group.

A **task group** is composed of several persons who work together, with or without a designated leader, and are charged with accomplishing specific time-limited assignments. A group of nurses selected by their colleagues to plan an orientation program for new staff constitute a task group. Usually, several task groups exist within a service area and may include representatives from several disciplines (e.g., nurse, physician, dietitian, social worker).

Other special groups include **committees or task forces** formed to deal with specific issues involving several service areas. A committee responsible for monitoring and improving patient safety or a task force assigned to develop procedures to adhere to patient privacy regulations are examples of special work groups. Health care organizations depend on numerous committees, which nurses participate in and often lead. Some of these committees are mandated by accrediting and regulatory bodies, such as committees for education, standards, disaster, and patient care evaluation. Others are established to meet a specific need (e.g., to formulate a new policy on substance abuse).

Teams are real groups in which individuals must work cooperatively with each other in order to achieve some overarching goal. They demonstrate healthy interdependence. According to Katzenbach and Smith (1993), a team is composed of "a small number of people with complementary skills who are committed to a common purpose, set of performance goals, and approach for which they hold themselves mutually accountable" (p. 112).

Teams have command or line authority to perform tasks, and membership is based on the specific skills required to accomplish the tasks. Similar to groups described above, teams may include individuals from a single work group or individuals at similar job levels from more than one work group, individuals from different job levels, or individuals from different work groups and different job levels in the organization. They may have a short life span or exist indefinitely.

Not all work groups, however, are teams. For example, groups of individuals who perform their tasks independently of each other are not teams. **Competing groups,** in which members compete with each other for resources to perform their tasks or compete for recognition, also are not teams.

A work group becomes a team when the individuals must apply group process skills to achieve specific results. They must exchange ideas, coordinate work activities, and develop an understanding of other team members' roles in order to perform effectively. Members appreciate the talents and contributions of each individual on the team and find ways to capitalize on them. Most work teams have a leader who maintains the integrity of the team's function and guides the team's activities, performance, and development. Teams may be self-directed, that is, led jointly by group members who decide together about work objectives and activities on an ongoing basis.

In a given service area, the entire staff might not function as a team, but a subgroup may. For example, case managers for the inpatient and ambulatory cystic fibrosis population in a children's medical center might be called a team. Individual members of an interdisciplinary team, such as this one, may report formally to different managers, but in delivering care to the cystic fibrosis population there is no designated individual in charge. In meetings, the team members discuss clients' problems and jointly decide on plans of action.

Many different types of groups and teams are used throughout the organization. Examples are ad hoc task groups, quality improvement teams, quality circles, self-directed work teams, councils, and focus groups.

KEY TERMS

Group   An aggregate of individuals who interact and mutually influence each other.

Formal groups   Clusters of individuals designated by an organization to perform specified organizational tasks.

Informal groups   Groups that evolve from social interactions that are not defined by an organizational structure.

Real (command) groups   Groups that accomplish tasks in an organization and are recognized as legitimate organizational entities.

Task group   Several individuals who work together to accomplish specific time-limited assignments.

Committees or task forces   Groups that deal with specific issues involving several service areas.

Teams   Real groups in which people work cooperatively with each other in order to achieve some goal.

Competing groups   Groups in which members compete for resources or recognition.

Most groups are considered **ordinary interacting groups.** These groups usually have a designated formal leader, but they may be leaderless. Most work teams, task groups, and committees are ordinary interacting groups. Discussions usually begin with a statement of the problem by the group leader followed by an open, unstructured conversation. Normally, the final decision is made by consensus (without formal voting; members indicate concurrence with a group agreement that everyone can live with and support publicly). The decision also may be made by the leader or someone in authority, majority vote, an average of members' opinions, minority control, or an expert member. Interacting groups enhance the cohesiveness and esprit de corps among group members. Participants are able to build strong social ties and will be committed to the solution decided on by the group.

Ordinary interacting groups often are dominated by one or a few members. If the group is highly cohesive, its decision-making ability may be affected by "groupthink." Members may spend excessive time dealing with socioemotional relationships, reducing the time spent on the problem and slowing consensus. Ordinary groups may reach compromise decisions that may not really satisfy any of the participants. Because of these problems, the functioning of ordinary groups is very dependent on the leader's skills. (See Chapter 7 for more about groupthink.)

Each type of group presents the nurse manager with unique opportunities and challenges. An important role of the nurse manager is to link service areas with groups at higher levels in the organization. This link facilitates problem solving, coordination, and communication throughout the organization. Leadership roles in work groups are important and also may be either formal or informal. For example, the nurse manager formally leads the unit or service area staff but may also informally lead a support group of nurse managers.

The leader's influence on group processes, formal or informal, and the ability of the group to work together as a team often determines whether the group accomplishes its goals. Nurse managers may effectively manage work groups and turn them into teams by understanding principles of group processes and applying them to group decision making, team building, and leading committees and task forces.

Group and Team Processes

The modified version of Homans' (1950, 1961) social system conceptual scheme presented in Figure 11-1 provides a framework for understanding group inputs,

processes, and outcomes. The schematic depicts the effects of organizational and individual background factors on group leadership, including dynamics (tasks, activities, interactions, attitudes) and processes (forming, storming, norming, performing, adjourning). Elements of the required group system and processes influence each other and the emergent group system and social structure.

This system determines the productivity of the group as well as members' quality of work life, such as job satisfaction, development, growth, and similarity in thinking. The framework distinguishes required factors that are imposed by the external system from factors that emerge from the internal dynamics of the group.

According to Homans' framework, the three essential elements of a group system are activities, interactions, and attitudes. Activities are the observable behaviors of group members. Interactions are the verbal or nonverbal exchanges of words or objects among two or more group members. Attitudes are the perceptions, feelings, and values held by individual group members, which may be both positive and negative. To understand and guide group functioning, a manager should analyze the activities, interactions, and attitudes of work group members.

Homans' framework indicates that background factors, the manager's leadership style, and the organiza-

---

KEY TERMS

Ordinary interacting groups Common types of groups; generally have formal leader and are run according to an informal structure with the purpose of solving a problem or making a decision.

Forming The initial stage of group development, in which individuals assemble into a well-defined cluster.

Storming The second stage of group development, in which group members develop roles and relationships; competition and conflict generally occur.

Norming The third stage of group development, in which group members define goals and rules of behavior.

Performing The fourth stage of group development, in which group members agree on basic purposes and activities and carry out the work.

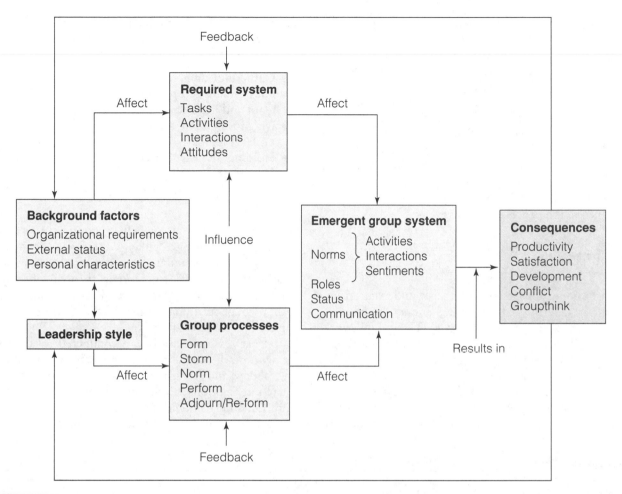

Figure 11-1   **Conceptual scheme of a basic social system. Adapted from *The Human Group* by G. Homans, 1950, New York: Harcourt Brace Jovanovich; and *Social Behavior: Its Elementary Forms* by G. Homans, 1961, New York: Harcourt Brace. By permission of Transaction Publishers.**

tional system influence the normal development of the group. Groups, whether formal or informal, typically develop in the phases: form, storm, norm, perform, and adjourn or reform. In the initial stage, **forming,** individuals assemble into a well-defined cluster. Group members are cautious in approaching each other as they come together as a group and begin to understand requirements of group membership. At this stage, the members often depend on a leader to define purpose, tasks, and roles.

As the group begins to develop, **storming** occurs. Members wrestle with roles and relationships. Conflict, dissatisfaction, and competition arise on important issues related to procedures and behavior. During this stage, members often compete for power and status, and informal leadership emerges. During the storming

stage, the leader helps the group to acknowledge the conflict and to resolve it in a win–win manner.

In the third stage, **norming,** the group defines its goals and rules of behavior. The group determines what are or are not acceptable behaviors and attitudes. The group structure, roles, and relationships become clearer. Cohesiveness develops. The leader explains standards of performance and behavior, defines the group's structure, and facilitates relationship building.

In the fourth stage, **performing,** members agree on basic purposes and activities and carry out the work. The group's energy becomes task-oriented. Cooperation improves, and emotional issues subside. Members communicate effectively and interact in a relaxed atmosphere of sharing. The leader provides feedback on the quality and quantity of work, praises achievement, critiques poor work and takes steps to improve it, and reinforces interpersonal relationships within the group.

The fifth stage is either **adjourning** (the group dissolves after achieving its objectives) or **re-forming**, when some major change takes place in the environment or in the composition or goals of the group that requires the group to refocus its activities and recycle through the four stages. When a group adjourns, the leader must prepare group members for dissolution and facilitate closure through celebration of success and leave-taking. If the group is to refocus its activities, the leader will explain the new direction and provide guidance in the process of re-forming.

Team Building

Team building focuses on both task and relationship aspects of a group's functioning and is intended to increase efficiency and productivity. The group's work and problem-solving procedures, member–member relations, and leadership are analyzed, and exercises are prescribed to help members modify their patterns of interaction or processes of decision making.

Team-building activities may include outside intervention to build team cohesiveness, use internal consultative services, be manager-driven, and/or involve the training and development of the group's members and/or leader.

Team building involves

- Gathering data through individual interviews, questionnaires, and/or group meetings about the team and its functioning;
- Diagnosing the team's strengths and areas in need of development; and
- Holding semistructured retreat sessions, usually directed by an experienced facilitator, aimed at addressing priority team problems.

Team building may occur over months during specially arranged retreats or may be confined to "quick fix" activities during regular work time. Most team building involves simulated real-life activities aimed at improving the team's functioning through observing and intervening in the team's actual performance rather than through training. Some of these strategies are depicted in Table 11-1.

Retreat sessions ideally are conducted away from the workplace over a period lasting from one day to several days and are insulated from professional or personal interruptions of the participants. Retreat-style team building is intended to create intense prolonged interactions that force conflicts and unhealthy group

Table 11-1　Strategies for Team Management

Problem	Solution
Member isn't a team player.	• Consider why you want person on team. • Approach person in an assertive manner. • Give person an opportunity to provide feedback on problematic situations. • If person is unable to communicate with other team members, leader might approach for one-to-one dialogue. • Listen actively, using all senses to assess both verbal and nonverbal messages. • Avoid blaming and shaming, which tend to create defensiveness and cause arguments.
Member lacks sense of personal accountability.	• Explain how failure to take responsibility affects team as a whole. (For example, "Mary, last week when you didn't present your part of the report, it set team goals back a week.") • Without blaming or shaming, provide feedback from all team members.
Team lacks clear goals.	• Brainstorm to clarify short-term goals and develop action plan. • Arrive at consensus regarding mission and goals. • Define member responsibilities. • Determine resources needed to accomplish goals, including staff, financial and administrative support, time, and equipment. • Periodically review team progress and goal attainment.
Roles and boundaries are unclear.	• With member input, leader must clarify boundaries. • All team members' roles and responsibilities must be defined, including leader's. • Periodically review team development.

From D. Antai-Otong, 1997, "Team building in a health care setting," *American Journal of Nursing, 97*(7), pp. 48–51.

processes to the surface so that they can be examined and improved under the guidance of an objective, skilled third party. Follow-up in the work setting is often overlooked, but it is an essential final step to ensure application of new collaborative behaviors and ongoing commitments to team development.

The most important initial activities in team building are data gathering and diagnosis. Questions must be asked about the group's context (organizational structure, climate, culture, mission, and goals); characteristics of the group's work, including group members' roles, styles, procedures, job complexity; and the team, its problem-solving style, interpersonal relationships, and relations with other groups.

The following questions may be asked:

1. To what extent do the team's members understand and accept the goals of the organization?
2. What, if any, hidden agendas interfere with the group's performance? **Hidden agendas** are members' individual unspoken objectives that interfere with commitment or enthusiasm.
3. How effective is the group's leadership?
4. To what extent do group members understand and accept their roles?
5. How does the group make decisions?
6. How does the group handle conflict? Are conflicts dealt with through avoidance, forcing, accommodating, compromising, competing, or collaborating?
7. What personal feelings do members have about each other?
8. To what extent do members trust and respect each other?
9. What is the relationship between the team and other units in the organization?

Only after diagnosing the problems of the team can the leader take actions to improve team functioning. A nurse manager may decide to assume personal responsibility for team building when the team is basically functional and simply needs some fine-tuning to deal more effectively with minor interpersonal issues or changing circumstances.

According to Antai-Otong (1997), four qualities are present in successful teams:

- Open and effective communication
- Involved members who are committed to the team, understand team dynamics, and are emotionally invested in the team
- Clearly defined goals that identify member roles and responsibilities
- Trust and collegiality

Thoughtful team-building strategies allow group members to acknowledge the developmental process and respond to it in constructive ways. Team-building activities may also be used to facilitate the normal stages of group development (forming, storming, norming, performing, and adjourning or re-forming), an important process in managing teams.

Team-building techniques also may be used to intervene in traditional work groups that are experiencing problems or in any other type of group, such as a task force or committee. Numerous techniques and commercial resources are available for managers or an intervention specialist to use.

Characteristics of Groups

Norms

Norms are the informal rules of behavior shared and enforced by group members. Norms emerge whenever humans interact. Groups develop norms that members believe must be adhered to for fruitful, stable group functioning. Nursing groups often establish norms related to how members deal with absences that affect the workload of colleagues. Norms may include not calling in sick on Fridays, readily accommodating requests for trading shifts, and returning from breaks in a timely manner. In a team environment, norms are

---

KEY TERMS

Adjourning The final stage of group development in which a group dissolves after achieving its objectives.

Re-forming A stage of group development in which the group reassembles after a major change in the environment or in the goals of the group that requires the group to refocus its activities.

Team building A group development technique that focuses on task and relationship aspects of a group's functioning in order to build team cohesiveness.

Hidden agendas A group member's individual, unspoken objectives that interfere with commitment or enthusiasm.

Norms Informal rules of behavior shared and enforced by group members.

more likely to be linked to each team member's expected contribution to the performance and products of the team's efforts. If an individual agrees to take on a specific assignment on the team's behalf and fails to complete the assignment on time, a group norm has been violated.

Group norms are likely to be enforced if they serve to facilitate group survival, ensure predictability of behavior, help avoid embarrassing interpersonal problems, express the central values of the group, and clarify the group's distinctive identity.

Groups go through several stages in enforcing norms with deviant members (Leavitt & Bahrami, 1988). First, members use rational argument, or present reasons for adhering to the norms to the deviant individual. Second, if rational argument is not effective, members may use persuasive or manipulative techniques, reminding the deviant of the value of the group. The third stage is attack. Attacks may be verbal or even physical and sometimes include sabotaging the deviant's work. The final stage is ignoring the deviant.

It becomes increasingly difficult for a deviant to acquiesce to the group as these strategies escalate. Agreeing to rational argument is easy, but agreeing after an attack is very difficult. When the final stage (ignoring) is reached, acquiescence may be impossible because group members refuse to acknowledge the deviant's surrender. A nurse manager has a responsibility to help groups deal with members who violate group norms related to performance, including counseling the employee and preventing destructive conflict.

Roles

Norms apply to all group members, whereas roles are specific to positions in the group. A **role** is a set of expected behaviors that fit together into a unified whole and are characteristic of persons in a given context (Biddle, 1979). Roles commonly seen in groups can be classified as either task roles or socioemotional (nurturing) roles (Bales, 1958). Often, individuals fill several roles. Individuals performing task roles attempt to keep the group focused on its goals.

Task roles include

- *Initiator-contributor.* Redefines problems and offers solutions, clarifies objectives, suggests agenda items, and maintains time limits.
- *Information seeker.* Pursues descriptive bases for the group's work.
- *Information giver.* Expands information given by sharing experiences and making inferences.

- *Opinion seeker.* Explores viewpoints that clarify or reflect the values of other members' suggestions.
- *Opinion giver.* Conveys to group members what their pertinent values should be.
- *Elaborator.* Predicts outcomes and provides illustrations or expands suggestions, clarifying how they could work.
- *Coordinator.* Links ideas or suggestions offered by others.
- *Orienter.* Summarizes the group's discussions and actions.
- *Evaluator critic.* Appraises the quantity and quality of the group's accomplishments against set standards.
- *Energizer.* Motivates group to accomplish, qualitatively and quantitatively, the group's goals.
- *Procedural technician.* Supports group activity by arranging the environment (e.g., scheduling meeting room) and providing necessary tools (e.g., ordering visual equipment).
- *Recorder.* Documents the group's actions and achievements.

Nurturing roles facilitate the growth and maintenance of the group. Individuals assuming these roles are concerned with group functioning and interpersonal needs. Nurturing roles include

- *Encourager.* Compliments members for their opinions and contributions to the group.
- *Harmonizer.* Relieves tension and conflict.
- *Compromiser.* Submits own position to maintain group harmony.
- *Gate-keeper.* Encourages all group members to communicate and participate.
- *Group observer.* Takes note of group processes and dynamics and informs group of them.
- *Follower.* Passively attends meetings, listens to discussions, and accepts group's decisions.

Status is the social ranking of individuals relative to others in a group based on the position they occupy. Status comes from factors the group values, such as achievement, personal characteristics, the ability to control rewards, or the ability to control information. Status is usually enjoyed by members who most conform to group norms. Higher-status members often exercise more influence in group decisions than others.

Status incongruence occurs when factors associated with group status are not congruent, such as when a younger, less experienced person becomes the group leader. Status incongruence can have a disruptive impact on a group. For example, isolates are members who have high external status and different backgrounds from regular group members. They usually work at acceptable levels but are isolated from the group because they do not fit the group member profile. Sometimes status incongruence occurs because the individual does not need the group's approval and makes no effort to obtain it.

The most important role in a group is the leadership role. Leaders are appointed for most formal groups, such as command groups, teams, committees, or task forces. Leaders in informal groups tend to emerge over time and in relation to the task to be performed. Some of the factors contributing to the emergence of leadership in small groups include the ability to accomplish the group's goals, sociability, good communication skills, self-confidence, and a desire for recognition. Guidelines for performing this leadership role are discussed later in this chapter.

Communication in Groups

Groups provide an important channel of communication in organizations. Members of high-performance work teams generally communicate openly, candidly, and clearly with one another about procedures, expectations, and plans. Communication is influenced by the status and roles of the individuals who dominate team discussions. High-status members who are fulfilling key roles in relation to a team's priorities are likely to exercise considerable control over communication in the group by determining topics, setting the tone of the discussion, and influencing how decisions are made.

Effective nurse managers can facilitate communication in groups by maintaining an atmosphere in which group members feel free to discuss concerns, make suggestions, critique ideas, and show respect and trust. An important leadership function related to communication is gate-keeping, that is, keeping communication channels open, refocusing attention on critical issues, identifying and processing conflict, fostering self-esteem, checking for understanding, actively seeking the participation of all group members, and suggesting procedures for discussing group problems.

How Groups Affect Individuals

Group relationships affect individual behavior in many ways. Organizational work groups affect the beliefs, knowledge, attitudes, values, emotions, and social behavior of individuals. Groups profoundly affect the nature and process of communication and interpersonal relationships. On the one hand, they may engender a higher degree of competition and political activity than individual behavior.

Group influence is greater than the sum of its parts. A group can bring out the best and the worst in individuals due to the stimulating presence of others. Frequently, this stimulation increases motivation, especially when an individual's potential contribution to the task is fairly clear or easily measured.

On the other hand, groups can lead to inordinate conformity among group members. Groups may be tyrannical toward members and ruthless toward nonmembers and thereby contribute to conflict in the organization. Some issues involved in intragroup, intergroup, and intraorganizational conflict are discussed in Chapter 20. The effect of groups on productivity, quality of work life (job satisfaction), and development and growth are discussed below.

Group Productivity and Cohesiveness

Productivity represents how well the work group or team uses the resources available to achieve its goals and produce its services. If patient care is satisfactorily completed at the end of each shift in relation to the levels of staffing, supplies, equipment, and support services used, the group has been productive. Productivity is influenced by work-group dynamics, especially a group's cohesiveness and collaboration.

Cohesiveness is the degree to which the members are attracted to the group and wish to retain membership

---

KEY TERMS

Role   A set of expectations about behavior ascribed to a specific position in society.

Status   The social ranking of individuals relative to others in a group based on the position they occupy.

Status incongruence   The disruptive impact that occurs when factors associated with group status are not congruent.

Productivity   A measure of how well the work group or team uses the resources available to achieve its goals and produce its services.

Cohesiveness   The degree to which the members are attracted to the group and wish to retain membership in it.

in it. Cohesiveness includes how much the group members enjoy participating in the group and how much they are willing to contribute. Cohesiveness is also related to homogeneity of interests, values, attitudes, and background factors. Strong group cohesiveness leads to a feeling of "we" as more important than "I" and ensures a higher degree of cooperation and interpersonal support among group members.

Group norms may support or subvert organizational objectives, depending on the level of group cohesiveness. High group cohesiveness may foster high or low individual performance, depending on the prevailing group norms for performance. When cohesiveness is low, productivity may vary significantly. Although groups, in general, tend toward lower productivity, nursing education and practice have especially high standards of performance that help to counter this tendency.

Groups are more likely to become cohesive when members

- Share similar values and beliefs,
- Are motivated by the same goals and tasks,
- Must interact to achieve their goals and tasks,
- Work in proximity to each other (on the same unit and on the same shift, for example), and
- Have specific needs that can be satisfied by involvement in the group.

Group cohesiveness is also influenced by the formal reward system. Groups tend to be more cohesive when group members receive comparable treatment and pay and perform similar tasks that require interaction among the members. Similarities in values, education, social class, gender, age, and ethnicity that lead to similar attitudes strengthen group cohesiveness.

Cohesiveness can produce intense social pressure. Highly cohesive groups can demand and enforce adherence to norms regardless of their practicality or effectiveness. In this circumstance, the nurse manager may have a very difficult time influencing individual nurses, especially if the group norms deviate from the manager's values or expectations. For example, operating room nurses may be used to arriving at the time their shift starts and then changing into scrubs. The nurse manager, in contrast, may expect the staff to be changed and ready for work by the time the shift starts. In addition, group dynamics can affect absenteeism and turnover. Groups with high levels of cohesiveness exhibit lower turnover and absenteeism than groups with low levels of cohesiveness.

For most individuals, the work group provides one of the most important social contacts in life; the experience of working on an effective work team contributes significantly to one's professional confidence and to the quality of work life and job satisfaction. The work group often provides the primary motivation for returning to the job day after day even when employees are dissatisfied with the employing organization or other working conditions.

Work groups not only perform tasks but also provide the context in which novices learn basic skills and become socialized and experts engage in clinical mentorship, standard setting, quality improvement, and innovation. Work-group relations influence the satisfaction of staff with their jobs, the overall quality of work life, and the quality of the environment for patient care. Managers play key roles in guiding the tasks of work groups and ensuring efficient and effective performance; managers also encourage relationships among members of work teams that will promote coordination and cooperation.

Development and Growth

Groups also can provide learning opportunities by increasing individual skills or abilities. The group may facilitate socialization of new employees into the organization by "showing them the ropes." The nurse manager must establish an atmosphere that encourages learning new skills and knowledge, creating a group-oriented learning environment by continuously encouraging group members to improve their technical and interpersonal skills and knowledge through training and development. Group cohesiveness and effectiveness improve as staff members take responsibility for teaching each other and jointly seeking new information or techniques.

The Nurse Manager as Team Leader

Influencing group processes toward the attainment of organizational objectives is the direct responsibility of the nurse manager. The nurse manager can do a great deal to foster effective individual and group performance by promoting the benefits of group membership and increasing interdependence. By publicizing group accomplishments, creating opportunities for group members to demonstrate new skills, and supporting group social activities, the manager can increase the perceived value of group membership. Indeed, this is one of the manager's primary functions in a nursing organization. Members of groups who have a history of success are attracted to each other more than those who have not been successful.

The manager's communication style also affects group cohesiveness. The nurse manager who maintains a high degree of information power, for instance, controls not only what information is received but also who receives it. Directing information to only a few staff nurses represents a highly centralized communication structure. In a decentralized structure, the nurse manager shares information freely, encouraging a high degree of mutual communication and participative problem solving. In participative groups, each individual has the opportunity, and is encouraged, to seek and share information and to communicate frequently with anyone and everyone in the group. Managers and staff alike check with each other to ensure that information is clear, to offer suggestions, and to provide feedback.

Group Task

The size of the group can influence its effectiveness, depending on the type of task: additive, disjunctive, divisible, or conjunctive (Steiner, 1972, 1976). The more people who work on an **additive task** (group performance depends on the sum of individual performance), the more inputs are available to produce a favorable result. For example, the game tug-of-war involves the combined effort of the team.

For a **disjunctive task** (the group succeeds if one member succeeds), the greater the number of people, the higher the probability that one group member will solve the problem. Consider the Olympics. The more athletes on one team, the greater the opportunity for a gold medal. Regardless of the event, a medalist from the United States team brings recognition to the country, and every citizen is able to share the honor.

With a **divisible task** (tasks that can break down into subtasks with division of labor), more people provide a greater opportunity for specialization and interdependence in performing the tasks. For instance, the construction of a car is a complex task. From design of the car to insertion of the last bolt, each individual involved has a specialized task. With a **conjunctive task** (the group succeeds only if all members succeed), more people increase the likelihood that one person can slow up the group's performance (e.g., jury trial).

On many tasks, interdependence is important (Thompson, 1967). There are three kinds:

- **Pooled interdependence,** in which each individual contributes but no one contribution is dependent on any other (e.g., a committee discussion)
- **Sequential interdependence,** in which group members must coordinate their activities with others in some designated order (e.g., an assembly line)
- **Reciprocal interdependence,** in which members must coordinate their activities with every other individual in the group (e.g., team nursing).

Group Size and Composition

Groups with five to ten members tend to be optimal for most complex organizational tasks, which require diversity in knowledge, skills, and attitudes and allow full participation. In larger groups, members tend to contribute less of their individual potential while the leader is called on to take more corrective action, do more role clarification, manage more disruption, and make recognition more explicit. Groups tend to perform better with competent individuals as members. However, coordination of effort and proper utilization of abilities and task strategies must occur as well. Homogeneous groups tend to function more harmoniously, whereas heterogeneous groups may experience considerable conflict.

Evaluating Team Performance

The manager may be accustomed to evaluating individual performance, but evaluating how well a team performs requires different assessments. Patient outcomes

---

KEY TERMS

Additive task   A task in which group performance depends on the sum of individual performance.

Disjunctive task   A task in which the group succeeds if one member succeeds.

Divisible task   Tasks that can be broken down into subtasks with division of labor.

Conjunctive task   A task in which the group succeeds only if all members succeed.

Pooled interdependence   A type of interdependence in which each individual contributes to the group but no one contribution is dependent on any other.

Sequential interdependence   A type of interdependence in which members must coordinate their activities with others in some designated order.

Reciprocal interdependence   A type of interdependence in which members must coordinate their activities with every other individual in the group.

and team functioning are the criteria by which teams can be evaluated (Barter, 2002). Using clinical pathway data, variances in critical paths, complication rates, falls, and medication errors are examples of outcome data that can help the manager evaluate team performance.

Group functioning can be assessed by the level of work-group cohesion, involvement in the job, and willingness to help each other. Conversely aggression, competition, hostility, aloofness, shaming, or blaming are characteristics of poorly functioning groups. Stability of members is an additional measure of group functioning.

See how one nurse handled his new assignment as manager for a multidisciplinary team in Case Study 11-1.

CASE STUDY 11-1: Introducing Multidisciplinary Teams

Bruce Shapiro was promoted 6 months ago to nurse manager for the stroke rehabilitation unit of a nationally owned rehabilitation hospital. Patient care delivery systems have been under intensive review at the corporate level, and major changes in staffing are underway. Previously, physical and occupational therapists were staffed out of a separate department and reported to the director of physical therapy. Now all therapists will be unit based and report to the nurse manager. Documentation will now be team centered instead of being split among nursing, therapists, and other care providers.

Janice Simpson has been a physical therapist for 25 years and has been at the rehab hospital for the past 6 years. She worked as a shift leader for physical therapy until the new unit-based staffing was implemented. Janice has been assigned to the stroke rehab unit and will report to Bruce. She is feeling uncomfortable in her new role and is concerned about how she will fit in with the established nursing staff. Janice is also concerned that with the new documentation system, the physical therapy patient evaluations will not be included in determining patient goals.

Bruce is eager for Janice to join the staff of the stroke rehabilitation unit. He schedules individual meetings with Janice and the three other therapists who will be assigned to his unit. Bruce outlines the roles and expectations of staff on the unit and listens attentively to their questions and concerns. He also reviews the physical and occupational therapy job descriptions and reviews their respective documentation standards. At the monthly staff meeting, Bruce

discusses the roles and responsibilities of the therapists with the nursing staff. A mentor is assigned to meet daily with each therapist for their first 2 weeks on the unit.

Manager's Checklist
The nurse manager is responsible for

- Understanding the new staffing policies and the impact on the unit,
- Gaining knowledge related to physical and occupational therapy practice,
- Easing the transition of new staff into the existing staff group to help build trust and respect,
- Educating all staff on the new staffing policies,
- Ensuring that all therapists and nurses attend mandatory documentation training and auditing patient records for compliance with new documentation standards,
- Communicating with human resources if there are any questions regarding performance evaluation, scheduling, or compensation,
- Reviewing the personnel files of new staff,
- Establishing roles for the therapists in the unit governance structure,
- Facilitating open communication with therapists and nurses to discuss concerns or suggestions, and
- Providing appropriate feedback to nursing management related to the new staffing changes.

Leading Committees and Task Forces

Committees are generally permanent and deal with recurring problems. Membership on committees is usually determined by organizational position and role. **Formal committees** are part of the organization and have authority as well as a specific role.

Informal committees are primarily for discussion and have no delegated authority. **Task forces** are ad hoc committees appointed for a specific purpose and a limited time. Task forces work on problems or projects that cannot be readily handled by the organization through its normal activities and structures. Task forces often deal with problems crossing departmental boundaries. They tend to generate recommendations and then disband.

Nurse managers often are selected for leadership roles on committees and task forces. In these leadership roles and as unit managers and team leaders, they conduct numerous meetings. The following section provides guidance for leading and conducting meetings.

Guidelines for Conducting Meetings

Although meetings are vital to the conduct of organizational work, they should be held principally for problem solving, decision making, and enhancing working relationships. Other uses of meetings, such as socializing, giving or clarifying information, or soliciting suggestions must be thoroughly justified. Meetings should be conducted efficiently and should result in relevant and meaningful outcomes. Meetings should not result in damaged interpersonal relations, frustration, or inconclusiveness.

Preparation The first key to a successful meeting is thorough preparation. Preparation includes clearly defining the purpose of the meeting. The nurse manager should prepare an agenda, determine who should attend, make assignments, distribute relevant material, arrange for recording of minutes, and select an appropriate time and place for the meeting. The agenda should be distributed well ahead of time, 7 to 10 days prior to the meeting, and it should include what topics will be covered, who will be responsible for each topic, what prework should be done, what outcomes are expected in relation to each topic, and how much time will be allotted for each topic.

Participation In general, the meeting should include the fewest number of stakeholders who can actively and effectively participate in decision making, who have the skills and knowledge necessary to deal with the agenda, and who adequately can represent the interests of those who will be affected by decisions made. Too few or too many participants may limit the effectiveness of a committee or task force.

Place and Time Meetings should be held in places where interruptions can be controlled and at a time when there is a natural time limit to the meeting, such as late in the morning or afternoon, when lunch or dinner make natural time barriers. Meetings should be limited to 50 to 90 minutes, except when members are dealing with complex, detailed issues in a one-time session. Meetings that exceed 90 minutes should be planned to include breaks at least every hour. Meetings should start

and finish on time. Starting late positively reinforces latecomers, while penalizing those who arrive on time or early. If sanctions for late arrival are indicated, they should be applied respectfully and objectively. If it is the leader who is late, the cost of starting meetings late should be reiterated and an appropriate designee should begin the meeting on time.

Member Behaviors The behavior of each member may be positive, negative, or neutral in relation to the group's goals. Members may contribute very little, or they may use the group to meet personal needs. Some members may assume most of the responsibility for the group action, thereby enabling less participative members to avoid contributing.

Group members should

- Be prepared for the meeting, having read pertinent materials ahead of time,
- Ask for clarification as needed,
- Offer suggestions and ideas as appropriate,
- Encourage others to contribute their ideas and opinions,
- Offer constructive criticism as appropriate,
- Help the discussion stay on track, and
- Assist with implementation as agreed.

These behaviors facilitate group performance. All attendees should be familiar with behaviors that they may employ to facilitate well-managed meetings. All meeting participants must be helped to understand that they share responsibility for successful meetings.

A leader can increase meeting effectiveness greatly by not permitting one individual to dominate the discussion; separating idea generation from evaluation; encouraging members to refine and develop the ideas of others (a key to the success of brainstorming); recording problems, ideas, and solutions on a blackboard or flip chart; checking for understanding; periodically summarizing information and the group's progress; encouraging further discussion; and bringing disagreements out into the open and facilitating their

---

KEY TERMS

Formal committees Committees in an organization with authority and a specific role.

Informal committees Committees with no delegated authority that are organized for discussion.

Task forces Ad hoc committees appointed for a specific purpose and a limited time.

Box 11-1 Guidelines for Leading Group Meetings

- Begin and end on time.
- Create a warm, accepting, and nonthreatening climate.
- Arrange seating to minimize differences in power, maximize involvement, and allow visualization of all meeting activities. (A U-shape is optimal.)
- Use interesting and varied visuals and other aids.
- Clarify all terms and concepts. Avoid jargon.
- Foster cooperation in the group.
- Establish goals and key objectives.
- Keep the group focused.
- Focus the discussion on one topic at a time.

- Facilitate thoughtful problem solving.
- Allocate time for all problem-solving steps.
- Promote involvement.
- Facilitate integration of material and ideas.
- Encourage exploration of implications of ideas.
- Facilitate evaluation of the quality of the discussion.
- Elicit the expression of dissenting opinions.
- Summarize discussion.
- Finalize the plan of action for implementing decisions.
- Arrange for follow-up.

---

reconciliation. The leader is also responsible for drawing out the members' hidden agendas (personal goals or needs). Revealing hidden agendas ensures that these agendas either contribute positively to group performance or are neutralized. Guidelines for leading group meetings are provided in Box 11-1.

Managing Task Forces

There are a few critical differences between task forces and formal committees. For example, members of a task force have less time to build relationships with each other, and, because task forces are temporary, there may be no desire for long-term positive relationships. Formation of a task force may suggest that the organization's usual problem-solving mechanisms have failed. This perception may lead to tensions among task force members and between the task force and other units in the organization. The various members of a task force usually come from different parts of the organization and, therefore, have different values, goals, and viewpoints. The leader will need to take specific action to efficiently familiarize task force members with each other and create bonds in relation to the task.

Preparing for the First Meeting Prior to the task force's first meeting, the leader must clarify the objectives of the task force in terms of specific measurable outcomes, determine its membership, set a task completion date, plan how often and to whom the task force should report while working on the project, and ascertain the group's scope of authority, including its budget, availability of relevant information, and decision-making power. The task force leader should communi-

cate directly and regularly with the administrator or governing body that commissioned the task force's work so that ongoing clarification of its charge and progress can be tracked and adjusted.

Task force members should be selected on the basis of their knowledge, skills, personal concern for the task, time availability, and organizational credibility. They should also be selected on the basis of their interpersonal skills. Those who relish group activities and can facilitate the group's efforts are especially good members. The group leader also should plan to include one or two individuals who potentially may oppose task force recommendations in order to solicit their input, involve them in the decision-making process, and win their support. By holding personal conversations with task force members before the first meeting, the group leader can explore individual expectations, concerns, and potential contributions. It also provides the leader with an opportunity to identify potential needs and conflicts and to build confidence and trust.

Conducting the First Meeting The goal of the first meeting is to come to a common understanding of the group's task and to define the group's working procedures and relationships. Task forces must rely on the general norms of the organization to function. The task force leader should legitimize the representative nature of participation on the task force and encourage members to discuss the task force's process with the other members of the organization.

During the first meeting, a standard of total participation should be well established. The leader should remain as neutral as possible and should prevent premature decision making. Working procedures and relationships among the various members, subgroups, and the rest of the organization need to be established. The frequency and nature of full task force meetings and the number of subgroups must be determined. Ground rules for communicating must be established, along with norms for decision making and conflict resolution.

Managing Subsequent Meetings and Subgroups In running a task force, especially when several subgroups are formed, the leader should hold full task force meetings often enough to keep all members informed of the group's progress. Unless a task force is small, subgroups are essential. The leader must not be aligned too closely with one position or subgroup. A work plan should be developed that includes realistic interim project deadlines. The task force and subgroups should be held to these deadlines. The leader plays a key role in coaching subgroups and the task force to meet its deadlines.

The leader also must be sensitive to the conflicting loyalties sometimes created by belonging to a task force. One of the leader's most important roles is to communicate information to both task force members and the rest of the organization in a timely and regular fashion. The leader should solicit feedback from other key organizational representatives during the course of the task force's work.

Completing the Task Force's Report In bringing a project to completion, the task force should prepare a written report for the commissioning administrators that summarizes the findings and recommendations. Drafts of this report should be shared with the full task force prior to presentation. To identify any overlooked or sensitive information and reduce defensive reactions, it is especially important that the task force leader personally brief key administrators prior to presenting the report. This gives administrators a chance to read and respond to the report before making recommendations. The leader should consider involving a few task force members in the administrative presentation.

Patient Care Conferences

Patient-related conferences are held to address the needs of individual patients or patient populations. The purpose of the conference determines the composition of the group. Patient-focused meetings are usually multidisciplinary and used for case management to discuss specific patient care problems. For example, a multidisciplinary team may form to discuss the failure of a rehabilitation regimen to help a home care patient and to develop new plans for intervention.

Often nurses also are involved in activities associated with improving the quality of care for various patient groups and their families. For example, a nurse manager might organize meetings with primary care physicians to discuss how to improve discharge planning, to explore strategies to reduce the length of inpatient stays, or to improve the coordination of care for ambulatory patients.

The team leader of a patient care conference often may not be a manager with line responsibility to supervise, evaluate, or hire employees. The team leader is, however, a coach, teacher, and facilitator. Thus the team leader needs to have excellent leadership skills. The task of a team leader varies according to the task and the skill level of the team members. Highly skilled registered nurses, for example, would not require, nor appreciate, a team leader who tries to micromanage their work, whereas less-experienced, technically trained individuals require more coaching and support (Barter, 2002).

What You Know Now

- A group is an aggregate of individuals who interact and mutually influence each other.
- Groups may be classified as real or task, formal or informal, permanent or temporary.
- A team is a group of individuals with complementary skills, a common purpose and performance goals, and a set of methods for which they hold themselves accountable.
- Groups have an impact on cohesiveness and productivity, as well as individual development and growth.
- A group's norms and roles directly influence the productivity and satisfaction of group members and their ability to develop and grow.
- Groups come together, build cohesiveness, complete their task, and disband or re-form.
- Leading teams requires good communication and conflict resolution skills as well as the ability to plan, organize, facilitate, and evaluate group performance.
- Managing meetings involves preparing thoroughly, facilitating participation, and completing the group's work.

Tools for Building and Managing Teams

1. Notice how groups around you function. Use the best ideas with your own groups.
2. Watch effective leaders. Identify skills you could incorporate into your own leadership repertoire.

3. Review the problem behaviors of team members discussed in Table 11-1 and adopt solutions as appropriate.

4. Recognize that you can develop good team leadership skills. Practice those discussed in the chapter.

5. At the next opportunity be prepared to follow the directions for leading meetings.

6. Make a development plan to enhance your leadership skills.

Questions to Challenge You

1. Identify the groups that include you in your work or school. How are they different? Similar? Explain.

2. Describe an example of effective group leadership and an example of poor leadership.

3. Evaluate your own leadership performance. How could you improve?

4. Have you been involved in team building at work or school? Was it effective? Explain.

5. What roles do you usually play in a group meeting (or class)? What role would you like to play? Describe it.

Explore 🌐 MediaLink

NCLEX review questions, essay activities, group activities, and other interactive resources for this chapter can be found on the Web site at http://www.prenhall.com/sullivan-decker. Click on "Chapter 11" to select activities for this chapter.

References

Antai-Otong, D. (1997). Team building in a health care setting. *American Journal of Nursing, 97*(7), 48–51.

Bales, R. F. (1958). Task roles and social roles in problem-solving groups. In E. E. Maccoby, T. M. Newcomb, & E. L. Hartley (Eds.), *Readings in social psychology.* New York: Holt, Rinehart & Winston.

Barter, M. (2002). Follow the team leader. *Nursing Management, 33*(10), 54–57.

Biddle, B. J. (1979). *Role theory: Expectations, identities, and behavior.* New York: Academic Press.

Homans, G. (1950). *The human group.* New York: Harcourt Brace Jovanovich.

Homans, G. (1961). *Social behavior: Its elementary forms.* New York: Harcourt Brace.

Katzenbach, J. R., & Smith, D. K. (1993). The discipline of teams. *Harvard Business Review, 71*(2), 111–120.

Leavitt, H. J., & Bahrami, H. (1988). *Managerial psychology* (5th ed.). Chicago: University of Chicago Press.

Steiner, I. D. (1972). *Group process and productivity.* New York: Academic Press.

Steiner, I. D. (1976). Task-performing groups. In J. W. Thibaut, J. T. Spence, & R. C. Carson (Eds.), *Contemporary topics in social psychology* (pp. 94–108). Morristown, NJ: General Learning Press.

Thompson, J. D. (1967). *Organizations in action.* New York: McGraw-Hill.

Budgeting and Managing Resources

Looking Ahead

This chapter examines one of the most important factors contributing to changes in health care and the role of the nurse manager: the economic climate. It is crucial that nurses be able to allocate resources effectively, plan and develop different types of budgets, and monitor expenditures. The challenge is to be able to juggle these responsibilities competently in an increasingly cost-conscious climate.

Objectives

In this chapter, you will learn

- How the budgeting process works.
- What different types of budgets exist.
- How to monitor and control budgetary performance.
- How to determine budget variance.
- How staff affect budgetary performance.

MediaLink 🔍 www.prenhall.com/ sullivan-decker

Additional resources for this chapter can be found on the Companion Website at www.prenhall.com/ sullivan-decker. Click on "Chapter 12" to select the activities for this chapter.

- NCLEX Review
- Critical Thinking Activities
- Current Events

- MediaLinks
- *Nursing Leadership & Management in Action:* Creating a Personnel Budget; Assessing Productivity; Identifying Variance

With the economic climate of health care in turmoil, greater attention is being given to cost containment and operational efficiency. Mergers, integrated health care systems, the nursing shortage, and the scarcity of financial resources are key forces behind the current focus on financial accountability. Because the nursing budget can account for as much as half of an organization's total expenses, nurse managers at all levels are facing significant pressure to become proficient in the budgeting process, to allocate resources, and to control and monitor expenditures. This level of fiscal accountability is new to many managers and comes at a time when nursing must compete with other departments within the organization for limited resources.

In today's competitive environment, a higher level of performance is necessary. A focus on efficiency and effectiveness is essential (Porter-O'Grady, 2003), and the manager must help design the work to reduce extraneous and redundant tasks, making the best use of each individual's time and effort. This is no small task. Attention to the budgeting process is the first step to understanding how to use resources most effectively.

This chapter explains the budgeting process, defines budget terms, and presents guidelines for developing a budget, including how to determine salary expenses as well as operating and capital equipment budgets. The chapter also explains how to monitor and control budgetary performance and how to project costs based on current and anticipated needs.

A **budget** is a quantitative statement, usually in monetary terms, of the plans and expectations of a defined area over a specified period of time. Budgets provide a foundation for managing and evaluating financial performance. Budgets detail how resources (money, time, people) will be acquired and used to support planned services within the defined time period. The budget's purpose is to allow management to project action plans and their economic impact on the future so that objectives of the organization are coordinated and met.

The budget process also helps ensure that resources necessary to achieve these objectives are available at the appropriate time and that operations are carried out within the resources available. The budgeting process increases the awareness of costs and also helps employees understand the relationships among goals, expenses, and revenues. As a result, employees are committed to the goals and objectives of the organization, and various departments are able to coordinate activities and collaborate to achieve the organization's objectives. Budgets also help management control the resources expended through an organizational awareness of costs. Finally, budget performance provides management with feedback about resources management and the impact on the budget.

The Budgeting Process

Budgeting is a process of planning and controlling future operations by comparing actual results with planned expectations. Planning first involves reviewing established *goals* and *objectives* of both nursing and the organization. Goals and objectives help identify the organization's priorities and direct the organization's efforts. To plan, the organization must anticipate the future by gathering information about the following:

- Demographics of the population served, community influences, and competitors
- Sources of revenue, especially managed-care contracts, as well as public payers such as Medicare, Medicaid, and commercial insurance companies, because payment arrangements and mechanisms determine the projected revenues of the organization
- Statistical data, including the number of admissions or patient visits, patient days, average length of stay, and projected occupancy or visits
- Projected salary increases and price increases, including inflation rate, for supplies and other costs
- Information about regulatory changes (e.g., Medicare regulations) for the budgetary period
- Organizational changes (e.g., decentralization of pharmacy or respiratory therapy services) that result in salary and benefit dollars being charged in portion to the unit

The organization may use sophisticated and complex forecasting methods, including statistical techniques, to assist in making projections related to the budgetary period. Management normally uses the past as the common starting point for projecting the future, but in today's volatile payment environment, the past may be a poor predictor of the future. This is one of the major drawbacks of the budgeting process. In a rapidly changing industry, basing budgets on historical data often requires readjustment during the actual budget period.

Controlling is the process of comparing actual results with the results projected in the budget. Two techniques for controlling budgetary performance are variance analysis and position control. By measuring the differences between the projected and the actual results, management is better able to make modifications and corrections. Therefore, controlling depends on planning.

Approaches to Budgeting

Budgets may be developed in various formats depending on how the department is viewed by administration (Contino, 2001). They may be considered:

- *Cost centers.* Managers are responsible for predicting, documenting, and managing the costs (staffing, supplies) of the department.
- *Revenue centers.* Managers are responsible for generating revenues (patient volumes).
- *Profit centers.* Managers are responsible for generating revenues and managing costs so that the department shows a profit (revenues exceed costs).
- *Investment centers.* Managers are responsible for generating revenues and managing costs and capital equipment (assets).

Nursing units are typically considered cost centers, but they may also be viewed as revenue centers, profit centers, or investment centers. How the unit is considered is crucial in determining the manager's approach to budgeting.

Also, some nursing managers are responsible for service lines, and their staff are from multiple disciplines and departments. Other nurse managers are responsible for a single unit, such as a telemetry unit or the staff in a multiple physician office.

The organization may choose various approaches, or combinations of them, for requesting departmental managers to prepare their budget requests. These approaches are incremental (line-by-line), zero-based, fixed, and variable.

Incremental Budget

With an **incremental,** or **line-by-line, budget,** the finance department distributes a budget worksheet listing each expense item or category on a separate expense line. The expense line is usually divided into salary and nonsalary items. A budget worksheet is commonly used for mathematical calculations to be submitted for the next year. It may include several columns for the amount budgeted for the current year,

the amount actually spent year-to-date, the projected total for the year based on the actual amount spent, increases and decreases in the expense amount for the new budget, and the request for the next year with an explanation attached.

The base or starting point for calculating next year's budget request may be either the previous year's actual results or projected expenditures for the current year. For salary expenses, the adjustment might be the average salary increase projected for next year. For nonsalary expenses, the finance department may provide an estimate of the average increase for supplies or opt to use a standard measure of cost increases, perhaps the consumer or medical price index projected for the next year.

For nurse managers to complete budget worksheets accurately, they must be familiar with expense account categories. The manager should understand what type of expenses, such as instruments and minor equipment, are included under each line item. In addition, the manager has to keep abreast of different factors that have affected the expenditure level for each expense line during the current year. The projected impact of next year's activities will be translated into increases or decreases in expense levels of the nursing unit's expenditures for the coming year.

The advantage of the line-by-line budget method is its simplicity of preparation. The disadvantage of this method is that it discourages cost efficiency. To avoid budget cuts for the next year, an astute manager learns to spend the entire budget amount established for the current year, because this amount becomes the base for the next year.

KEY TERMS

Budget A quantitative statement, usually in monetary terms, of the expectations of a defined area of the organization over a specified period of time in order to manage financial performance.

Budgeting The process of planning and controlling future operations by comparing actual results with planned expectations.

Controlling The process of comparing actual results with the results projected in the budget.

Incremental (line-by-line) budget A budget worksheet listing expense items on separate lines that is usually divided into salary and nonsalary expenses.

Zero-Based Budget

The **zero-based budget** approach assumes the base for projecting next year's budget is zero. Managers are required to justify all activities and programs as if they were being initiated for the first time. Regardless of the level of expenditure in previous years, every proposed expenditure for the new year must be justified under the current environment and its fit with the organization's objectives. Because zero-based budgeting is time consuming, organizations may not use this process every year. An adaptation of the zero-based budget is to start the budget with a lower base, for example, 80 percent of the current expenses. Managers then have to justify any budgetary expenses requested above the 80 percent base.

Fixed or Variable Budgets

Budgets also can be categorized as fixed or variable. Budgets are considered **fixed budgets** when the budgeted amounts are set without regard to changes that may occur during the year, such as patient volume or program activities, that have an impact on the cost assumptions originally used for the coming year. In contrast, **variable budgets** are developed with the understanding that adjustments to the budget may be made during the year based on changes in revenues, patient census, utilization of supplies, and other expenses.

The Operating Budget

The **operating budget**, also known as the annual budget, is the organization's statement of expected revenues and expenses for the coming year. It coincides with the **fiscal year** of the organization, a specified 12-month period during which the operational and financial performance of the organization is measured. The fiscal year may correspond with the calendar year—January to December—or another time frame. Many organizations use July 1 to June 30; the federal government begins its fiscal year on October 1. The operating budget may be further broken down into smaller periods of 6 months or 4 quarters; each quarter may be further separated into three 1-month periods. The revenues and expenses are organized separately, with a bottom-line net profit or loss calculated.

The Revenue Budget

The **revenue budget** represents the patient care income expected for the budget period. Most commonly health care payers pay a predetermined rate based on discounts or allowances. In many cases, actual payment generated by a given service or procedure will not equal the charges that appear on the patient bill. Instead, the health care provider will be reimbursed based on a variety of methods. These include

- Reimbursement of a predetermined amount, such as fixed costs per case (Medicare recipients);
- Negotiated rates, such as per diems (a specified reimbursement amount per patient, per day);
- Negotiated discounts; and
- Capitation (one rate per member, per month, regardless of the service provided).

Revenue projections for the next year are based on the volume and mix of patients, rates, and discounts that will prevail during the budget period. Projections are developed from historical volume data, impact of new or modified clinical programs, shifts from inpatient to outpatient procedures, and other influences. The impact of the payers' mix and the percentage that each of them contributes to projected revenues of the organization also is taken into consideration, such as the percentage of revenues derived from Medicare, Medicaid, commercial insurance companies, HMOs, and other third-party payers.

Medicare payments for inpatient services are made at a predetermined specific rate for each Medicare recipient based on the patient's diagnosis. Care is classified into diagnosis-related groups (DRGs). Payments are made based on the assumption that patients with the same DRG use similar resources.

DRGs are based on primary and secondary diagnoses, age, and treatment received. Within each DRG is the assumption that a certain number of resources are required for a specific patient treatment. It also is assumed that the use of resources varies according to the patient's age, sex, primary and secondary diagnosis, and discharge status. The health care organization has a financial incentive to provide care at a cost below the fixed DRG price because it can keep the difference between the cost of treating the patient and the amount the organization is paid. Because of this incentive, organizations have used different methods to minimize the costs of caring for that patient, including reducing the patient's length of stay.

The Expense Budget

The **expense budget** consists of salary and nonsalary items. Expenses should reflect patient care objectives and activity parameters established for the nursing unit.

The expense budget should be comprehensive and thorough; it should also take into consideration all available information regarding the next year's expectations. Described below are several concepts and definitions related to the budgetary process in a health care setting.

Cost Centers   In health care organizations, nursing units are typically considered cost centers. A **cost center** is described as the smallest area of activity within an organization for which costs are accumulated. Cost centers may be revenue producing, such as laboratory and radiology, or non–revenue producing, such as environmental services and administration. Nursing managers are commonly given the responsibility for costs incurred by their department, but they have no revenue responsibilities.

In contrast, if managers are responsible for controlling both costs and revenues and if their financial performance is measured in terms of **profit** (the difference between revenues and expenses), then the manager is responsible for a profit center. Customarily, nursing is not directly reimbursed for its services. Nursing-related costs usually are included in the room charge. In addition, nursing lacks a method to categorize its activities, although work has been done in developing a taxonomy and minimum data set for nursing.

Classification of Costs   Costs are commonly classified as fixed or variable. **Fixed costs** are costs that will remain the same for the budget period regardless of the activity level of the organization, such as rental payments and insurance premiums. **Variable costs** depend on and change in direct proportion to patient volume and patient acuity, such as patient care supply expenses. If more patients are admitted to a nursing unit, more supplies are used, causing higher supply expenses.

Expenditures also may be direct or indirect. **Direct costs** are expenses that directly affect patient care. For example, salaries for nursing personnel who provide hands-on patient care are considered direct costs. **Indirect costs** are expenditures that are necessary but don't affect patient care directly. Salaries for dietary or housekeeping personnel, for example, are classified as indirect costs.

Determining the Salary (Personnel) Budget

The **salary budget,** also known as the **personnel budget,** projects the salary costs that will be paid and charged to the cost center in the budget period (see Table 12-1). Managing the salary budget is directly related to the manager's ability to supervise and lead the staff. Better managers tend to have more stable staff with fewer resources spent on supplementary staff,

---

KEY TERMS

Zero-based budget   A budgetary approach that assumes the base for projecting next year's budget is zero; managers are required to justify all activities and every proposed expenditure.

Fixed budget   A budget in which budgeted amounts are set regardless of changes that occur during the year.

Variable budget   A budget developed with the understanding that adjustments to the budget may be made during the year.

Operating budget   The organization's statement of expected revenues and expenses for the upcoming year.

Fiscal year   A specified 12-month period during which operational and financial performance is measured.

Revenue budget   A projection of expected income for a budget period based on volume and mix of patients, rates, and discounts.

Expense budget   A comprehensive budget that lists salary and nonsalary items that reflect patient care objectives and activity parameters for the nursing unit.

Cost center   The smallest area of activity within an organization for which costs are accumulated.

Profit   The difference between revenues and expenses.

Fixed costs   Expenses that remain the same for the budget period regardless of the activity level of the organization.

Variable costs   Expenses that depend on and change in direct proportion to patient volume and acuity.

Direct costs   Expenses that directly affect patient care.

Indirect costs   Necessary expenditures that do not affect patient care directly.

Salary (personnel) budget   A budget that projects salary costs to be paid and charged to the cost center during the budget period.

MEDIALINK   Creating a Personnel Budget

Table 12-1 Monthly Salary Budget and Year-to-Date Budget Comparison Report Fiscal Year Ending June 30

Position	June Actual Salary	June Budgeted Salary	June Variance	Year-to-Date Actual Salary	Year-to-Date Budgeted Salary	Year-to-Date Variance
Nurse Manager	$ 6,250	$ 6,250	$ 0	$ 68,750	$ 75,000	$ 6,250
Registered Nurses	95,722	93,825	(1,897)	1,048,813	1,125,878	77,065
Licensed Practical Nurses	19,025	20,800	1,775	231,426	249,600	18,174
Nursing Assistants	14,886	13,200	(1,686)	159,500	158,400	(1,100)
Unit Clerks	5,483	5,495	12	60,391	65,273	4,882
Float Pool RNs	1,426	1,000	(426)	16,800	12,500	(4,300)
TOTAL SALARY:	$142,792	$140,570	($2,222)	$1,585,680	$1,686,651	$100,971

turnover, or absenteeism. Managing personnel costs are challenges for all managers, and a system to track needs and expenses is essential (Walsh, 2003).

In addition to anticipated salary expenses, factors such as benefits, shift differentials, overtime, on-call expenses, and bonuses and premiums may affect the salary budget as well.

Benefits After the number of required full-time equivalents (FTEs) is determined (see Chapter 17 on scheduling), it is also necessary to determine how many FTEs are necessary to replace personnel for **benefit time** (vacations, holidays, personal days, and so on). This factor can be calculated by determining the average number of vacation days, paid holidays, personal days, bereavement days, or other days off with pay that the organization provides and the average number of sick days per employee as experienced by the cost center. By definition, replacement time is not calculated for indirect staff.

To determine FTEs required for replacement:

1. Determine hours of replacement time per individual.

Benefit time	Hours/shift	Replacement hours
15 vacation days	× 8 hours	= 120
8 holidays	× 8 hours	= 64
4 personal days	× 8 hours	= 32
5 sick days	× 8 hours	= 40
	Total	= 256

2. Then determine FTE requirement. Divide replacement time by annual FTE base

$$\frac{256}{2,080} = 0.12$$

From the FTE calculations an FTE budget is calculated (Table 12-1). This budget provides the base for the salary budget. However, shift differentials,

overtime, and bonuses or premiums also may affect budget performance and need to be considered.

Shift Differentials Most facilities use a set percentage to determine shift differential. For example, 10 percent for evenings, 15 percent for nights, and 20 percent for weekends and holidays. If the hourly rate is $18.00, for instance, then the cost for a nurse working evenings would be $18.00 plus $1.80 for each hour worked. On an eight-hour shift, the total cost would be $158.40 and for the year, $41,184.

Overtime Fluctuations in workload, patient volume, variability in admission patterns, and temporary replacement of staff due to illness or time off all create overtime in the nursing unit. A projection of overtime for the next year can be calculated by determining by staff classification (RN, LPN, nursing assistant, and other employee classifications) the historical or typical number of hours of overtime worked and multiplying that number by 1.5 times the hourly rate. For example, if the average number of overtime hours paid in a unit for RNs is 35 hours per 2-week pay period and the average hourly rate is $18.00, the projected overtime cost for the year would be $ 24,570 for the RN category.

To determine overtime costs:

1. Multiply average salary for classification $18.00
     by factor   ×   1.50
     to obtain overtime rate $27.00

2. Multiply average overtime hours   35
     by overtime rate   × $27.00
     to obtain expenditure per pay period $945.00

3. Multiply number of pay periods   26
     by overtime expenditure   × $945.00
     to obtain annual overtime costs $24,570.00

Clearly, overtime can rapidly deplete finite budget dollars allocated to a nursing unit. The nurse manager should explore options to overtime such as using part-time or per diem workers in order to keep the cost per hour more in line with the regular hourly rates. A competent manager certainly would also evaluate unit productivity to decrease overtime.

On-Call Hours   If the nursing unit uses a paid on-call system, the approximate number of hours that employees are put on call for the year should be estimated and that cost added to the budget. Typically under the on-call system, staff are requested to be available to be called back to work if patient need arises, and the number of hours on call are paid at a flat rate per hour.

Premiums   Some organizations offer premiums for certifications or clinical ladder steps. In this situation, a fixed dollar amount may be added to the base hourly rate of eligible personnel; for example, an additional $1.00 per hour paid for professional certifications. This would result in the hourly rate of the employee being adjusted from a base of $18.00 to $19.00. In this case, if the employee is full time and works 2,080 hours a year (40 hours a week multiplied by 52 weeks a year), the annual new salary would be $39,520, or $19.00 multiplied by 2,080.

Salary Increases   Merit increases or cost-of-living raises also need to be factored into budget projections. These increases are usually calculated on base pay. For example, if a 3 percent cost-of-living raise is projected and the base salary for an RN is $40,000, then the new base becomes $41,200.

Additional Considerations   Other important factors to consider when developing the salary budget are changes in technology, clinical supports, delivery systems, clinical programs or procedures, and regulatory requirements. Changes in patient care technology or introduction of new equipment may influence the number, skill, or time that unit personnel may spend in becoming oriented to the new equipment and, later, operating and maintaining it. If significant, the projected number of additional labor hours for the new budgetary period should be incorporated into the request.

The Joint Commission on Accreditation for Healthcare Organizations (JCAHO) and government regulations help establish the number and level of nursing personnel for specific clinical units to maintain safety requirements. For example, in critical care units and some other specialty units, a minimum of two staff members are required at all times, regardless of patient number or acuity. This may mean that even during times when no patients are in the unit, two employees must be paid to stay there.

Departments such as environmental services, dietary, escort, or laboratory may provide the nursing unit with support in performing certain tasks, such as transporting patients or specimens. Any change in the level of support they provide should be reviewed, and the effect of such change on the unit's staffing levels should be quantified for the next year's budget request. Changes in the method of delivering care (primary, team, differentiated practice, or functional nursing) or staff mix (RNs, LPNs, unlicensed assistive personnel) also will affect staffing patterns for the next year. Any changes in staffing can place new demands on the unit. Therefore, orientation and additional workload needs also should be considered.

In addition, changes might be made to the way the organization charges costs. For example, some direct or indirect costs formerly charged under other departments might now be allocated to the various units. You might find your unit charged its fair share of the heating or security budget. Major changes, of course, are planned ahead of time but some changes occur during the budget year and the unit might be expected to absorb those additional costs within its original budget.

Managing the Supply and Nonsalary Expense Budget

The supply and nonsalary expense budget identifies patient-related supplies needed to operate the nursing unit. In addition to supplies, other operating expenses, such as office supplies, rental fees, maintenance costs, and equipment service contracts, also may be paid out of the nursing unit's nonsalary budget.

An analysis of the current expense pattern and a determination of its applicability for the next budget period should be performed first. Any projected changes in patient volume, acuity, and patient mix also should be considered because they will affect next year's supply use and other nonsalary expenses. As an example, if patient days for a particular type of patient

KEY TERMS

Benefit time   Paid time, such as vacation, holidays, and sick days for which there is no work output.

are projected to multiply and cause a 5 percent increase in the use of intravenous solutions, this increase should be addressed in the budget request by requesting an additional 5 percent for intravenous solution supplies for the next year.

Increases due to an inflation rate index, or at a rate estimated by the finance or purchasing department, are included as part of the budget request. A simple way of calculating the effect of a price increase is to take the estimated total ending expense for the year and multiply it by the inflationary factor.

To determine projected price increases

Multiply current total line item expense	$12,758
by inflation factor plus 1.0	× 1.05
	$13,396

Increases in expenses, such as maintenance agreements and rental fees, should also be incorporated as part of the budget request. The introduction of new technology and changes in programs and regulatory requirements may require additional resources for supplies as well as increased salaries.

The Capital Budget

The **capital budget** is an important component of the plan to meet the organization's long-term goals. This budget identifies physical renovations, new construction, and new or replacement equipment planned within the budget period. Organizations define capital items based on certain conditions or criteria. Usually, capital items must have an expected performance of 1 year or more and exceed a certain dollar value, such as $500 or $1,000. Capital budgets also may be designed with a time horizon longer than 1 year, such as 3, 5, 10, or more years.

Today few nurse managers are asked to prepare a capital budget because most organizations are buying through consortiums or negotiated agreements with one supplier. Many health care organizations have departments that coordinate bringing in selected vendors and items and limit equipment choices to those. The nurse manager would then be responsible for assisting in selecting and determining the amount of equipment needed. The capital pool is expensed out across all units who use the equipment.

The impact of the new equipment on the unit's expenses, such as the number of staff needed to run the equipment, use of supplies, and maintenance costs, needs to be considered as part of the operating budget,

however. For example, if monitoring equipment is being requested, the cost of electrocardiogram paper and electrodes should be determined, documented, and included in the supply budget. Likewise, the need for additional nursing and nonnursing personnel to operate the new equipment, additional workload, and training of personnel should be quantified for the next year's budget.

Timetable for the Budgeting Process

Depending on the size and complexity of the organization, the budgeting process takes 3 to 6 months. The process begins with the first-level manager. The individual at this level of management may or may not have formalized budget responsibilities, but he or she is key to identifying needed resources for the upcoming budget period.

The manager seeks information from staff about areas of needed improvement or change and reviews unit productivity and the need for updated technology or supplies. The manager uses this information to prepare the first draft of the budget proposal.

Depending on the levels of organizational management, this proposal ascends through the managerial hierarchy. Each subsequent manager evaluates the budget proposal, making adjustments as needed. By the time the budget is approved by executive management, significant changes to the original proposal usually have been made.

The final step in the process is approval by a governing board, such as a board of directors or designated shareholders. Typically, the budget process timetable is structured so that the budget is approved a few months before the beginning of the new fiscal year.

Nurse managers must recognize the importance of clearly articulating their budgetary needs. Senior management must prioritize budget requests for the entire organization, and they base those decisions on strong supporting documentation. Nurse managers should not expect to receive all of their budget requests, but they need to be prepared to defend their priorities.

Monitoring Budgetary Performance during the Year

In many organizations, nurse managers receive a monthly report prepared by the accounting department summarizing the expenses for the department (see Table 12-1). This report shows expense line items with the budgeted amount, actual expenditure, variance from budget, and the percentage from the budgeted amount that such variance represents. Commonly these monthly reports also show the comparison between actual year-to-date results and the year-to-date budget.

The difference between the amount that was budgeted for a specific revenue or cost and the actual revenue or cost that resulted during the course of activities is known as the **variance**. In the case of nursing units, variance might occur in the actual cost of delivering patient care for a certain expense line item in a specified period of time. Nurse managers are commonly asked to justify the reason for variances and present an action plan to reduce or eliminate these variances.

Variance Analysis

In the daily course of events, it is unlikely that projected budget items will be completely on target in all situations. One of the manager's most important jobs is to manage the financial resources for the department and to be able to respond to variances in a timely fashion (Kirkby, 2003).

When expenses occur that differ from the budgeted amounts, organizations usually have an established level at which a variance needs to be investigated and explained or justified by the manager of the department. This level may be a certain dollar amount, such as $500, or it may be a percentage, such as a 5 percent or 10 percent increase above the budget.

In determining causes for variance, the nurse manager must review the activity level of the unit for the same period. There may have been increases in census or patient acuity that generated additional expense in salary and supplies.

Also, in many situations, variances might not be independent of one another. Variances may result from expenses that follow a seasonal pattern, occurring only at determined times in the year; renewal of a maintenance agreement is one example. Expenses may also follow a tendency or trend either to increase or to decrease during the year. Even if the situation is outside the manager's usual responsibility or control, the manager needs to understand and be able to identify the cause or reason for the variance.

To determine when a variance is favorable or unfavorable, it is important to relate the variance to its impact on the organization in terms of revenues and expenses. If more earnings came in than expected, the variance is favorable; if less, the variance is negative. Likewise, if less was spent than expected, the variance is favorable; if more was spent, the variance is negative.

For instance, the nurse manager might receive the following expense report:

MEDICAL/SURGICAL SUPPLIES

Budgeted expenditures	Actual expenditures	Variance (in $)	Percent (in %)
$34,560	$36,958	(2,398)	(6.9)

This expense variance is considered unfavorable because the actual expense was greater than the budget. In this example, more money was spent on medical/surgical supplies than was projected in the budget.

If the variance percentage of the actual budget amount is not presented in the reports, it can be calculated as follows:

Divide the dollar variance by the budget amount, then multiply by 100:

$$\frac{\$2,398}{\$34,560} = 0.069$$
$$0.069 \times 100 = 6.9\% \text{ over budget}$$

Salary Variances With salary expenditures, variances may occur in volume, efficiency, or rate. Typically these factors are related and have an impact on each other. **Volume variances** result when there is a difference in the budgeted and actual workload requirements as would occur with increases in patient days. An increase in the actual number of patient days will increase the salary expense, resulting in an unfavorable volume variance. Although the variance is unfavorable, concomitant increases in revenues for the organization should be apparent. Thus, the impact to the organization should be welcomed, even though it generated higher salary costs at the nursing unit level.

Efficiency variance, also called quantity or use variance, reflects the difference between budgeted and actual nursing care hours provided. Patient acuity,

---

KEY TERMS

Capital budget   A component of the budget plan that includes equipment and renovations needed by an organization in order to meet long-term goals.

Variance   The difference between the amount that was budgeted for a specific cost and the actual cost.

Volume variances   Differences in the budget as a result of increases or decreases in patient volume.

Efficiency variance   The difference between budgeted and actual nursing care hours provided.

nursing skill, unit management, technology, and productivity all affect the number of patient care hours actually provided versus the original number planned or required. At the same time, if the census had been higher than expected, it would be understandable if more hours of nursing care were provided and paid. A favorable efficiency, or fewer nursing care hours paid, could suggest that patient acuity was lower than projected, that staff was more efficient, or that higher-skilled employees were used. An unfavorable efficiency may be due to greater patient acuity than allowed for in the budget, overstaffing of the unit, or the use of less experienced or less efficient employees.

Rate variances, also known as price or spending variance, reflect the difference in budgeted and actual hourly rates paid. A favorable rate variance may reflect the use of new employees who were paid lower salaries. Unfavorable rate variance may reflect unanticipated salary increases or increased use of personnel paid at higher wages, such as agency personnel.

Nonsalary Expenditure Variances Nonsalary expenditure variances may be due to changes in patient volume, patient mix, supply quantities, or prices paid. New, additional, or more expensive supplies used at the nursing unit because of technology changes or new regulations also could influence expenditure totals.

Position Control

Another monitoring tool used by nurse managers is the position control. The **position control** is used to compare actual numbers of employees to the number of budgeted FTEs for the nursing unit. The position control is a list of approved, budgeted FTE positions for the nursing cost center. The positions are displayed by category or job classification, such as nurse manager, RNs, LPNs, and so on. The nurse manager updates the position control with employee names and FTE factors for each individual with respect to personnel changes, new hires, and resignations that take place during the year.

Staff Impact on Budgetary Performance

Staff can acutely affect the organization's finances. Misuse of sick time, excessive overtime or turnover, and wasteful use of resources can result in negative variance. The manager plays a key role in explaining the unit's goals, the organization's financial goals, and how each individual is responsible for helping the organization meet those goals.

Organizations have implemented a number of different programs and incentives for increasing employee

> ### KEY TERMS
>
> *Rate variance*   The difference between budgeted and actual hourly rates paid.
>
> *Nonsalary expenditure variance*   Deviation from the budget as a result of changes in patient volume, supply quantities, or prices paid.
>
> *Position control*   A monitoring tool used to compare actual numbers of employees to the number of budgeted FTEs for the nursing unit.

awareness and minimizing costs. Techniques to decrease absenteeism and turnover may be instituted (see Chapters 22 and 23). Displaying equipment costs on supply stickers or requisitions and indicating medication costs on medication sheets increase staff awareness of costs. Participation in quality improvement and action teams also serves to inform staff of cost factors. Bonuses based on net gains have been shared with employees, in addition to cost-of-living raises.

Future Trends

A major trend in financial management of health care organizations is the shift from a revenue-based to a cost-based accounting system. Formerly, hospitals emphasized generating revenues to cover the costs of health care. With the shift to managed care, however, the focus is on decreasing costs to maintain adequate profit margins in an era of diminishing compensation. In the managed-care environment, payment is prospectively determined in a competitive arrangement between provider and payer.

In an effort to be a low-cost provider of health care, organizations are strongly motivated to be cost effective. This trend has serious implications for nursing. Nursing has always been considered a cost, not a source of revenue. It is nursing's challenge to be consistently cost-conscious and to measure, manage, and document nursing's cost-effectiveness in this financial environment.

What You Know Now

- A budget is a quantitative statement, usually written in monetary terms, of plans and expectations over a specified period of time.

- The operating or annual budget is the organization's statement of expected revenues and expenses for the coming year.

- The revenue budget represents the patient care revenues expected for the budget period based on volume and mix of patients, rates, and discounts that will prevail during the same period of time.

- Nursing units are typically considered cost centers, but may be considered revenue centers, profit centers, or investment centers.

- Nurse managers may be responsible for service lines and staff from multiple disciplines and departments.

- Nurse managers have input into capital expenses and are responsible for salary and operating costs related to new equipment.

- A full-time equivalent (FTE) is a full-time position that can be equated to 40 hours of work per week for 52 weeks, or 2,080 hours per year.

- The position control is a list of approved, budgeted FTEs that compares the budgeted number of FTEs by classification (RN, LPN), shift, and status to the actual available employees of the unit.

- Variance is the difference between the amount that was budgeted for a specific revenue or cost and the actual revenue or cost that resulted during the course of activities.

- The shift from a revenue- to a cost-based accounting system requires nurses to remain cost-conscious and to demonstrate nursing's cost-effectiveness.

Tools for Budgeting and Managing Resources

1. Understand the budgeting process in your organization.

2. Determine the number of full-time equivalents necessary to staff the unit.

3. Compute the salary and nonsalary budget, including salary increases and various additional factors.

4. Monitor variances over the budget period and identify negative variances, responding promptly as appropriate.

5. Understand that factors out of your control, such as changes in technology or indirect or direct costs that may be assigned to your budget, affect your budget and its performance.

6. Encourage staff to monitor resource use, including time and supplies.

Questions to Challenge You

1. Do you have a budget for your personal and professional income and expenses? If so, how well do you manage it? If not, begin next month to track your income and expenses for one month. See if you are surprised at the results.

2. How well does your organization manage its resources? Can you make suggestions for improvement?

3. Are there tasks or functions in your work that you believe are redundant, unnecessary, or repetitive or that could be done by a lesser-paid employee? Explain.

4. Does your organization waste salary or nonsalary resources? If not, think of ways that organizations could waste resources. Describe them.

Explore ⊕ MediaLink

NCLEX review questions, essay activities, group activities, and other interactive resources for this chapter can be found on the Web site at http://www.prenhall.com/sullivan-decker. Click on "Chapter 12" to select activities for this chapter.

References

Contino, D. S. (2001). Budget training: It's overdue. *Nursing Management, 32*(8), 16–17.

Kirkby, M. P. (2003). Number crunching with variable budgets. *Nursing Management, 34*(2), 28–33.

Porter-O'Grady, T. (2003). A different age for leadership, Part 1: New context, new content. *Journal of Nursing Administration, 33*(2), 105–110.

Walsh, E. (2003). Get real with workload measurement. *Nursing Management, 34*(2), 38–42.

Managing and Improving Quality

Looking Ahead

We now move into a more specific discussion of the implementation of quality management in health care. Chapter 13 examines the role of nursing management in relationship to the concepts of quality and risk. Quality management is a prevention-focused philosophy seeking to balance cost-effectiveness with quality patient care. Risk management, a component of quality management, focuses on problems and their solutions.

Objectives

In this chapter, you will learn

- What total quality management, continuous quality management, and Six Sigma are.
- How the principles of quality management apply to health care.
- What the nurse's role in risk management is.
- How incident reports are used.
- How to handle complaints.

MediaLink 🌐 www.prenhall.com/
sullivan-decker

Additional resources for this chapter can be found on the Companion Website at www.prenhall.com/ sullivan-decker. Click on "Chapter 13" to select the activities for this chapter.

- NCLEX Review
- Critical Thinking Activities
- Current Events
- MediaLinks
- *Nursing Leadership & Management in Action:* Defining Quality; Application of the CQI Process

In today's highly competitive health care environment, each member of the health care organization must be accountable for the quality and cost of health care. Concern about quality gained national attention after publication of the Institute of Medicine's (IOM) reports on medical errors in 1999 (IOM, 1999) and their later recommendations for health professionals' education (IOM, 2003). Additionally, concern about cost continues unabated. Both quality and cost containment are found in the concept of total quality management, which has evolved into a model continuous quality improvement designed to improve system and process performance. Risk management is integrated within a quality management program.

Quality Management

Quality management moved health care from a mode of identifying failed standards, problems, and problem people to a proactive organization in which problems are prevented and ways to improve care and quality of care are sought. This paradigm shift involves all in the organization and promotes problem solving and experimentation.

A quality management program is based on an integrated system of information and accountability. Clinical information systems (described in Chapter 14) can provide the information needed to enable organizations to track activities and outcomes. Methods to discover problems in the system without blaming the last individual in the chain to act (e.g., the nurse gives a wrong medication) must be established, and the system must be accepted and used by the entire staff.

Total Quality Management

Total quality management (TQM) is a management philosophy that emphasizes a commitment to excellence throughout the organization. The creation of Dr. W. Edwards Deming, TQM was adopted by the Japanese and helped transform their industrial development after World War II. Dr. Deming based his system on principles of quality management that were originally applied to improve quality and performance in the manufacturing industry. They are now widely used to improve quality and customer satisfaction in a number of service industries, including health care.

TQM Characteristics Four core characteristics of total quality management are

- Customer/client focus,
- Total organizational involvement,

- Use of quality tools and statistics for measurement, and
- Identification of key processes for improvement.

Customer/Client Focus. An important theme of quality management is to address the needs of both internal and external customers. Internal customers include employees and departments within the organization, such as the laboratory, admitting office, and environmental services. External customers of a health care organization include patients, visitors, physicians, managed-care organizations, insurance companies, and regulatory agencies, such as the Joint Commission on Accreditation of Healthcare Organizations (JCAHO) and public health departments.

Under the principles of TQM, the nurse manager must know who the customers are and endeavor to meet their needs. Providing flexible schedules for employees, adjusting routines for A.M. care to meet the needs of patients, extending clinic hours beyond 5 P.M., and putting infant changing tables in restrooms are some health care examples. Putting the customer first requires creative and innovative methods to meet the ever-changing needs of internal and external customers.

Total Organizational Involvement. The goal of quality management is to involve all employees and empower them with the responsibility to make a difference in the quality of service they provide. This means all employees must have knowledge of the TQM philosophy as it relates to their job and the overall goals and mission of the organization. Knowledge of the TQM process breaks down barriers between departments. The phrase "That's not my job" is eliminated. Departments work together as a team. On occasion, nursing personnel might clean a bed for a new admission from the emergency room or a physician might transport a patient to the radiology department.

Use of Quality Tools and Statistics for Measurement. A common management adage is, "You can't manage what you can't (or don't) measure" (Chaiken & Holmquest, 2003). There are many tools, formats, and designs that can be used to build knowledge, make decisions, and improve quality. Tools for data analysis and display can be used to identify areas for process and

KEY TERMS

Total quality management (TQM) A management philosophy that emphasizes a commitment to excellence throughout the organization.

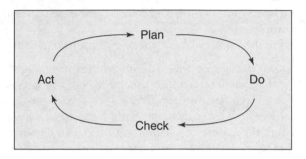

Figure 13-1 **PDCA cycle. From** *Improving Quality Performance,* **by P. Schroeder, 1994, St. Louis: Mosby.**

quality improvement, and then to benchmark the progress of improvements. Deming applied the scientific method to the concept of TQM to develop a model he called the PDCA cycle (Plan, Do, Check, Act) depicted in Figure 13-1.

Identification of Key Processes for Improvement. All activities performed in an organization can be described in terms of processes. Processes within a health care setting can be

- Systems-related (e.g., admitting, discharging, and transferring patients),
- Clinical (e.g., administering medications, managing pain), or
- Managerial (e.g., risk management and performance evaluations).

Processes can be very complex and involve multidisciplinary or interdepartmental actions. Processes involving multiple departments must be investigated in detail by members from each department involved in the activity so that they can proactively seek opportunities to reduce waste and inefficiencies and develop ways to improve performance and promote positive outcomes.

Continuous Quality Improvement

TQM is the overall philosophy, whereas **continuous quality improvement (CQI)** is the process used to improve quality and performance. TQM and CQI often are used synonymously. In health care organizations, CQI is the process used to investigate systematically ways to improve patient care. As the name implies, continuous quality improvement is a never-ending endeavor.

CQI means more than just meeting standards and thresholds or solving problems. It involves evaluation, actions, and a mind-set to strive constantly for excellence. This concept is sometimes difficult to grasp

because patient care involves the synchronization of activities in multiple departments. Therefore, the importance of developing and implementing a well-thought-out process is key to a successful CQI implementation.

There are four major players in the CQI process:

- Resource group
- Coordinator
- Team leader
- Team

The resource group is made up of senior management (e.g., CEO, vice presidents, department directors). It establishes overall CQI policy, vision, and values for the organization and actively involves the board of directors in this process, thereby ensuring that the CQI program has sufficient emphasis and is provided with the training resources needed. The CQI coordinator is often appointed by the CEO to provide day-to-day management of the CQI process and related activities (e.g., training programs).

CQI teams are designated to evaluate and improve select processes. They are formally established and supported by the resource group. CQI teams range in size from 5 to 10 people, representing all major functions of the process being evaluated.

Each CQI team is headed by a team leader who is familiar with the process being evaluated. The leader organizes team meetings, sets the agenda, and guides the group through the discussion, evaluation, and implementation process.

Continuous quality improvement was integrated with patient feedback in one study (Hyrkas & Lehti, 2003). Results revealed that nurses and patients were more satisfied when the evaluations of the quality of their care agreed. The researchers concluded that integrating CQI with team supervision improved the quality of patient care as well.

Components of Quality Management

A comprehensive quality management program includes

- *A comprehensive quality management plan.* A quality management plan is a systematic method to design, measure, assess, and improve organizational performance. Using a multidisciplinary approach, this plan identifies processes and systems that represent the goals and mission of the organization, identifies the customers, and specifies opportunities for improvement. Critical paths, which are described in Chapter 3, are an example of a quality management plan. Critical paths identify expected outcomes within a specific time frame. Then variances are tracked and accounted for.

- *Set standards for benchmarking.* **Standards** are written statements that define a level of performance or a set of conditions determined to be acceptable by some authorities. Standards relate to three major dimensions of quality care:
  - Structure
  - Process
  - Outcome

Structure standards relate to the physical environment, organization, and management of an organization. **Process standards** are those connected with the actual delivery of care. **Outcome standards** involve the end results of care that has been given.

An **indicator** is a tool used to measure the performance of structure, process, and outcome standards. It is measurable, objective, and based on current knowledge. Once indicators are identified, **benchmarking,** or comparing data with other reliable sources internally and externally, is the key to quality improvement.

In nursing, both generic and specific standards are available from the American Nurses Association and specialty organizations; however, each organization and each patient care area must designate standards specific to the patient population being served. These standards are the foundation on which all other measures of quality are based.

An example of a standard is: Every patient will have a written care plan within 12 hours of admission.

- *Performance appraisals.* Based on requirements of the job, employees are evaluated on their performance. This feedback is essential for employees to be professionally accountable. (See Chapter 20 for more on performance appraisals.)
- *A focus on intradisciplinary assessment and improvement.* There will always be a need for groups to assess, analyze, and improve their own performance. Methods to assess performance should, however, focus on the CQI philosophy, which involves group or intradisciplinary performance. Peer review is an example of intradisciplinary assessment. (Peer review is discussed later in the chapter.)
- *A focus on interdisciplinary assessment and improvement.* Multidisciplinary, patient-focused teamwork emphasizing collaboration, communication, coordination, and integration of care is the core of CQI in health care. It is important not to disband departmental quality functions, such as patient satisfaction, utilization review, or infection

control, but rather to refocus information on improving the process.

Resources are used to collect data, such as the number of postoperative infections or the number of return clinic visits, to guide the decision-making process. Throughout the evaluation and implementation process, the team's focus is the patient. Implementation is continually evaluated using a patient satisfaction survey, which is just one of the methods used to monitor nursing care. Other methods include the nursing audit, peer review, and utilization review.

Nursing Audits   A nursing audit can be retrospective or concurrent. A **retrospective audit** is conducted after a patient's discharge and involves examining records of a large number of cases. The patient's entire course of care is evaluated and comparisons made across cases. Recommendations for change can be based on the experiences of many patients with similar care problems as well as on the spectrum of care considered.

A **concurrent audit** is conducted during the patient's course of care; it examines the care being

---

KEY TERMS

Continuous quality improvement (CQI)   The process used to improve quality and performance.

Standards   Written statements that define a level of performance or a set of conditions determined to be acceptable by some authority.

Structure standards   Standards that relate to the physical environment, organization, and management of an organization.

Process standards   Standards connected with the actual delivery of care.

Outcome standards   Standards that reflect the desired result or outcome of care.

Indicator   A tool used to measure the performance of structure, process, and outcome standards.

Benchmarking   The process of comparing data with reliable internal and external sources.

Retrospective audit   A nursing audit conducted after a patient's discharge that involves examining records of a large number of cases.

Concurrent audit   A nursing audit conducted during the patient's course of care.

given to achieve a desired outcome in the patient's health and evaluates the nursing care activities being provided. Changes can be made if patient outcomes so indicate.

Peer Review **Peer review** occurs when practicing nurses determine the standards and criteria that indicate quality care and then assess performance against these. In this case, nurses are the experts at determining what the indicators of quality care are and when such care has been provided. Their expertise is especially useful in complicated cases; sometimes more than one expert's opinion is used for comparisons.

Utilization Review **Utilization reviews** are based on the appropriate allocation of resources and are mandated by the JCAHO. Such a review is not specifically directed toward nursing care, but it may provide information on nursing practices that require further investigation.

Once standards have been set, criteria established, and methods for evaluating adherence to the standards determined, the organization is prepared to examine its risk in relation to its accountability. Risk management programs in health care organizations involve two important areas: patient and/or family incident review, and employee and visitor safety.

Outcomes Management **Outcomes management** is a new technology in which costs and quality are concurrently and retrospectively measured and evaluated in order to improve clinical practice. Internal or external data from the literature or other health care providers are used as benchmarks against which process, quality, and financial goals can be set and achieved. Collaborative practice teams consisting of physicians, nurses, dietitians, pharmacists, social workers, and finance experts develop research-based standardized practice models such as order sets or critical pathways. These models are implemented and patient outcomes measured. The outcomes are statistically analyzed. Care is redesigned based on the outcomes analysis and the new processes implemented. The cycle continues, constantly evaluating whether desired outcomes have been achieved.

Six Sigma

Six Sigma is another quality management program that uses, primarily, quantitative data to monitor progress (Pande & Holpp, 2002). Six Sigma is a *measure*, a *goal*, and a *system of management*.

- *As a measure*. Sigma is the Greek letter—σ—for standard, meaning how much performance varies from a standard. This is similar to how CQI monitors results against an outcome measure.
- *As a goal*. One goal might be accuracy. How many times, for example, is the right medication given in the right amount to the right patient at the right time by the right route?
- *As a management system*. Compared to other quality management systems, Six Sigma involves management to a greater extent in monitoring performance and ensuring favorable results.

The system has six themes:

- Customer (patient) focus
- Data driven
- Process emphasis
- Proactive management
- Boundaryless collaboration
- Aim for perfection; tolerate failure

The first three themes are similar to other quality management programs. The focus is on the object of the service, in nursing's case—the patient. Data provide the evidence of results and the emphasis is on the processes used in the system.

The latter three themes, however, differ from other programs. Management is actively involved and boundaries breached (e.g., the disconnect between departments). More radically, Six Sigma tolerates failure (a necessary condition for creativity) while striving for perfection.

Allowing for Variance and Fostering Innovation

TQM, CQI, and Six Sigma are quantifiable systems that measure performance against set standards. If the organization embraces these systems to a such an extent that all variance is discouraged, then innovation is also suppressed (Harris & Zeisler, 2002). Improvement in the quality of care may have been sacrificed at the expense of innovative ideas and processes. Ultimately, then, organizations fail to allow input, become stagnant, and cease to be effective. This is the danger of all living systems that depend on outside input for survival. This is not to say that quality systems are not essential. They are. Organizations must find ways to foster creativity and innovation without compromising quality management.

Risk Management

Risk management is a program directed toward identifying, evaluating, and taking corrective action against potential risks that could lead to the injury of patients, staff, or visitors. Risk management is problem-focused, whereas quality management is a prevention-focused approach. Risk management is a planned program of loss prevention and liability control. It is a component of a quality program. Its purpose is to identify, analyze, and evaluate risks and then to develop a plan for reducing the frequency and severity of accidents and injuries. Risk management is a continuous daily program of detection, education, and intervention.

A Risk Management Program

A risk management program involves all departments of the organization. It must be an organization-wide program, with the board of directors' approval and input from all departments. The program must have high-level commitment, including that of the chief executive officer and the chief nurse.

A risk management program

1. Identifies potential risks for accident, injury, or financial loss. Formal and informal communication with all organizational departments and inspection of facilities are essential to identifying problem areas.
2. Reviews current organization-wide monitoring systems (incident reports, audits, committee minutes, oral complaints, patient questionnaires), evaluates completeness, and determines additional systems needed to provide the factual data essential for risk management control.
3. Analyzes the frequency, severity, and causes of general categories and specific types of incidents causing injury or adverse outcomes to patients. To plan risk intervention strategies, it is necessary to estimate the possible loss associated with the various types of incidents.
4. Reviews and appraises safety and risk aspects of patient care procedures and new programs.
5. Monitors laws and codes related to patient safety, consent, and care.
6. Eliminates or reduces risks as much as possible.
7. Reviews the work of other committees to determine potential liability and recommend prevention or corrective action. Examples of such committees are infection, medical audit, safety/security, pharmacy, nursing audit, and productivity.
8. Identifies needs for patient, family, and personnel education suggested by all of the foregoing and implementing the appropriate educational program.
9. Evaluates the results of a risk management program.
10. Provides periodic reports to administration, medical staff, and the board of directors.

The establishment of a risk management program starts at the top. The board of directors commits the necessary resources and directs the administrator to establish the program. The administrator then appoints a risk management committee, whose members are responsible for the overall planning and decision making that are involved in risk management. A risk manager should be appointed to manage the day-to-day operation of the program.

Nursing's Role in Risk Management

In the organizational setting, nursing is the one department involved in patient care 24 hours a day; nursing personnel are therefore critical to the success of a risk management program. The chief nursing administrator must be committed to the program. Her or his attitude will influence the staff and their participation. After all, it is the staff, with their daily patient contact, who actually implement a risk management program.

KEY TERMS

Peer review An evaluation by practicing nurses who have determined the standards and criteria that indicate quality care.

Utilization reviews JCAHO-mandated reviews based on the appropriate allocation of resources.

Outcomes management A system in which costs and quality are concurrently and retrospectively measured and evaluated in order to improve clinical practice.

Six Sigma Six Sigma is a quality management program that uses measures, goals, and management involvement to monitor performance and ensure progress.

Risk management A program directed toward identifying, evaluating, and taking corrective action against potential risks that could lead to injury.

 MEDIALINK Health Professions Education: A Bridge to Quality

High-risk areas in health care fall into five general categories:

- Medication errors
- Complications from diagnostic or treatment procedures
- Falls
- Patient or family dissatisfaction with care
- Refusal of treatment or refusal to sign consent for treatment

Nursing is involved in all areas, but the medical staff may be primarily responsible in cases involving refusal of treatment or consent to treatment.

Medical records and incidence reports serve to document organizational, nurse, and physician accountability. For every reported occurrence, however, many more are unreported. If records are faulty, inadequate, or omitted, the organization is more likely to be sued and more likely to lose. **Incident reports** are used to analyze the severity, frequency, and causes of occurrences within the five risk categories. Such analysis serves as a basis for intervention.

Incident Reports Accurate and comprehensive reporting on both the patient's chart and in the incident report is essential to protect the organization and caregivers from litigation. Incident reporting is often the nurse's responsibility. Reluctance to report incidents is usually due to fear of the consequences. This fear can be alleviated by

- Holding staff education programs that emphasize objective reporting,
- Omitting inflammatory words and judgmental statements,
- Having a clear understanding that the purposes of the incident reporting process are documentation and follow-up, and
- Never using the report, under any circumstances, for disciplinary action.

A **reportable incident** should include any unexpected or unplanned occurrence that affects or could potentially affect a patient, family member, or staff. The report is only as effective as the form on which it is reported, so attention should be paid to the adequacy of the form as well as to the data required. Figure 13-2 is a sample incident report form.

Reporting incidents involves the following steps:

1. *Discovery.* Nurses, physicians, patients, families, or any employee or volunteer may report actual or potential risk.

2. *Notification.* The risk manager receives the completed incident form within 24 hours after the incident. A telephone call may be made earlier to hasten follow-up in the event of a major incident.
3. *Investigation.* The risk manager or representative investigates the incident immediately.
4. *Consultation.* The risk manager consults with the referring physician, risk management committee member, or both to obtain additional information and guidance.
5. *Action.* The risk manager should clarify any misinformation to the patient or family, explaining exactly what happened. The patient should be referred to the appropriate source for help and, if needed, be assured that care for any necessary service will be provided free of charge.
6. *Recording.* The risk manager should be sure that all records, including incident reports, follow-up, and actions taken, if any, are filed in a central depository.

Examples of Risk

The following are some examples of actual events in the various risk categories.

Medication Errors A reportable incident occurs when a medication or fluid is omitted, the wrong medication or fluid is administered, or a medication is given to the wrong patient, given at the wrong time, in the wrong dosage, or by the wrong route. Here are some examples.

Patient A. *Weight was transcribed incorrectly from emergency room sheet. Medication dose was calculated on incorrect weight; therefore, patient was given double the dose required. Error discovered after first dose and corrected. Second dose omitted.*

Patient B. *Tegretol dosage written in Medex as "Tegretol 100 mg chewable tab—50 mg po BID." Tegretol 100 mg given po at 1400. Meds checked at 1430 and error noted. 50 mg Tegretol should have been given. Doctor notified. Second dose held.*

KEY TERMS

Incident report An accurate and comprehensive report on unplanned or unexpected occurrences that could potentially affect a patient, family member, or staff.

Reportable incident Any unexpected or unplanned occurrence that affects or could potentially affect a patient, family member, or staff.

Privileged and Confidential

–Not a part of Hospital Record–

Hospital Report of Incident to Counsel

Complete this report in the event of an accident, discovery of a hazardous condition, or any occurrence which is not consistent with the routine operation of the hospital or routine care of a patient.

1. Name:

   Address:

Unit #:

(Use addressograph if available)

2. ☐ Inpatient
   ☐ Outpatient
   ☐ Visitor
   ☐ Employee
   ☐ Other ____

3. Sex
   ☐ M
   ☐ F

4. Age

5. If patient admission date

6. Occurrence information:

   Date: _____ Time: _____ ☐ am ☐ pm

   Location: Bldg. _____ Floor _____

   Room ____

7. Reason for being in hospital: _____

8. Type of occurrence and/or related factors:
   ☐ Fall   ☐ Blood transfusion   ☐ Equipment   ☐ Patient behavior
   ☐ Medication   ☐ Diagnostic procedure   ☐ Communication   ☐ Visitor: faint/fall (Circle one)
   ☐ IV Therapy   ☐ Therapeutic procedure ☐ Support services ☐ Other: _____

9. If fall from bed, siderails position: ☐ One up—full ☐ Two up—full ☐ One up—1/2 ☐ None up
   Bed position: ☐ Locked ☐ Fixed ☐ High ☐ Low

10. Were any of the following medications given in the past four (4) hours: ☐ No   ☐ Yes
    ☐ Sedative ☐ Laxative ☐ Diuretic ☐ Insulin ☐ Narcotic ☐ Other: _____

11. Ambulation privilege:
    ☐ Unlimited   ☐ Limited w/o assistance   ☐ Limited w/assistance   ☐ Bed rest   ☐ Not specified

12. Description of incident (state significant facts in chronological order): _____
    _____
    _____
    _____
    _____

13. Physician of record: _____   Dept.: _____
    R.N. or L.P.N. assigned
    to patient at time of occurrence: _____   N.C./Charge nurse: _____
    Resident (year): _____
    Others present during the time of occurrence:
    Name: _____   Status: _____

14. Pertinent findings by examining physician: _____
    _____

15. Patient/family aware of incident ☐ Yes ☐ No   Examination or follow-up refused ☐ Yes ☐ No

16. Follow-up treatment ☐ Yes ☐ No   X-rays ☐ Yes ☐ No

                        Print last name   Signature   Date
17. Examining physician _____

Reported by _____
Staff member present at time
of incident (if other than above) _____

Figure 13-2 Sample incident report.

Patient C. *During rounds at 3:30 P.M. found .9% sodium chloride at 75 c.c.'s per hour hanging. Order was D5W. Fluids last checked at 2:00 P.M. Changed to correct fluid. Doctor notified.*

Diagnostic Procedure Any incident occurring before, during, or after such procedures as blood sample stick, biopsy, X-ray examination, lumbar puncture, or other invasive procedure is categorized as a diagnostic procedure incident.

Patient A. *When I checked the IV site, I saw that it was red and swollen. For this reason, I discontinued the IV. When removing the tape, I noted a small area of skin breakdown where the tape had been. There was also a small knot on the medial aspect of the left antecubital above the IV insertion site. Doctor notified. Wound dressed.*

Patient B. *Patient found on the floor after lumbar puncture. Right side rail down. Examined by a physician, BP 120/80, T 98.6, P 72, R 18. No injury noted on exam.*

Medical-Legal Incident If a patient or family refuses treatment as ordered and prescribed or refuses to sign consent forms, the situation is categorized as a medical-legal incident.

Patient A. *After a visit from a member of the clergy, patient indicated he was no longer in need of medical attention and asked to be discharged. Physician called. Doctor explained potential side effects if treatment was discontinued. Patient continued to ask for discharge. Doctor explained "against medical advice" (AMA) form. Patient signed AMA form and left at 1300 without medications.*

Patient B. *Patient refused to sign consent for bone marrow biopsy. States side effects not understood. Doctor reviewed reasons for test and side effects three different times. Doctor informed the patient that without consent he could not perform the test. Offered to call in another physician for second opinion. Patient agreed. After doctor left, patient signed consent form.*

Patient or Family Dissatisfaction with Care When a patient or family indicates general dissatisfaction with care and the situation cannot be or has not been resolved, then an incident report is filed.

Patient A. *Mother complained that she had found child saturated with urine every morning (she arrived around 0800). Explained to mother that diapers and linen are changed at 0600 when 0600 feedings*

and meds are given. Patient's back, buttocks, and perineal areas are free of skin breakdown. Parents continue to be distressed. Discussed with primary nurse.

Patient B. *Mr. Smith obviously very angry. Greeted me at the door complaining that his wife had not been treated properly in our emergency room the night before. Wanted to speak to someone from administration. Was unable to reach the administrator on call. Suggested Mr. Smith call administrator in the morning. Mr. Smith thanked me for my time and assured me that he would call the administrator the next day.*

Role of the Nurse Manager

The nurse manager plays a key role in the success of any risk management program. Nurse managers can reduce risk by helping their staff view health and illness from the patient's perspective. Usually, the staff's understanding of quality differs from the patient's expectations and perceptions. By understanding the meaning of the course of illness to the patient and the family, the nurse will manage risk better because that understanding can enable the nurse to individualize patient care. This individualized attention produces respect and, in turn, reduces risk.

A patient incident or a patient's or family's expression of dissatisfaction regarding care indicates not only some slippage in quality of care but also potential liability. A distraught, dissatisfied, complaining patient is a high risk; a satisfied patient or family is a low risk. A risk management or liability control program should therefore emphasize a personal approach. Many claims are filed because of a breakdown in communication between the health care provider and the patient. In many instances, after an incident or bad outcome, a quick visit or call from an organization's representative to the patient or family can soothe tempers and clarify misinformation.

In the examples given, prompt attention and care by the nurse manager protected the patients involved and may have averted a potential liability claim. Once an incident has occurred, the important factors in successful risk management are

- Recognition of the incident,
- Quick follow-up and action,
- Personal contact, and
- Immediate restitution (where appropriate).

It is estimated that 90 percent of patients' concerns can and should be handled at the unit level. When that first line of communication breaks down, however, the nurse manager needs a resource—usually the risk manager or nursing service administrator.

Handling Complaints

Handling a patient's or family member's complaints stemming from an incident can be very difficult. These confrontations are often highly emotional; the patient or family member must be calmed down, yet have their concerns satisfied. Sometimes just an opportunity to release the anger or emotion is all that is needed.

The first step is to listen to the person to hear concerns and to help defuse the situation. Arguing or interrupting only increases the person's anger or emotion. After the patient or family member has had his or her say, the nurse manager can then attempt to solve the problem by asking what is expected in the form of a solution. The nurse manager or other organizational representative should then explain what can and cannot be done and try to negotiate with the injured party an agreement or a solution. It is important to be specific. Offering vague solutions (e.g., "everything will be taken care of") may only lead to more problems later on if expectations as to solution and timing differ.

All incidents must be properly documented. Information on the incident form should be detailed and include all the factors relating to the incident, as demonstrated in the previous examples. The documentation in the chart, however, should be only a statement of the facts and of the patient's physical response; no reference to the incident report should be made, nor should words such as *error* or *inappropriate* be used.

When a patient receives 100 mg of Demerol instead of 50 mg as ordered, the proper documentation in the chart is, "100 mg of Demerol administered. Physician notified." The remainder of the documentation should include any reaction the patient has to the dosage, such as "Patient's vital signs unchanged." If there is an adverse reaction, a follow-up note should be written in the chart, giving an update of the patient's status. A note related to the patient's reaction should be written as frequently as the status changes and should continue until the patient returns to his or her previous status.

The chart must never be used as a tool for disciplinary comments, action, or expressions of anger. Notes such as "Incident would never have occurred if Doctor X had written the correct order in the first place" or "This carelessness is inexcusable" are totally inappropriate and serve no meaningful purpose. Carelessness and incorrect orders do indeed cause errors and incidents, but the place to address and resolve these issues is in the risk management committee or in the nurse manager's office, not on the patient chart.

Handling a complaint without punishing a staff member is a delicate situation. The manager must determine what happened in order to prevent another occurrence, but using an incident report for discipline might result in fewer or erroneous incident reports in the future. Learn how one manager handled a situation of this kind in Case Study 13-1.

CASE STUDY 13-1: Risk Management

Sandy Cannors is the nurse manager for the cardiac catheterization lab and special procedures unit in a suburban hospital. The hospital has an excellent reputation for its cardiac care program, including the use of cutting-edge technology. The cath lab utilizes a specialized computer application that records the case for the nursing staff, requiring little handwritten documentation at the end of a procedure.

Last month, a 56-year-old woman was brought from the ER to the cath lab at approximately 1900 for placement of a stent in her left anterior descending coronary artery. During the procedure, the heart wall was perforated, the patient coded and was taken in critical condition to the OR, where she died during surgery.

Two days following the incident, the patient's husband requested a review of his wife's medical records. During his review, he pointed out to the medical records clerk that the documentation from the cath lab stated that his wife "... tolerated the procedure well and was taken in satisfactory condition to the recovery area." The documentation was

signed, dated, and timed by Elizabeth Clark, RN. The medical records director notified the hospital's risk manager of the error. The risk manager investigated the incident and determined that Elizabeth Clark's charting was in error.

Following her meeting with the risk manager, Sandy met with Elizabeth to discuss the incident. She showed Elizabeth a copy of the cath lab report. Elizabeth asked Sandy if she could have the chart from medical records so she could correct her mistake. Sandy informed Elizabeth that she couldn't correct her charting at this point in time. But, she could, however, write an addendum to the chart, with today's date and time, to clarify the documentation. Sandy also told Elizabeth that the addendum would be reviewed by the risk manager and the hospital's attorney prior to inclusion in the chart.

To ensure compliance with the hospital's documentation standards and to determine if Elizabeth or any other cath lab nurse had committed any similar charting errors, Sandy requested charts for all patients in the past 12 months who had been sent to surgery from the cath lab due to complications during a procedure. She conducted a retrospective audit and determined that this had been an isolated incident.

Manager's Checklist

The nurse manager is responsible for

- Meeting with the risk manager and hospital attorney to review documentation and determine staff to be interviewed regarding an incident,
- Providing any requested information to administration in a timely manner,

- Auditing documentation and processes to determine if an incident is part of a pattern or an isolated incident,
- Providing the results of any audits or discussions with staff to appropriate administrators,
- Educating staff as appropriate,
- Determining if disciplinary action is required,
- Following up with risk management, nursing administration, and human resources as appropriate, and
- Continuing to cooperate with the hospital attorney if the incident results in litigation.

A Caring Attitude

The nurse manager sets the tone with employees that contributes to a safe and low-risk environment. One of the most important ways to reduce risk is to instill a sense of confidence in both patients and families by emphasizing and recognizing that they will receive personalized attention and that their needs will be attended to with competence. This confidence is created environmentally and professionally.

Examples of environmental factors include cleanliness, attention to patients' privacy, an orderly looking unit, and minimal social conversations in front of patients. One example of portraying professional confidence is to provide patients and families with the name of the person in charge. A sincere visit by that person is reassuring. Also, a thorough orientation creates independence for the patient and confidence in an efficient unit.

The nurse manager needs to foster the attitude that any mistake that does occur is perceived as an opportunity to improve a system or a process rather than to punish an individual. If the nurse manager has developed a patient-focused atmosphere in which patients believe their best interests are a priority, the potential for risk will be reduced.

Evaluating Risk Management

Identifying and reducing risks involves close monitoring and analysis of incident reports (see Figure 13-2). Incident reports that include statements of blame should be discussed. A risk management program needs support and participation from all staff. To elicit their commitment, the nurse manager must limit the use of incident reports to risk reduction only. This policy must be emphasized and practiced.

A risk management program requires resources. In times of budget reductions, it may be one of the first

programs to be cut, but the purpose of risk management is to reduce losses; it is a case of spending money to save it. Return on the investment takes time, however, and it is difficult to estimate what might have been lost had risk management activities not been in place. Most organizations are convinced that a risk management program is cost-effective and provides a safer environment for patients, visitors, and employees.

An additional benefit of a risk management program may be an increase in positive attitudes toward the organization from employees, physicians, insurers, and the community. When implemented in a spirit of concern and responsibility, a risk management program can be a visible means of responding to patient needs. Health care organizations, physicians, and nurses have had their share of negative press in the past—sometimes with good reason. The courts, insurance carriers, and legislative action have mandated that organizations respond to patient demands. Risk management helps meet this obligation.

Risk management makes sense. It improves the quality of patient care and reduces liability claims. It represents the outstanding characteristic of health care professionals: care and concern for people. It provides the best care possible at the most reasonable cost.

What You Know Now

- Quality management is the method by which performance of care is evaluated and improved.
- The principles of quality management in health care include a focus on the patient, empowerment of employees, and the collective work of the team.
- A continuous quality improvement program is a prevention-focused approach that provides the basis for managing risk.

- Outcomes management develops research-based models that are implemented, analyzed, and adapted based on identified benchmarks.
- Successful quality management improves patient care, reduces liability, and is cost effective.
- Six Sigma is another quality management program that uses measures, has goals, and is a system of management.
- The key ingredients in a successful risk management program are an organized program of incident reporting, review and follow-up, and most important, an environment that the patient and family perceive as friendly and caring.
- The nurse manager's support of the risk management program is essential to its success.
- Risk management programs help reduce costs and demonstrate the organization's concern for its patients, visitors, and employees.

Tools for Managing and Improving Quality

1. Remember: quality management is a system. When something goes wrong, it is usually a flaw in the system.
2. Become familiar with standards and outcome measures and use them to guide and improve your practice.
3. Strive for perfection but be prepared to tolerate failure in order to encourage innovation.
4. Be sure that performance appraisals and incident reports are not used for discipline but rather are the bases for improvements to the system and/or development of individuals.
5. Remind yourself and your colleagues that a caring attitude is the best preventative of problems.

Questions to Challenge You

1. Do you know what standards and outcome measures are used in the organization where you work or have your clinical experiences? How are the data handled? Are they shared with employees?
2. What comparable groups, both internal and external, are used for benchmarking performance in your organization?
3. Universities also use benchmarking. What institutions does your college or university use to benchmark its performance? Find out.
4. Imagine that an organization is debating among several quality management programs. What would you recommend? Why?
5. Have you, a family member, or a friend ever had a serious problem in a health care organization that resulted in injury? What was the outcome? Is this how you would have handled it? What will you do in the future in a similar situation?

Explore 🌐 MediaLink

NCLEX review questions, essay activities, group activities, and other interactive resources for this chapter can be found on the Web site at http://www.prenhall.com/sullivan-decker. Click on "Chapter 13" to select activities for this chapter.

References

Chaiken, B. P., & Holmquest, D. L. (2003). Patient safety: Modifying processes to eliminate medical errors. *Nursing Outlook, 51*(3), S21–S24.

Harris, S. D., & Zeisler, S. (2002). Weak signals: Detecting the next big thing. *The Futurist, 36*(6), 21–28.

Hyrkas, K., & Lehti, K. (2003). Continuous quality improvement through team supervision supported by continuous self-monitoring of work and systematic patient feedback. *Journal of Nursing Management, 11*(3), 177–188.

Institute of Medicine. (1999). *To err is human: Building a safer health system.* Washington, DC: National Academy Press.

Institute of Medicine. (2003). *Health professions education: A bridge to quality.* Washington, DC: National Academy Press.

Pande, P., & Holpp, L. (2002). *What is Six Sigma?* New York: McGraw-Hill.

Using Health Care Technology Systems

Looking Ahead

Over the past few decades, our society has moved into an age of technologic wizardry. These rapid advances have altered approaches to health care. The applications are endless: Computers can monitor and care for patients, store vast amounts of information, teach and research, and connect people from around the world. This chapter introduces the various health care technology systems that are currently used and offers predictions about the future in technology.

Objectives

In this chapter, you will learn

- How information technology has changed nursing and health care practice.
- How technology can reduce errors and improve efficiency and effectiveness.
- What technology applications are used in patient care.
- Why technology benefits nurses.
- What obstacles to using technology exist.
- What concerns about privacy have emerged with information technology.
- What is predicted for the future of technology in health care.

MediaLink 🌐 **www.prenhall.com/ sullivan-decker**

Additional resources for this chapter can be found on the Companion Website at www.prenhall.com/sullivan-decker. Click on "Chapter 14" to select the activities for this chapter.

- NCLEX Review
- Critical Thinking Activities
- Current Events
- MediaLinks
- *Nursing Leadership & Management in Action:* Letting Technology Work for You; Health Care Technology into the Future

To achieve its goals and maintain efficiency and effectiveness, the organization uses a variety of tools to collect information, analyze data, and make predictions about outcomes. Information technology and its integration with patient care technology has changed forever how health care is delivered, monitored, and evaluated. This chapter provides an overview of technology used in health care and possibilities for the future.

Information Systems

Information systems are complex automated systems that are integrated through networked computers to process data in order to answer questions, solve problems, or make decisions. Information technology can link separate entities into a seamless system of information available to all users, obviating the need for multiple record keeping.

Management Information Systems

A **management information system** (MIS) is a defined set of techniques to capture and collect data, analytical tools, operating policies and procedures, and reporting and communicating protocols that support management decision making. Management information systems generally provide data about an organization's operations, services, employees, and clients.

A **hospital information system** (HIS) is an integrated system used in health care settings to manage patient information. Originally, the HIS was an add-on to the hospital accounting system. Today the HIS is a patient-centered collaborative care delivery framework (Harsanyi, Allan, Anderson, Valo, Fitzpatrick, Schofield, Benjamin, & Simundza, 2000;

see Figure 14-1). The system provides the infrastructure for the patient record and integrates it with information from emerging technologies, initiatives, and health care networks.

The patient record includes admission data, laboratory and X-ray test results, pharmacy orders, billing information, previous services, care planning or critical pathways, and patient acuities. This type of information is shared not only among a number of different departments within a hospital but also with clinics and other health care providers through vast networks.

Recently additional products and innovations have made even better use of information systems. Computerized order entry, pharmacy orders, laboratory services, point-of-care devices (e.g., personal data assistants [PDAs]), and expert systems are being integrated into the health care organization's information system. **Expert systems,** also known as artificial intelligence, offer inference-generated solutions to aid decision makers (Nelson, 2003).

Benefits of Using Information Systems

Information systems are becoming more and more valuable in all business operations and especially so in health care. The demand to reduce mistakes in hospitals and other care settings has grown.

A comprehensive information system can help a health care organization

- Reduce errors,
- Lower costs,
- Speed care,
- Coordinate services and records,
- Improve quality of services,

KEY TERMS

Management information system A defined set of techniques to capture and collect data, analytical tools, operating policies and procedures, and reporting and communicating protocols that support decision making.

Hospital information system An integrated system used in health care settings to manage patient information.

Expert systems Computer programs that provide inference-generated solutions to aid decision makers.

MEDIALINK 🌐 Letting Technology Work for You

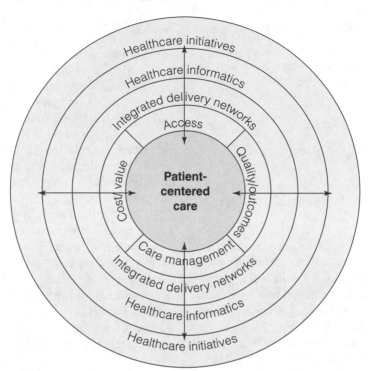

Figure 14-1 **Patient-centered collaborative care delivery framework. From "Healthcare information systems"** **(p. 265), by B. E. Harsanyi, K. C. Allan, J. Anderson, C. R. Valo, J. M. Fitzpatrick, E. A. Schofield, S. Benjamin, and B. W. Simundza, in** ***Nursing Informatics: Where Caring and Technology Meet,*** **3rd ed., by M. J. Ball, K. J. Hannah, S. K. Newbold, and J. V. Douglas (Eds.), 2000, New York: Springer.**

- Increase accuracy, and
- Make nursing more accountable with fewer resources (O'Neil, 2003).

At the same time that information technology has expanded, biomedical technology used to examine, intervene, and monitor patients likewise has grown. Integrating the two into a care management system is the most recent advancement in automation technology (O'Neil, 2003).

Obstacles to Using Information Systems

Although information systems offer many benefits to nursing, there are also a number of obstacles. One is user resistance, including concern about loss of control over practice, depersonalization of care, previous negative experiences, and resistance to change. Time to learn, problems with faulty systems, and cost are also obstacles. As hardware and software continue to improve and become more user friendly, user resistance diminishes somewhat. Also widespread consumer use of computers and the Internet improves user ability and comfort in using the technology.

Technology Applications in Patient Care

Clinical Information Systems

Clinical information systems are used to collect, integrate, and distribute information to the appropriate areas of responsibility. This component of the HIS allows information to be gathered in such a way that it can be manipulated for an infinite number of purposes, such as billing, inventory control, research, scheduling, and planning. The system allows health care providers to have valuable information that is difficult to collect manually in a timely manner.

Nurses use clinical information systems to

- Assess patient acuity and condition,
- Prepare a plan of care or critical path,
- Specify interventions,
- Document care, and
- Track outcomes and quality control.

The clinical information system is a great time saver and efficient tool. Let's say, for example, that gentamicin is ordered for a neonate in the nursery. The order automatically and instantaneously

- Notifies the pharmacy to send the drug,
- Places the medication on the automated medicine record,
- Schedules the time for administration,
- Notifies the laboratory to expect the blood samples,
- Notifies the nurse of the need to draw blood on the neonate at specified times, and
- Sends the appropriate charges for pharmacy, laboratory, and nursing services to the accounting department.

Such a system is not only efficient but also more accurate than any other method that uses multiple entry points.

Nursing Information System A **nursing information system** is a component of the integrated hospital system. It standardizes nursing records across the system, reduces reporting workloads, and improves the quality of patient care (Kurihara, Kusunose, Okabayashi, Nyu, Fujikawa, Miyai, & Okuhara, 2001). Figure 14-2 illustrates a computerized nursing records system (CNRS).

Taxonomy for Nursing One problem nursing continues to experience is how to describe what nurses do, how to measure nursing activities, and how to determine nursing's outcomes. Several efforts have been made to standardize nursing language, including the Nursing Minimum Data Set (NMDS), the North American Nursing Diagnosis Association (NANDA), the Nursing Interventions Classification (NIC), and other systems used for public health and community health nursing.

For outcome information to become standardized across health care, much research is still needed to identify what nursing assessments, diagnoses, and treatments must be included. Until the creation of such a database, data analysis for the purposes of outcomes research will be difficult to perform. Although nursing has not come to consensus as to what should be included, there is general agreement that such a database is urgently needed to measure nursing's effectiveness more broadly.

Monitoring Devices Monitoring devices can be integrated with the clinical information system. They provide surveillance, freeing the nurse from routine, repetitive tasks while providing precise measurements that also alert the nurse to abnormal values. Most devices, especially cardiac and invasive line monitors,

ventilators, and pulse oximeters, for example, have cards that allow data to flow from the device into the clinical system, saving documentation time.

Computerized Physician Order Entry Computerized physician order entry (CPOE) systems are automated systems for physicians to enter orders and access decision support. CPOE systems reduce errors, improve efficiency, and protect patients (Parker, 2003). They were developed in response to the Institute of Medicine's report "To Err is Human" (IOM, 1999) that unleashed an outcry from consumers. The Leapfrog Group, a consortium of large health care purchasers, has targeted CPOE as one of its three safety standards they leverage their purchasing power to encourage hospitals to adopt. The cost of implementation, the newness of the systems, and physician resistance to using the systems continue to make the widespread use of CPOE a challenge (Clinical Advisory Board, 2001).

Point-of-Care Devices Point-of-care devices, such as **personal data assistants** (PDAs) or wireless laptops on movable carts, allow nurses and others to access information, enter orders, monitor patients, and complete record keeping (Sensmeier, Raiford, Taylor, & Weaver, 2003). These devices contain power comparable to desktop and laptop computers and can be integrated with the clinical information system. Nurses at one Visiting Nurse Association report that the time they spent with record keeping was reduced from 3 or 4 hours to 90 minutes when they used PDAs (Houck, 2001).

KEY TERMS

Clinical information systems Systems used to collect, integrate, and distribute information to the appropriate areas of responsibility.

Nursing information system A component of the integrated hospital system that standardizes nursing records across the system.

Computerized physician order entry (CPOE) Automated systems for physicians to enter orders and access decision support.

Personal data assistants (PDAs) Hand-held devices that can be used to access information, enter orders, monitor patients, and complete record keeping.

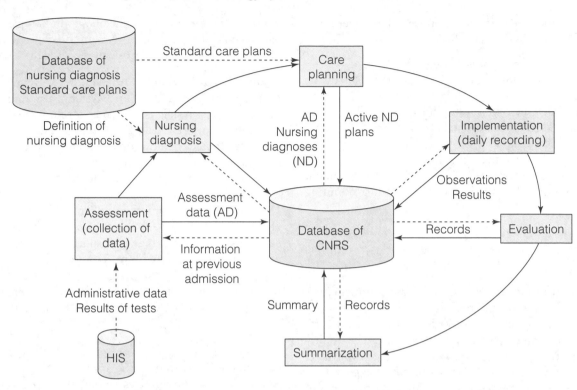

Figure 14-2 The data flow and workflow of a designed CNRS. The full-line and the dash-line arrows indicate registering data into database and referring data from database, respectively. From "Full implementation of a computerized nursing records system at Kochi Medical School Hospital in Japan," by Y. Kurihara, T. Kusunose, Y. Okabayashi, K. Nyu, K. Fujikawa, C. Miyai and Y. Okuhara, 2001, *Computers in Nursing, 19*(3), p. 127.

Patient Care Technologies

Biomedical technologies continue to expand, specifically offering less invasive examinations (e.g., imaging) and interventions (e.g., lasers). In addition, nanotechnology, genetics, replacement organs and tissues, targeted medications, and vaccines are just a few of the many patient care technologies in development or in use today. Sensors that monitor bodily functions as well as the effects of treatments can also monitor room conditions.

Minimally invasive surgery in the operating room has proved to be an advantage to nurses (Perry, 2003). The integration of technology with surgical procedures has resulted in a more egalitarian setting because nurses have their hands on the technology as much as surgeons do. The environment is now more peer-to-peer, according to the author.

Telehealth

Telehealth is the use of telecommunications technology to provide health care at a distance. Medical and nursing care can be delivered using various video, audio, and communications technologies. Radiological, visual, and audio examinations and even telesurgery is now possible (Johnson, 2002). Information can be exchanged between providers and patients in real time or they can communicate by voice mail or e-mail.

Technology in Education and Research

Educational Applications

Distance Learning The earliest use of technology in distance learning occurred through the use of video and/or audio connections. Today distance education is online, using Web-based technology that may include video and audio applications. Most Web-based learning is asynchronous, that is, exchanges do not occur in real time. This is a tremendous advantage to both instructors and students, allowing them to access and respond at their convenience.

With **online instruction,** instructors provide lectures, case studies, and sometimes clinical slides, graphics, or video; monitor discussion; and answer questions.

Students can register for classes, order textbooks and supplementary material, use the library, submit assignments, and take tests, all from a location far from campus. Adult, working students, such as those enrolled in baccalaureate programs for registered nurses and master's degree programs for nurse practitioners, are among those targeted for online instruction.

In addition, other forms of computer-assisted technology can be used to teach nurses, students, patients, or their families essential information about their conditions, treatments, and their care. This technology uses CD-ROMs, the Internet, or Web-based kiosks and typically involves tutorials or simulations, allowing individuals to interact with the system at their own pace. Other applications useful in education are graphics packages that allow the use of clip, live, or graphic art to develop figures; and presentation packages, such as PowerPoint, to develop slides and overheads.

Simulation   The increasing sophistication of simulators to mimic human conditions and responses are revolutionizing clinical education. Simulators allow students to practice on computerized models, repeating techniques as often as necessary without jeopardizing live patients.

A teaching-simulation program has been developed at the University of Kansas in collaboration with a provider of hospital information systems, the Cerner Corporation. Called the Simulated E-health Delivery System (SEEDS), the program uses a live-production, clinical information system based on best practices in education (Connors, Weaver, Warren, & Miller, 2002).

Use in Research

Computerized literature searches have radically changed the time involved in searching the literature for research studies. Whatever is not available online is often available for purchase as a download or a document that can be mailed or faxed. Databases make subject selection accurate and rapid, and contact with subjects can sometimes be accomplished by e-mail. Statistical packages speed analysis of data.

Consumer Health Information

With the expansion of the Internet and the accompanying growth of computer hardware and software as well as communications technology, consumers can easily access unprecedented amounts of information about any subject of interest, including health information. The accuracy of the information is, however,

unknown, and consumers may be unable to interpret information correctly. Nevertheless it is common today to have an informed consumer who is able, at the least, to pose pointed questions.

The paternalistic system of the past is fast disappearing as consumers become partners in their care. All health care professionals are challenged to be as current regarding the latest information as their patients are likely to be cognizant of research results. Providers must be prepared to collaborate with their patients in care decisions.

Privacy Considerations

Malicious intruders such as viruses, worms, and logic or time bombs are threats to the automation and integration of patient records into wide area networks. These threats have provoked a number of concerns: How can integrity of the data be maintained? Can more than one individual access the record at the same time? Who maintains ownership of the record? Who is responsible for information in transit? Many of these questions have yet to be answered; however, a secure system should have the following characteristics:

- Allow only authorized users
- Limit access based on the need to know
- Ensure security at each access point

The Health Information Portability and Accountability Act of 1996 (HIPAA) demands more rigorous standards of privacy of patient medical information than earlier regulations required. Computerized records are no exception; in fact, they are at greater risk of exposure due to multiple users, password exposure, and computer hackers. Health care organizations must guard against unauthorized access of records under penalty of federal law. In addition, staff need to be trained not to give out passwords or leave unattended a computer that has been logged on.

KEY TERMS

Telehealth   The use of network technology to provide medical, nursing, and other health care through electronic linkages.

Online instruction   A method of instruction that uses the Internet for teaching and learning. It is the fastest-growing method of distance education.

Although most attention has been given to protecting patient records, ensuring the privacy of student records is also essential. Similarly the records of subjects participating in research must remain confidential.

The Nurse Informatics Specialist

Nursing informatics focuses on the processes of nursing information rather than the substance of nursing (American Nurses Association, 2001). Nursing informatics is a growing specialty, combining clinical knowledge and skills with informatics expertise. Nursing informatics supports the work of nurses by integrating science with technology and also supports the work of nurse educators, researchers, and administrators. Several universities offer advanced degrees in nursing informatics.

The Nurse Manager's Role

The nurse manager's responsibilities vis-à-vis technology include helping select a system or system redesign, implementing a system, preparing and training staff for information technology or patient care technology, and monitoring performance and effectiveness of the technology and systems in use. The steps to adopt a new technical system are similar to the nursing process, as shown in Table 14-1. The manager's belief in the value of the new technology can help the staff accept the difficult, and sometimes frustrating, process of learning how to use it. Remind staff that the technologies that make their work easier today were once awkward to learn and that learning requires persistence and patience to yield results they desire, such as rapid access to accurate information.

Table 14-1 Similarities of System Development Process with the Nursing Process

Nursing Process	System Development Process
Assess	Analyze needs
Plan	Design system
	Train staff
Implement	Test simulated system
	Implement integrated system
Evaluate	Evaluate performance and outcomes

Future Trends in Health Care Technology

Technology advances will continue into the future, offering heretofore unknown solutions as well as problems. Voice-input interfaces, virtual reality, robotics, bar codes, and augmented technology (computers embedded in a variety of products) are a few examples of future expectations (Turley, 2000).

Just as the model T began the automobile age so have computers initiated the technology age. Similarly it is no more possible for people today to imagine the future of technology than it was for our long-ago relatives early in the 20th century to imagine what automobiles would do. Although we may not be able to envision what lies ahead, what we do know is that technology will continue to be essential in our lives and practice.

What You Know Now

- Information technology helps nurses to care for patients, manage information and records, teach, perform research, and communicate.
- Technology applications include clinical information systems, patient care technologies, and telehealth.
- Clinical information systems can be integrated with patient care technologies to make nurses' work more accurate and efficient.
- Although nursing outcomes can be compared across a system that uses standardized measures, nursing outcomes and effectiveness cannot be determined until a standardized database is available for use across the expanse of health care.
- Knowledgeable consumers are becoming partners with their health care providers.
- Confidentiality and security are major concerns associated with automated patient records.
- The nurse manager may be involved in selecting technology, preparing staff in its use, and monitoring the effectiveness of the technology.
- Advances in technology and information systems can be anticipated well into the future.

Tools for Using Health Care Technology Systems

1. Become familiar with the clinical information system used in your facility.
2. Take advantage of every opportunity to update and upgrade your skills to use technology.

3. Keep up to date on clinical research in your field; your patients surely are.

4. Maintain strict adherence to privacy standards and regulations.

5. Welcome the future of technology.

Questions to Challenge You

1. What experiences have you had using information systems? What were the problems? Benefits?

2. What patient care technologies connect with information systems in your experience? Are they reliable? Explain. Hint: patient monitors.

3. What obstacles have you seen in using technology? Describe how those could be overcome.

4. How have privacy regulations affected how you or your organization does its work? Are you/they successful in adhering to the law?

Explore 🌐 MediaLink

NCLEX review questions, essay activities, group activities, and other interactive resources for this chapter can be found on the Web site at http://www.prenhall.com/sullivan-decker. Click on "Chapter 14" to select activities for this chapter.

References

American Nurses Association. (2001). *The scope and standards of nursing informatics practice.* Washington, DC: Author.

Clinical Advisory Board. (2001). *Computerized physician order entry: Lessons from pioneering institutions.* Washington, DC: Author.

Connors, H. R., Weaver, C., Warren, J., & Miller, K. L. (2002). An academic-business partnership for advancing clinical informatics. *Nursing Education Perspectives, 23*(5), 228–233.

Harsanyi, B. E., Allan, K. C., Anderson, J., Valo, C. R., Fitzpatrick, J. M., Schofield, E. A., Benjamin, S., & Simundza, B. W. (2000). Healthcare information systems (pp. 264–283). In M. J. Ball, K. J. Hannah, S. K. Newbold, & J. V. Douglas (Eds.), *Nursing informatics: Where caring and technology meet* (3rd ed., pp. 264–283). New York: Springer.

Houck, J. B. (2001). PDAs—stat—for busy nurses. Retrieved October 10, 2003, from http://www.wirelessnewsfactor.com

Institute of Medicine. (1999). *To err is human: Building a safer health system.* Washington, DC: National Academy Press.

Johnson, D. (2002). Technology: The telesurgery revolution. *The Futurist, 36*(1), 6–7.

Kurihara, Y., Kusunose, T., Okabayashi, Y., Nyu, K., Fujikawa, K., Miyai, C., & Okuhara, Y. (2001). Full implementation of a computerized nursing records system at Kochi Medical School Hospital in Japan. *Computers in Nursing, 19*(3), 122–129.

Nelson, A. (2003). Using simulation to design and integrate technology for safer and more efficient practice environments. *Nursing Outlook, 51*(3), S27–S29.

O'Neil, E. (2003). A strategic workforce framework for considering the use of technology to address the current and future shortage of nurses. *Nursing Outlook, 51*(3), S2–S4.

Parker, P. J. (2003). Computerized order entry goes beyond safety net. *Nursing Management, 34*(2), 45–46.

Perry, G. (2003). Nurses in the new OR. *Excellence in Clinical Practice, 4*(3), Retrieved October 10, 2003, from http://www.nursingsociety.org/publications

Sensmeier, J., Raiford, R., Taylor, S., & Weaver, C. (2003). Improved operational efficiency through elimination of waste and redundancy. *Nursing Outlook, 51*(3), S30–S32.

Turley, J. P. (2000). Nursing future: Ubiquitous computing, virtual reality and augmented reality. In M. J. Ball, K. J. Hannah, S. K. Newbold, & J. V. Douglas (Eds.), *Nursing informatics: Where caring and technology meet* (3rd ed., pp. 305–328). New York: Springer.

Managing Stress and Time

The Nature of Stress

Causes of Stress
Role Conflict and Role Ambiguity
Consequences of Stress

Managing Stress

Personal Methods
Organizational Methods

Time Management

Goal Setting
Delegation
Time Analysis
Setting Priorities
Daily Planning and Scheduling
Grouping Activities and
    Minimizing Routine Work
Implementation
Personal Organization
    and Self-Discipline
Controlling Interruptions
Paperwork
Respecting Time

Looking Ahead

Do you ever feel as if there aren't enough
hours in a day for the work you need to do?

We all know how it feels to be stressed and not
have enough time to get things done. How do
we deal with the constant demands of our
environment? Learning to cope with stress and
manage time wisely is important to becoming
an effective leader and manager. This chapter
contains proven strategies to help you identify
and manage stress so you can plan and accomplish the endless number of tasks and goals
you want to accomplish.

Objectives

In this chapter, you will learn

- What factors cause stress.
- What consequences result from stress.
- How stress can be managed by personal
  and organizational methods.
- How to identify goals and set priorities.
- How to identify time wasters and minimize
  them.

MediaLink www.prenhall.com/ sullivan-decker

Additional resources for this chapter can be found
on the Companion Website at www.prenhall.com/
sullivan-decker. Click on "Chapter 15" to select the
activities for this chapter.

- NCLEX Review
- Critical Thinking Activities
- Current Events
- MediaLinks

- *Nursing Leadership & Management in Action:* Reducing Organizational Stress; Recognizing Time Wasters

Consider the following scenario. Keandra is a medical nurse with 10 years of experience. She is married and has two children under the age of six who attend preschool while Keandra is at work. As a nurse manager, Keandra has 24-hour responsibility for supervision of two 30-bed medical units. She frequently receives calls from the unit nurses during the evenings and nights, and approximately once a week she has to return to the unit to intervene in a situation or to replace nurses who are absent. Keandra is responsible for scheduling all nurses on her unit and has no approval to use agency nurses, in spite of a 20 percent vacancy rate. In addition, Keandra serves on four departmental committees and the hospital task force on consumer relations. She consistently takes work home, including performance appraisals, quality assessment reports, and professional journals. Although provided with an office, Keandra has little opportunity to use it because of constant interruptions from nurses, physicians, other departmental leaders, and her clinical director. Recently, Keandra saw her family physician, complaining of persistent headaches, weight loss, and a feeling of constant fatigue. After a complete diagnostic workup, Keandra was found to have a slightly elevated blood pressure, with a resting pulse of 100. Her physician prescribed an exercise program, and she was advised to lighten her workload, take a vacation, and reduce her stress level.

Steers (1991) defines **stress** as the nonspecific reaction that people have to demands that pose a threat from the environment. Stress results when two or more incompatible demands on the body cause a conflict. Selye (1978), recognized as the pioneer of stress research, suggests that the body's wear and tear results from its response to normal stressors. The rate and intensity of damage increase when an organism experiences greater stress than it is capable of accommodating.

Selye maintains that the physiological response to stress is the same whether the stressor is positive, *enstress*, or negative, *distress*. It is easy to see how negative events, such as job loss, can cause stress. However, positive events also may cause stress.

Anthony was the director of nursing for critical care in a 400-bed hospital. He was offered the opportunity to develop a hyperbaric unit. In assuming the additional responsibility, Anthony began putting in long hours and working weekends. As the project progressed, Anthony became unable to sleep and gained 10 pounds. After the unit opened, Anthony's sleep pattern and weight returned to normal. Clearly, Anthony displayed emotional and physical signs of stress although he was experiencing a "positive" promotion and career opportunity.

A certain amount of stress is essential to sustain life, and moderate amounts serve as stimuli to performance, but overpowering stress can cause a person to respond in a maladaptive physiological or psychological manner.

This chapter describes the causes and consequences of stress and proposes several techniques for managing stress. In addition, the chapter provides guidelines to help you use time effectively.

The Nature of Stress

A balance must exist between stress and the capability to handle it. When the degree of stress is equal to the degree of ability to accommodate it, the organism is in a state of equilibrium. Normal wear and tear occur, but sustained damage does not. When the degree of stress is greater than the available coping mechanism, the individual experiences negative aspects of stress. The situation is often described metaphorically through such statements as "carrying a load on one's shoulders" or "bearing a heavy burden." This often leads to physiological and psychological problems for the person and poor performance for the organization. When the degree of stress is not stimulating enough, lack of interest, apathy, boredom, low motivation, and even poor performance can result.

The experience of stress is subjective and individualized. One person's stressful event is another's challenge. One individual can experience an event, positive or negative, that would prove overwhelming for someone else. Even a minor change in organizational policy may cause some individuals to experience stress, whereas others welcome it. Some nurses seem to thrive on the demands of work, family, school, and community involvement, whereas others find even minimal changes in their expectations a source of great discomfort. In the current health care environment, where constant change is the norm, some nurse managers may choose a less demanding position because they find the stress level too high in their current position.

For nurses, stress in the workplace can develop from several sources and may be due to organizational, interpersonal, or individual (intrapersonal) factors.

KEY TERMS

Stress The nonspecific reaction that people have to threatening demands from the environment.

Causes of Stress

Organizational Factors Stress can result from job-related factors, such as task overload, conflicting tasks, inability to do the tasks assigned because of lack of preparation or experience, and unclear or insufficient information regarding the assignment. Nurses' jobs are often performed in life-or-death situations; emergencies may cause periods of extreme overload.

The physical environment may also be stressful. Consider the intensive care unit with its constant alarms, beeps, and other noises. Besides noise levels, lighting and other comfort factors may increase stress within the environment. Tight quarters, poorly organized work environments, and lack of equipment also augment stress levels.

The manager's behavior also can be a factor in stress. Authoritarian or punitive supervisory behavior is closely related to stress levels. Participative management, in contrast, can reduce job stress.

Other organizational factors that can lead to stress include organizational norms and expectations that conflict with an individual's needs. Managers trying to do more with less, overworked staff, and more acutely ill patients can lead to an organizational environment that by its very nature is stressful.

Managed care, cost containment, the creation of integrated organizations, and downsizing are creating dramatic changes in health care that are contributing to stress in nursing. New technology, increased expectations from patients and their families, liability concerns, and competition among health care providers (and the increased pressures for efficiency that are associated with it) have made the role of nurses more difficult, conflicting, and stressful.

Interpersonal Factors To add to the pressures created by organizational changes, nurses must contend with strained interpersonal relationships within the nursing profession and between nursing and other professions (e.g., medicine, administration). Relationships are strained even further as pressures mount. Shorter lengths of stay for patients, supervision of assistive personnel, job redesign, and case management challenge relationships among nursing care providers.

Interdisciplinary difficulties may precipitate tension. For example, in one rehabilitation setting, therapists expect the patients to be bathed, to have eaten breakfast, and to be dressed and ready to start therapy by 8:30 A.M. This expectation places undue stress on rehabilitation nurses, who must motivate patients who complain that they have had far too little sleep.

Another example of stress due to interdisciplinary conflict is: A radiology technician responds to a 9:00 P.M. page for a chest x-ray examination and informs the registered nurse that the patient will have to be brought back down because the radiology department is understaffed.

Interactions between physicians and nurses often are not characterized by open communication. Most nurses have experienced an irate response from a physician who is awakened during the night for something the physician thinks should have been handled earlier or might have waited until morning. In one small community hospital, an internist was well known for his outbursts during middle-of-the-night calls. One experienced nurse dealt with necessary calls to him by directly stating when he answered the phone, "This is Jane Jones from St. Matthew's. I have two important things to tell you about Mrs. Smith...." This helped the internist focus on the problem at hand and reduced his outbursts.

The need to fulfill multiple roles is another source of stress. A **role** is a set of expectations about behavior ascribed to a specific position in society (e.g., nurse, spouse, parent). Conflict between family roles and professional ones results in stress. Adding to stress is the shift and weekend work required in nursing jobs in hospitals that must be staffed 24 hours a day, 7 days a week. Nurses who work on evening or night shifts may experience family problems if their spouse and children are on different schedules, especially if the nurse rotates shifts. It takes several weeks to adjust physiologically to a change in shifts, however, most rotation patterns require nurses to change shifts several times a month. Managers can reduce the physiological pressure through ensuring that nurses receive adequate rest and work breaks, rotating staff only between two shifts, and never scheduling "double backs" (working 8 hours, off 8 hours, working 8 hours).

Individual Factors Stress can result from personal factors as well. One of these factors is the rate of life change. Changes throughout life, such as marriage, pregnancy, or purchasing a new home, generate stress. Each individual responds to stress differently, but the cumulative effects of stress often lead to the onset of disease or illness. The ways people interpret events ultimately determine whether the person sees the event as stressful or as a positive challenge.

Deficiency focusing is the habit of focusing on the negatives at the expense of the positives. There is a tendency to exaggerate weaknesses and disregard strengths. Deficiency focusing can lead to an increased sense of threat and a diminished sense of optimism, immobilizing individuals and limiting their ability to solve problems. They become so overwhelmed with what might go wrong that they don't look at options and opportunities that also are present.

As resources in health care continue to shrink, nurses are being asked or told to assume responsibility for tasks that had been performed by other departments (e.g., phlebotomy, electrocardiography, respiratory therapy). Nurses can see these responsibilities as an overwhelming amount of work that can't possibly be accomplished given the existing number of staff or as work that is not appropriate for nurses to do. But if nurses approach the task as a means to improve continuity of care or deliver patient-focused care, they can focus energy on skills in which nurses excel: managing patient care.

Necessitating is the belief that it is imperative or necessary that a particular task be done by a specific person; it is a belief structure that limits choice. Tasks become inflexible demands that must be met. Nurses are especially prone to this type of thinking. Many nurse managers continue to believe that it is necessary to be as clinically competent as their staff. There are many tasks that nursing staff believe only nurses can do. Then, as patient care loads become heavier, their stress level increases.

Nurse managers must begin to question old ways of thinking and to evaluate what tasks should belong to the nursing profession in the future. Core competencies for nurse managers include a different set of managerial skills (e.g., facilitation, negotiation, team building), not excelling at clinical skills. By continually questioning whether the usual activity continues to be appropriate, both the manager and members of the staff can reduce stress.

Low skill recognition is perhaps the least stress-producing of the three habits but may be the one that needs the most attention in an unstable and unpredictable environment. Low skill recognition is a tendency not to recognize the role one's own ability has played in producing one's successes; it affects both managers and staff nurses when they face something unfamiliar.

New graduates, for example, often do not recognize that they have demonstrated a definitive set of skills and knowledge in having passed all the requirements to become a registered nurse. The stress they experience when changing from the student role to the professional practitioner role has been labeled **reality shock**. It is the surprise and disequilibrium experienced when moving from the familiar school culture to the work culture, where values, rewards, and sanctions are different and often seem illogical.

Moving from a staff nurse position to a management position also creates surprise and disequilibrium. The reward structure is totally different for managers. New managers often experience a sense of isolation from the peer group of staff nurses who previously provided support. In each of these cases, the individual often questions her or his abilities to make the transition to the new role. Therefore, low skill recognition is not to be overlooked as a key element in developing stress resiliency.

Stress can also result from incongruence between one's expectations for performance and one's perception of the resulting performance (**intrarole conflict**). Similarly, conflict between the roles of nurse manager and nurse can be a source of stress (**interrole conflict**). Doing a job and directing others to do the job are different. Directing others is stressful, and a person may be tempted to believe that it will be faster to complete a task by doing it herself or himself.

KEY TERMS

Role   A set of expectations about behavior ascribed to a specific position.

Deficiency focusing   The habit of focusing on the negatives at the expense of the positives.

Necessitating   The belief that it is imperative or necessary that a particular task be done by a specific person.

Low skill recognition   The tendency not to recognize the role one's own ability has played in producing one's successes.

Reality shock   The stress, surprise, and disequilibrium experienced when shifting from a familiar culture into one whose values, rewards, and sanctions are different (e.g., from school culture to work culture).

Intrarole conflict   Conflict resulting from incongruence between one's expectations for performance and one's perception of the resulting performance.

Interrole conflict   Conflict resulting from incongruence between the different roles an individual might play, such as doing a job and directing others to do the job.

MediaLink ⊕ National Institute for Occupational Safety and Health

Past experience in coping with stress provides insight into an individual's ability for successful coping in current experiences. People tend to repeat coping behaviors in similar situations, regardless of whether the initial behavior reduced stress.

One's self-esteem also affects coping. Individuals with low self-esteem often have difficulty coping with role conflict and role ambiguity. **Role ambiguity** results from unclear expectations for one's performance. Individuals with high tolerances for ambiguity can deal better with the strains that come from uncertainties and, therefore, are likely to be able to cope with role ambiguity.

Certain personality traits either positively or negatively influence one's responses to stress. Individuals who believe that their life is controlled largely by events external to themselves often perceive less stress and are less likely to react negatively to surrounding events. However, those who perceive factors as being internal react more negatively to situations that are beyond their control. They are more likely to be proactive to situations within their control and engage in positive coping behaviors to change the environment and reduce stresses on themselves.

Role Conflict and Role Ambiguity

Role conflicts occur when an individual has two competing roles, such as when a nurse manager both assumes a patient care assignment and needs to attend a leadership meeting. Another example is the conflict between nurses' personal roles as parents or spouses versus their roles as professional nurses.

Individual role conflict is the result of incompatibility between the individual's perception of the role and its actual requirements. Novice nurse managers experience this type of conflict when they find that administration expects primary loyalty to the organization and its goals, whereas the staff expects the nurse manager's first loyalty to be to their needs.

Role conflict within the profession places nursing at a distinct disadvantage in its relationship with other health care workers. Strife within the profession, differences in educational preparation, the structure of practice settings, and the role of labor and professional organizations contribute to the environment in which nurses must function. This conflict has its roots in a perceived poor regard for nurses. The felt lack of worth is complicated by divisiveness within the profession and the image nursing presents to others.

Role underload and *underutilization* can also occur. Being underutilized or not having much responsibility may be seen as stressful by a person who is a high achiever or who has high self-esteem.

Consequences of Stress

What happens to a person when stress overload occurs? Both physiological and psychological responses can cause structural or functional changes or both. Warning signs of too much stress are

- Undue, prolonged anxiety, phobias, or a persistent state of fear or free-floating anxiety that seems to have many alternating causes;
- Depression, which causes people to withdraw from family and friends, to be unable to experience emotions, and to feel helpless to change the situation;
- Abrupt changes in mood and behavior, which may be exhibited as erratic behavior;
- Perfectionism, which is the setting of unreasonably high standards for oneself and thereby being under constant stress; and
- Physical illnesses, such as an ulcer, arthritis, colitis, hypertension, myocardial infarction, and migraine headaches.

Ineffective coping methods for reducing stress include excessive use of alcohol and other mood-altering substances, which can result in substance abuse or dependence. Some people become workaholics in an attempt to cope with real or imagined demands.

The term **burnout** refers to the perception that an individual has used up all available energy to perform the job and feels that he or she doesn't have enough energy to complete the task. Burnout is a combination of physical fatigue, emotional exhaustion, and cognitive weariness. As a result, the individual may reduce hours worked or change to another profession. One director of nursing at a 120-bed nursing home stated that she could no longer handle the overwhelming needs of the patients; the ever-present shortage of qualified, caring nurses; and consistently dwindling resources. When a for-profit chain purchased the home and further reduced economic resources, the director of nursing left to become a real estate agent.

The results of employee stress are increased absenteeism and turnover. Although there are various causes of absenteeism (see Chapter 23) and turnover (see Chapter 22), both may result when the individual attempts to withdraw from a stressful situation.

Job performance suffers during times of high stress, so much energy and attention are needed to manage the stress that little energy is available for performance.

MEDIALINK ☙ Burnout

Such a situation is financially costly in industry but even more costly in human health and well-being.

Managing Stress

We will always have factors in our lives that create stress. To manage those factors effectively and keep stress at levels that enhance one's performance rather than deplete energy, the key is to develop some resiliency. To accomplish this requires a comprehensive approach to managing stress, which involves planning, time, and energy.

Personal Methods

One of the first steps in managing stress is to recognize stressors in the environment and control them. Nurses tend to think they can be "all things to all people." Therefore, it is important to improve one's self-awareness regarding stressors.

Caring for yourself physically (e.g., eating a well-balanced diet, exercising regularly, getting adequate sleep) and developing effective mental habits are also important for coping with stress. These effective habits include role redefinition, improved time-management techniques, and relaxation. Development of interpersonal skills and identifying and nurturing social supports can also facilitate stress management.

Role redefinition involves clarifying roles and attempting to integrate or tie together the various roles individuals play. If there is role conflict or ambiguity, it is important to confront others by pointing out conflicting messages. Role redefinition may also involve renegotiation of roles in an attempt to lessen overload.

Much of the stress nurse managers experience results from the perception that staff, patient, and work-group needs must be met immediately and simultaneously. A common feeling is the need to slow down or "get off the train." A notable method of coping with and reducing the stress of time is through time management. We determine how, where, and when our time is used. Time is the essence of living, and it is the scarcest resource. Because the nurse manager has a limited amount of time, it is essential that time be used expeditiously. One lost hour a day every day for a year results in 260 hours of waste, or 6.5 weeks of missed opportunity, annually. (Time management is discussed later in the chapter.)

It also is important to use positive self-talk and to learn how to relax. This is not easy, especially for an individual with a high-stress job. Some relaxation methods are listening to music, reading, and socializing with friends. Developing outside interests, such as hob-bies and recreational activities, can provide diversion and enjoyment and also can be a source of relaxation. Taking regular vacations, regardless of job pressures, is important for renewal and revitalization.

Organizational Methods

Nurse managers are often in the position of helping others identify their level of stress and stressors. If staff appear to be under a great deal of stress, the manager must help identify the source and decide how these can be reduced or eliminated. In addition to suggesting the techniques previously delineated, the manager should explore work-related sources of stress.

The manager must ask these questions:

- Is role ambiguity or conflict creating the stress?
- Can the manager help clarify individual staff members' roles, thereby reducing the conflict or ambiguity?
- Is the manager using an appropriate leadership style? (See Chapter 4.)
- Does the manager need to clarify a staff member's goals and eliminate barriers that are interfering with goal attainment? Involving staff in decision making is one way to identify and reduce such stress.
- Is the stress due to feelings of low self-worth?
- Would additional training or education help reduce the stress?
- Can I help by recognizing and reinforcing positive behaviors and accomplishments?
- Can other sources of support, such as the work group, help the individual deal with stress?
- Are counseling services available in the organization?

When stress is job-related, several strategies can be used. First, proper matching of the job with the applicant during the selection and hiring process is an important step in reducing stress (see Chapter 18). Skills training

MediaLink How to Deal with Stress

KEY TERMS

Role ambiguity The frustrations that result from unclear expectations for one's performance.

Burnout The perception that an individual has used up all available energy to perform the job and feels that he or she doesn't have enough energy to complete the task.

Role redefinition The clarification of roles and an attempt to integrate or tie together the various roles individuals play.

also reduces stress and promotes better performance and less turnover (see Chapter 22). Developing a program of job enrichment matched to the individual's goals and desires often increases autonomy and participation. In turn, greater participation in decisions increases job commitment and reduces stress.

Communication and social support are additional factors in reducing stress. Both upward and downward communication channels should be open. Keeping personnel informed about what is going on in an organization helps reduce suspicion and rumor. Team building encourages staff to build a network of support with each other.

Policies that reduce the stress of shift work also are important. The number of hours in the night shift, weekend, and holiday work assignments also can reduce stress. Providing adequate opportunities for breaks and meals is an important function of the organization. (See Chapter 23 for more about how to help employees with stress-related problems.)

Time Management

Time management is a misnomer. No one manages time: What is managed is how time is used. Box 15-1 shows some of the constraints on an individual's ability to manage time effectively. These patterns of behavior must be understood and dealt with to achieve effective time management.

In addition to these patterns of behavior, certain time wasters prevent the nurse manager from effectively managing time. A **time waster** is something that prevents a person from accomplishing the job or achieving the goal. Common time wasters include

1. Interruptions, such as telephone calls and drop-in visitors;
2. Meetings, both scheduled and unscheduled;
3. Lack of clear-cut goals, objectives, and priorities;
4. Lack of daily and/or weekly plans;
5. Lack of personal organization and self-discipline;
6. Lack of knowledge about how one spends one's time;
7. Failure to delegate, working on routine tasks;
8. Ineffective communication;
9. Waiting for others, not using transition time effectively; and
10. Inability to say no.

Techniques to deal with these time-management constraints and time wasters are discussed in detail later in the chapter.

Goal Setting

Nurses are accustomed to setting both long- and short-range goals, although typically such goals are stated in terms of what patients will accomplish

---

Box 15-1   Potential Constraints on the Ability to Manage Time Effectively

- We do what we like to do before we do what we don't like to do.
- We do things we know how to do faster than things we do not know how to do.
- We do things that are easiest before things that are difficult.
- We do things that require a little time before things that require a lot of time.
- We do things for which resources are available.
- We do things that are scheduled (for example, meetings) before nonscheduled things.
- We sometimes do things that are planned before things that are unplanned.
- We respond to demands from others before demands from ourselves.
- We do things that are urgent before things that are important.

- We readily respond to crises and emergencies.
- We do interesting things before uninteresting things.
- We do things that advance our personal objectives or that are politically expedient.
- We wait until a deadline approaches before we really get moving.
- We do things that provide the most immediate closure.
- We respond on the basis of who wants it.
- We respond on the basis of the consequences to us of doing or not doing something.
- We tackle small jobs before large jobs.
- We work on things in the order of their arrival.
- We work on the basis of the squeaky-wheel principle (the squeaky wheel gets the grease).
- We work on the basis of consequences to the group.

rather than what the nurse will achieve. A critical component of time management is establishing one's own goals and time frames. **Goals** provide direction and vision for actions as well as a timeline in which activities will be accomplished. Defining goals and time frames helps reduce stress by preventing the panic people often feel when confronted with multiple demands. Although time frames may not be as fast as the nurse manager would like (the tendency is to expect change yesterday), necessary actions have been identified.

Individual or organizational goals encourage thinking about the future and what might happen. **Goal setting** helps to relate current behavior, activities, or operations to the organization's or individual's long-range goals. Without this future orientation, activities may not lead to the outcomes that will help achieve the goals and meet the ideals of the individual or organization. The focus should be to develop measurable, realistic, and achievable goals. Specific goal setting is discussed more extensively in Chapter 19.

It is useful to think of individual or personal goals in categories, such as

- Department or unit,
- Interpersonal (at work),
- Professional,
- Financial,
- Family and friends (outside of work),
- Vacation and travel,
- Physical,
- Lifestyle,
- Community, and
- Spiritual.

This partial listing is a guide to stimulate thinking about goals. In considering individual goals, nurses should think about long-term goals, lifetime goals, and short-term goals. These should be divided into job-related goals and personal goals. Job-related goals may revolve around unit or departmental changes, whereas personal goals may include personal life and community involvement.

Short-term goals should be set for the next 6 to 12 months but need to be related to long-term goals. To manage time effectively, the nurse manager must answer five major questions about these goals:

1. What specific objectives are to be achieved?
2. What specific activities are necessary to achieve these objectives?
3. How much time is required for each activity?
4. Which activities can be planned and scheduled for concurrent action, and which must be planned and scheduled sequentially?
5. Which activities can be delegated to staff?

Delegation

Delegating tasks to others can be an efficient time-management tool. **Delegation** involves assigning tasks, determining expected results, and granting authority to the individual expected to accomplish these tasks. Delegation is perhaps the most difficult leadership skill for nurses to acquire. Today, when more and more assistive personnel are being used to carry out the nurse's work, appropriate delegation and supervisory skills are essential for success. Chapter 10 discusses delegation in detail.

Time Analysis

The first step in time analysis is to identify how time is being used. The second is to determine whether time use is appropriate to the manager's role. Nurse managers find much of their time is taken up doing things that seem to be "busy work" rather than activities that contribute to a particular outcome. Job redesign places emphasis on ensuring that time is spent wisely and that the right individual is correctly assigned the responsibility for tasks.

Time logs, typically kept in intervals of 30 to 60 minutes, are useful in analyzing the actual time spent

KEY TERMS

Time waster Something that prevents a person from accomplishing a job or achieving a goal.

Goals Specific statements of achievement that provide direction; in an organization, goals follow the mission and vision.

Goal setting The relating of current behavior, activities, or operations to the organization's or individual's long-range goals.

Delegation A time-management tool that involves assigning tasks, determining expected results, and transferring responsibility to another individual.

Time logs Journals of activities that are useful in analyzing actual time spent on specific activities.

on various activities. These logs can be reviewed to determine which activities are essential to the nurse manager's job and which activities can be delegated to others or eliminated. Instead of a separate log, the nurse manager's schedule book also may be used to review patterns of time use.

A significant difficulty in moving from a staff nurse position to a leadership position is the need to develop different time-management and organizational skills. In a staff nurse role, the registered nurse has little, if any, free or uncommitted time. Almost every minute of the shift is assigned to a task. For example, at 6:45 A.M., report is taken; at 7:00 A.M., insulin is administered; at 7:15 A.M., breakfast trays are distributed; from 8:00 A.M. to 10:30 A.M., morning care is administered; and so on. No planning is required, because every minute is taken. In contrast, when the nurse moves to a leadership position, she or he is responsible for defining how time will be spent. Learning to focus on priorities and evaluating time use is an important part of the analysis.

Setting Priorities

Nurse managers should establish priorities, taking into consideration both short- and long-term goals as well as the importance and urgency of each activity. Table 15-1 illustrates examples of five types of activities. Activities can be identified as

- Urgent and important,
- Important but not urgent,
- Urgent but not important,
- Busy work, or
- Wasted time.

Activities that are both urgent and important, such as the example described in Table 15-1, must be completed. Activities that are important but not urgent may be those that make the difference between career progression or maintaining the status quo. Urgent but not important activities must be completed immediately but are not considered important or

significant. Busy work and wasted time are self-explanatory.

Daily Planning and Scheduling

Once goals and priorities have been established, the nurse manager can concentrate on scheduling activities. A **to-do list** should be prepared each day, either after work hours the previous day or early before work on the same day. The list is typically planned by workday or workweek. Because nurse managers combine many responsibilities, a weekly to-do list may be more effective. Flexibility must be a major consideration in this plan; some time should remain uncommitted to allow the manager to deal with emergencies and crises that are sure to happen. The focus is not on activities and events, but rather on the outcomes that can be achieved in the time available.

A system to keep track of regularly scheduled meetings (staff meetings), regular events (annual or quarterly report due dates), and appointments is also necessary. This system should be used when establishing the to-do list; it should include both a calendar and files. The calendar might include information on the purpose of the meeting, who will be attending, and the time and place. Several commercial planning systems are available, including computer software packages for desktop or personal data assistants (PDAs). Any such system includes a daily, weekly, or monthly calendar; a to-do section; a memo or note section; and an address component. An additional consideration is to have a calendar that is small enough to be taken to meetings or home. Files are maintained on the correspondence or reports related to the meeting. These files can be arranged by date so that they are readily retrievable when needed.

> **KEY TERMS**
>
> **To-do list**   A list of responsibilities to be accomplished within a specific time frame.

| Table 15-1 | Importance-Urgency Chart |

Category of Time Use	Examples
Important and urgent	Replacing two call-offs and ensuring sufficient staffing for the upcoming shift.
Important, not urgent	Drafting an educational program for nurses on the changes in Medicare reimbursement.
Urgent, not important	Completing and submitting the "beds available" list for a disaster drill.
Busy work	Compiling new charts for future patient admissions.
Wasted time	Sitting by the phone waiting for return calls.

Grouping Activities and Minimizing Routine Work

Work items that are similar in nature and require similar environmental surroundings and resources for their accomplishment should be grouped within divisions of the work shift. Set aside blocks of uninterrupted time for the really important tasks, such as preparing the budget. Routine tasks, especially those that are not important or urgent and contribute little to overall objectives, should be minimized. If you insist on doing them, group them together and do them in your least productive time. List a few 5- to 10-minute discretionary tasks. This helps to use the small bits of time that become available.

Much time is spent in transition or waiting. Using time effectively can increase the time available. Commuting time can be used for self-development or planning work activities. We all have to wait sometimes; waiting for a meeting to start or waiting to talk to someone are just two examples. Bring along materials to read or work on in case you are kept waiting. View waiting or transition time as an opportunity.

If you are having difficulty completing important tasks and are highly stressed, doing routine tasks for a while often helps to reduce stress. Pick a task that can be successfully completed and save it for the end of the day. Reaching closure on even a routine task at the end of the day can reduce the sense of overload and stress.

Implementation

Implementation of the daily plan and daily follow-up is essential to time management. In addition, you should repeat your time analysis at least semiannually to see how well you are managing your time, whether the job or the environment has changed, and which requires changes in planning activities. This can help prevent reverting to poor time-management habits.

Personal Organization and Self-Discipline

Some other time wasters are lack of personal organization and self-discipline, including the inability to say no, waiting for others, and excessive or ineffective paperwork. Effective personal organization results from clearly defined priorities based on well-defined, measurable, and achievable objectives. Because the nurse manager does not work alone, priorities and objectives are often related to those of many professionals, as well as to objectives of patients and their families.

How time is used is often a matter of resolving conflicts among competing needs. It is easy for the nurse manager to become overloaded with responsibilities and with more to do than should be expected in the time available. This is typical. There is never sufficient time for all the activities, situations, and events in which one might like to become involved.

To be effective, the nurse manager must be personally well organized and possess self-discipline. This often includes the ability to say no. Taking on too much work can lead to overload and stress. Being realistic about the amount of work to which you commit is an indication of effective time management. If a superior is overloading you, make sure the person understands the consequences of additional assignments. Be assertive in communicating your own needs to others.

A cluttered desk, working on too many tasks at one time, and failing to set aside blocks of uninterrupted time to do important tasks also indicate a lack of personal self-discipline. Clean your desk, get out the materials you need to complete your highest-priority task, and start working on it immediately. Focus on one task at a time, making sure to start with a high-priority task.

Controlling Interruptions

An interruption occurs any time the nurse manager is stopped in the middle of one activity to give attention to something else. Interruptions can be an essential part of the nurse manager's job, or they can be a time waster. An interruption that is more important and urgent than the activity in which the nurse manager is involved is a positive interruption; it deserves immediate attention. An emergency or crisis, for instance, may cause the nurse manager to interrupt daily rounds.

Some interruptions interfere with achieving the nurse manager's job and are less important and urgent than current activities. As the nurse manager's role expands to a broader span of responsibility, more decision making is placed on the staff nurse. When a manager is interrupted to solve problems within the staff nurse's scope of accountability, the manager should not become responsible for solving the problem. Gently but firmly directing the individual to search for solutions begins to break old patterns of behavior and helps develop individual responsibility. Although time consuming in the beginning, this practice eventually reduces the number of unnecessary interruptions.

Keeping an **interruption log** on an occasional basis may help. The log should show who interrupted, the nature of the interruption, when it occurred, how long it lasted, what topics were discussed, the importance of the topics, and time-saving actions to be taken. Analysis of these data may identify patterns that the nurse manager can use to plan ways to reduce the frequency and duration of interruptions. These patterns may indicate that certain staff members are the most frequent interrupters and require individual attention to develop problem-solving skills.

Telephone Calls Telephone calls are a major source of interruption, and the interruption log will provide considerable insight for the nurse manager regarding the nature of telephone calls received. Although it is not possible to function today without a telephone, some people do not use the telephone effectively. A ringing telephone is highly compelling; few people can allow it to go unanswered. Nurse managers receive many telephone calls, some of them time wasters. Handling telephone calls effectively is a must:

- Minimize socializing and small talk. If you answer the phone with, "Hello, what can I do for you?" rather than, "Hello, how are you?" the caller is encouraged to get to business first. Be warm, friendly, and courteous, but do not allow others to waste time with inappropriate or extensive small talk. Calls placed and returned just prior to lunchtime, at the end of the day, and on Friday afternoons tend to result in more business and less socializing.
- Plan calls. The manager who plans telephone calls does not waste anyone's time, including that of the person called. Write down topics to be discussed before making the call. This prevents the need for additional calls to inform the other party of an important point or to ask a forgotten question.
- Set a time for calls. The nurse manager may have a number of calls to return as well as calls to initiate. It is best to set aside a time to handle routine phone calls, especially during "downtime." Try not to interrupt what is being done at the moment. If an answer is necessary before a project can be continued, phone immediately; if not, phone for the information at a later time.
- State and ask for preferred call times and the purpose of the call. If a party is not available, state the purpose of the call, and provide several time frames when you will be available for a return call. Have those accepting messages ask for the same

information. This makes it easier for the responder to be prepared for the call and helps to prevent "telephone tag."

Voice mail is an excellent way to send and receive messages when a real-time interaction is not essential. For example, one person or a large group of people can be informed about an upcoming meeting in one voice mail message. They can phone their responses at their convenience, thus obviating the need for continuing to try to reach each other directly. Like other forms of communication, voice mail must be used appropriately. Long messages or sensitive information are better conveyed one-on-one. Also, another person (e.g., unit clerk) may be responsible for taking voice mail messages off the system, so it is important to state the message in a professional manner, omitting personal or confidential information.

E-mail is another tool that enhances time management. E-mail (electronic mail) minimizes time wasted trying to contact individuals and provides a means whereby the urgency of the message can be coded. Tone, however, is difficult to convey by e-mail. Therefore it is advisable to use more personal forms of communication, such as the telephone or in-person contact, for potentially sensitive or troublesome issues.

Drop-In Visitors Although often friendly and seemingly harmless, the typical "got-a-minute?" drop-in visit can last several minutes. Rather than eliminate drop-in visits, the nurse manager should skillfully direct the visit by identifying the issue or question, arranging an alternative meeting, referring the visitor to someone else, or redirecting the visitor's problem-solving efforts. An additional strategy is to stand up to greet the visitor and remain standing. The gesture appears gracious yet is obvious enough to encourage a short visit.

The nurse manager who is fortunate enough to have an office will find that open doors are open invitations for interruption. Although it is essential that nurse managers be available and accessible, concentration time also is necessary. The manager can obtain concentration time by informing the staff that a specific block of time (a few hours at most) will be available to address issues.

KEY TERMS

Interruption log Journal of specific information regarding interruptions, analysis of which may help identify ways to reduce interruptions.

Interruptions also can be controlled by the arrangement of furniture. The nurse manager whose desk is arranged so that immediate eye contact is made with passers-by or drop-in visitors is asking for interruptions. A desk turned 90 or even 180 degrees from the door minimizes potential eye contact.

Encouraging appointments to deal with routine matters also reduces interruptions. Regularly scheduled meetings with those who need to see the nurse manager allow them to hold routine matters for those appointments. Holding such meetings in the other person's office places the nurse manager in charge of keeping the time. It is easier to leave someone's office than to remove an individual from yours.

Paperwork

Health care organizations cannot function effectively without good information systems. In addition to telephone calls and face-to-face conversations, nurse managers spend considerable time writing and reading communications. Increasing government regulations, measures to avoid legal action, stronger privacy requirements, new treatments and medications, data processing, work processing, and electronics place pressure on the nurse manager to cope with increasing paperwork (including electronic "paperwork"). Some basic principles can help the nurse manager process information while reducing it as a waster of time.

1. *Plan and schedule paperwork.* Writing and reading reports, forms, e-mail, letters, and memoranda are essential elements of the nurse manager's job. They cannot be ignored. They will, however, become a major source of frustration if their processing is not planned and scheduled as an integral part of the nurse manager's daily activities. Nurse managers should learn the organization's information system and requirements, analyze the paperwork requirements of the position, and make significant progress on that part of the job daily.

2. *Sort paperwork for effective processing.* A system of file folders either for paper mail or for e-mail can be very helpful. Here is one way to handle it.
   • Place all paperwork (or e-mail) requiring personal action in a red file or in an "action" folder on your computer's hard drive. It can then be handled according to its relative importance and urgency.
   • Place work that can be delegated in a separate pile, and distribute it appropriately.
   • Place all work that is informational in nature and related to present work in a yellow file folder or in an "informational" folder on the hard drive.
   • Place other reading material, such as professional journals, technical reports, and other items that do not relate directly to the immediate work, in a blue file folder or a file labeled "R."

   The informational file contains materials that must be read immediately, whereas the reading file materials are not as urgent and can be read later.

   Do not be afraid to throw things away or erase them from the memory of your electronic information system. When they no longer have value, do not let them become clutter. Use trash receptacles in the office and on the electronic system.

3. *Use the computer for all letters, memos, reports, and messages.* The computer revolutionized communications; take advantage of it.

4. *Analyze paperwork frequently.* Review filing policies and rules regularly, and purge files at least once each year. All standard forms, reports, and memos should be reviewed annually. Each should justify its continued existence and its present format. Do not be afraid to recommend changes and, when possible, initiate those changes.

5. *Do not be a paper shuffler.* "Handle a piece of paper only once," is a common adage, but impossible to follow if taken literally. It really means that each time a piece of paper or e-mail message is handled, some action should be taken to further processing it. Paper shufflers are those who continually move things around on their desks or accumulate unread e-mails. They delay action unreasonably, and the problem mounts. A desktop is a working surface; it is not for files and piles.

Respecting Time

The key to using time-management techniques is to respect one's own time as well as that of others. Nurse managers who respect their time are likely to find others respecting it also. The same values and attitudes indicate respect for one's own time and for that of others. Using the above suggestions regarding time management communicates to those who interact with the nurse manager that respect for time is demanded.

The manager, however, must reciprocate by respecting the time needs of others. If you need to talk to someone, it is appropriate to arrange an appointment, particularly for routine matters. One should continually ask, "What is the best use of my time right now?" and should answer in three ways:

- For myself and my goals
- For my staff and their goals
- For the organization and its goals

One manager who felt stressed by all of her responsibilities used the strategies shown in Case Study 15-1 to help her solve her problems.

CASE STUDY 15-1: Time Management

For the past 6 years, Jane Schumann has been manager of staff development for three hospitals in a Catholic health care system. After the health care system suffered record operating losses last fiscal year, many middle management positions were eliminated. Jane was retained but had several other departments assigned to her. Now Jane has four hospitals and responsibility for staff development, utilization review staff, in-house float pool, night nursing supervisors, agency staffing, coordination of student nurse clinical rotations, and training of all nursing staff for the new hospital information system.

Jane has been overwhelmed with her new responsibilities. Wanting to establish trust and learn more about her staff, Jane has adopted an "open-door policy" resulting in many drop-in visits each day. She has been working much longer hours and most weekends. Frequently she has had to fill in for night supervisors, stretching her workday to 18 hours. Her desk is stacked with paperwork and her voice mail box is full of messages to be returned. On average, she returns 40 of the 60 e-mails received each day. Although Jane is pleased she was chosen for the additional responsibilities, she has difficulty sleeping and is concerned about the effect of career responsibilities on her family life.

Jane decides to take 2 vacation days and turns off her pager. She makes a list of priorities for each of her departments and a time frame for completing each project. She makes daily plans for the next 2 weeks and a 3-month plan for the upcoming quarter. Jane also determines who

among her new staff members can assume additional responsibilities and notes tasks that can be delegated. She sorts through paperwork and establishes a filing system for each department. Jane's administrative assistant will be trained to file routine paperwork and route other paperwork to Jane or delegated personnel. Jane also decides that at each departmental meeting she will establish specific times she will be available for drop-in visitors. Jane schedules a meeting with the senior nursing executive to discuss the staffing implications for training nurses at four hospitals to use the new hospital information system. Finally, she takes advantage of her 4-day weekend to catch up on some well-deserved rest.

Manager's Checklist

The nurse manager is responsible for

- Recognizing the impact of stress, both positive and negative, on professional and personal life,
- Prioritizing workload and determining the best use of resources,
- Effectively delegating tasks and projects to staff,
- Identifying major issues that require communication with administrators before problems or delays arise,
- Respecting their own time and the time of others, and
- Knowing how to best request assistance when appropriate.

What You Know Now

- Stress is a person's reaction to demands from the environment that pose a threat.
- Causes of stress come from job and organizational factors, from interpersonal factors, and from individual factors.
- The consequences of stress are physiological and psychological problems for the individual, poor job performance, low job satisfaction, and high absenteeism.
- Strategies to help individuals, as well as organizations, manage stress include clarifying goals and roles; providing support, including training and education on

stress management; using participative management techniques; and practicing personal stress management techniques.

- Nurse managers must use time wisely to accomplish everything that is expected of them; this takes planning.
- The nurse manager's work is subject to many interruptions. An interruption log helps identify patterns that the manager can use to plan ways to reduce unnecessary interruptions.
- Telephone calls are a major source of interruption. They can be controlled by minimizing small talk, planning calls, setting aside time for calls, stating preferred call times, and using voice mail.

- Drop-in visitors are also a source of interruption. One should meet visitors outside the office, keep visits short, encourage appointments, keep staff informed, and arrange furniture to discourage unscheduled visitors.
- Written communication also can cause interruptions. These can be minimized by planning and scheduling paperwork, sorting, delegating, writing effectively, and using an effective filing system.
- Nurse managers who respect their own time are likely to find others respecting it also.

Tools for Managing Stress and Time

1. If you are experiencing an exceptional amount of stress, try to identify the source and find various ways to reduce your stress.
2. Pay attention to your stress levels and try to create opportunities to help deal with stress.
3. Study the chapter for time-management strategies, including goal setting, time analysis, setting priorities, planning, and dealing with time wasters. This information may be new to you, and it may take a while to integrate these practices into your work life. Be patient with yourself during the learning curve.
4. Pay special attention to handling paperwork, e-mail, and voice mail messages. Mail piling up contributes to stress. Practice skimming materials, including voice mail, to decide which messages and mail need further attention.

Questions to Challenge You

1. Have you experienced any of the consequences of stress described in the chapter? How did you handle it? Explain.
2. Have you experienced role ambiguity or role conflict? Describe the situation. How did you handle it?
3. Make a list for yourself using the individual goal categories in the chapter. During the next week try to complete it.
4. Identify three time wasters that are problems for you. Explain how you can minimize them.

Explore 🌐 MediaLink

NCLEX review questions, essay activities, group activities, and other interactive resources for this chapter can be found on the Web site at http://www.prenhall.com/sullivan-decker. Click on "Chapter 15" to select activities for this chapter.

References

Selye, H. (1978). *The stress of life* (2nd ed.). New York: McGraw-Hill.

Steers, R. (1991). *Introduction to organizational behavior* (4th ed.). Santa Monica, CA: Goodyear.

Initiating and Managing Change

Looking Ahead

How do you view change? Does it bring up feelings of anxiety and distrust? Or do you see it as a challenge? Today's health care environment is changing rapidly; as we've shown in the opening chapters, it pervades every aspect of our work environment. How can nurses learn to view this transformation as positive and even go so far as to initiate change? This chapter examines the theoretical approach to the process of change and offers insights into planning, implementing, and evaluating change while developing the skills necessary to become an effective change agent.

Objectives

In this chapter, you will learn

- What the change process involves.
- How different theorists explain change.
- What steps it takes to make change.
- What skills a change agent needs.
- How to handle resistance to change.

MediaLink 🌐 **www.prenhall.com/ sullivan-decker**

Additional resources for this chapter can be found on the Companion Website at www.prenhall.com/ sullivan-decker. Click on "Chapter 16" to select the activities for this chapter.

- NCLEX Review
- Critical Thinking Activities
- Current Events
- MediaLinks
- *Nursing Leadership & Management in Action:* Developing Strategies for Change; Managing Resistance to Change; Responses to Change: A Personal Experience

In today's health care environment, organizational change is essential for adaptation; creative change is mandatory for growth. This climate for change produces new opportunities for nurses. Nurses are rethinking the way health care is organized and delivered. Innovation is in. The participatory approach is popular because status quo management will not work when a whole system is in transition. Transitional times demand new ways of thinking, creative strategies, and fresh opinions.

Change is inevitable, if not always welcome. Change is necessary for growth, although it often produces anxiety and fear. Even when planned, it can be threatening and a source of conflict because **change** is the process of making something different from what it was. There is a sense of loss of the familiar, the status quo. This is particularly true when change is unplanned or beyond human control. Even when change is expected and valued, a grief reaction still may occur. Those who initiate and manage change often encounter resistance from those experiencing unease and, possibly, symptoms of anxiety and grief.

Change is a continually unfolding process rather than an either/or event. The process begins with the present state, is disrupted, moves through a transition period, and ultimately comes to a desired state. Once the desired state has been reached, however, the process begins again.

Although nurse managers should understand and anticipate these reactions to change, they need to develop and exude a different approach. They can view change as a challenge and encourage their colleagues to participate. They can become uncomfortable with the status quo and be willing to take risks.

Leaders initiate change; followers survive it. Porter-O'Grady (2003, p. 177) suggests that leaders must "help the staff close the door" on the old way of thinking and doing, going so far as to disrupt the status quo. Today's realities require that nurses stop trying to do more and more of the same activities, expecting a different result. Hawke (2003) suggests that nurses must adopt a different mindset to negotiate the changes in health care.

Nurse managers must become skilled in implementing organizational change and in initiating change within the organization. Nurse leaders must initiate the changes they believe are necessary to strengthen nursing practice, provide quality care, and create a better system.

The Nurse as Change Agent

A **change agent** is one who works to bring about a change. The notion of the nurse as change agent is not new. The nurse often acts as an insider, a change agent

who is part of the system being altered (managing a unit or team). But nurses can also be outsiders or consultants for change in other systems. There has never been a better time for the nursing profession to take the initiative. As the largest health profession, nurses make the health care system run; they have concrete ideas about how to make it run better. Nurses who can suggest changes to control costs, improve quality, or offer new services will be in great demand, especially for management positions.

Changes will continue at a rapid pace with or without nursing's expert guidance. Nurses, like organizations, cannot afford merely to survive changes. If they are to exist as a distinct profession that has expertise in helping individuals respond to actual or potential health problems, they must be proactive in shaping the future. Opportunities exist now for nurses, especially those in management positions, to change the system about which they so often complain. On the other hand, managers should not initiate change just for the sake of change or to show that they are "managing" (McConnell, 2002).

Change Theories

Lewin's Force-Field Model

Lewin (1951) provides a social-psychological view of the change process. He sees behavior as a dynamic balance of forces working in opposing directions within a field (such as an organization). **Driving forces** facilitate change because they push participants in the desired direction. **Restraining forces** impede change because they push participants in the opposite direction. To plan change, one must analyze these forces and shift the balance in the direction of change through a

---

KEY TERMS

Change   The process of making something different from what it was.

Change agent   One who works to bring about change.

Driving forces   Behaviors that facilitate change by pushing participants in the desired direction.

Restraining forces   Behaviors that impede change by discouraging participants from making specified changes.

three-step process: unfreezing, moving, and refreezing. Change occurs by adding a new force, changing the direction of a force, or changing the magnitude of any one force. Basically, strategies for change are aimed at increasing driving forces, decreasing restraining forces, or both.

Lewin's force-field model and an example are diagrammed in Figure 16-1. This scheme shows how a system's driving and restraining forces oppose each other. These forces, which are part of the system's maintenance and adaptive mechanisms, are balanced at the present, or status quo, level. To achieve change, first an imbalance must occur between the driving and restraining forces, which unfreezes the present patterned behavior. Behavior moves to a new level, at which the opposing forces are brought into a new state of equilibrium. Once participants integrate new patterns of behavior into their personalities and relationships with others, a refreezing takes place. The new level becomes institutionalized into formal and informal behavioral patterns.

Lewin's change strategies fall within this three-step process:

1. *Unfreeze the existing equilibrium.* Motivate participants by getting them ready for change. Build trust and recognition for the need to change. To thaw attitudes, actively participate in identifying problems and generate alternative solutions.
2. *Move the target system to a new level of equilibrium.* Get participants to agree that the status quo is not beneficial to them. Encourage participants

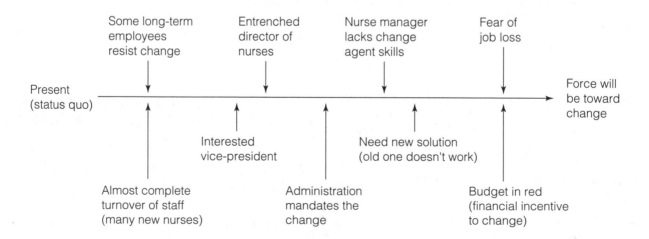

Figure 16-1   Lewin's force-field model of change. Adapted from *Field Theory in Social Science* by K. Lewin, 1997, New York: Harper & Row.

to view the problem from a new perspective. Stimulate identification by linking group views to those of a respected or powerful leader who supports the change. Help them scan the environment to search for relevant information.

3. *Refreeze the system at the new level of equilibrium.* Reinforce the new patterns of behavior. Institutionalize them through formal and informal mechanisms (e.g., policies, communications channels).

Lewinian thinking is fundamental to the views of later theorists. Clearly, it is a behavioral approach that nurses find consistent with their theoretical understanding of human behavior, and it has been used successfully in health care settings (Baulcomb, 2003). The image of people's attitudes thawing and then refreezing is conceptually useful. This symbolism helps to keep theory and reality in mind simultaneously.

Lippitt's Phases of Change

Lippitt and colleagues (1958) extended Lewin's theory to a seven-step process and focused more on what the change agent must do than on the evolution of change itself. (See Table 16-1 for a comparison of four change theories.) They emphasized participation of key members of the target system throughout the change process, particularly during planning. Communication skills, rapport building, and problem-solving strategies underlie their phases.

The seven steps are

1. *Diagnose the problem.* Involve key people in data collection and problem solving.
2. *Assess the motivation and capacity for change.* What are the financial and human resources and constraints? Are the structure and function of the organization conducive to change? What are the possible solutions, and which are preferred?
3. *Assess the change agent's motivation and resources.* This assessment is important. Consider the change agent's own commitment to change, energy level, future ambitions, and power bases. Starting a change and dropping it midstream can waste valuable personal energy and undermine the confidence of colleagues and subordinates.
4. *Select progressive change objects.* Develop the action plan, evaluation criteria, and specify strategies.
5. *Choose a change agent role.* The change agent can act as cheerleader, expert, consultant, or group facilitator. Whichever role is selected, all participants should recognize it so that expectations are clear.
6. *Maintain the change.* Communication, feedback, revision, and coordination are essential components of this phase.
7. *Terminate the helping relationship.* The change agent withdraws from the selected role gradually as the change becomes institutionalized.

Havelock's Model

Havelock (1973) described a six-step process, also a modification of Lewin's model (see Table 16-1). Havelock describes an active change agent as one who uses a participative approach.

Havelock emphasizes the unfreezing or planning stage as:

- Building a relationship
- Diagnosing the problem
- Acquiring resources

| Table 16-1 | Comparison of Change Models |

Lewin	Lippitt	Havelock	Rogers
1. Unfreezing	1. Diagnose problem	1. Building a relationship	1. Knowledge
2. Moving	2. Assess motivation	2. Diagnosing the problem	2. Persuasion
3. Refreezing	3. Assess change agent's motivations and resources	3. Acquiring resources	3. Decision
	4. Select progressive change objects	4. Choosing the solution	4. Implementation
	5. Choose change agent role	5. Gaining acceptance	5. Confirmation
	6. Maintain change	6. Stabilization and self-renewal	
	7. Terminate helping relationships		

This stage is followed by the moving stage:

- Choosing the solution
- Gaining acceptance

Refreezing is referred to as:

- Stabilization
- Self-renewal

Rogers's Diffusion of Innovations

Rogers (1983) takes a broader approach than Lewin, Lippitt, or Havelock (see Table 16-1). His five-step innovation-decision process details how an individual or decision-making unit passes from first knowledge of an innovation to confirmation of the decision to adopt or reject a new idea. His framework emphasizes the reversible nature of change: Participants may initially adopt a proposal but later discontinue it, or the reverse—they may initially reject it but adopt it at a later time. This is a useful distinction. If the change agent is unsuccessful in achieving full implementation of a proposal, it should not be assumed the issue is dead. It can be resurrected, perhaps in an altered form or at a more opportune time. However, if it is accepted, one also cannot assume permanence.

Rogers's five steps to the diffusion of innovation are

1. *Knowledge.* The decision-making unit is introduced to the innovation and begins to understand it.
2. *Persuasion.* A favorable (or unfavorable) attitude toward the innovation forms.
3. *Decision.* Activities lead to a decision to adopt or reject the innovation.
4. *Implementation.* The innovation is put to use, and reinvention or alterations may occur.
5. *Confirmation.* The individual or decision-making unit seeks reinforcement that the decision was correct. If there are conflicting messages or experiences, the original decision may be reversed.

Finally, Rogers stresses two important aspects of successful planned change: Key people and policymakers must be interested in the innovation and committed to making it happen.

The Change Process

The change process follows the same path as the nursing process: assessment, planning, implementation, and evaluation.

Assessment

Emphasis is placed on the assessment phase of change for two reasons. First, without thorough data collection and analysis, planned change will not proceed past the "wouldn't it be a good idea if" stage. Second, nurses often are not familiar with the kind of data they need to collect or with the method by which to analyze data to manage and initiate change.

Identify the Problem or the Opportunity Change is often planned to close a discrepancy between the desired and actual state of affairs. Discrepancies may arise because of problems in reaching performance goals or because new goals have been created. Opportunities demand change as much as (or more than) problems do, but they are often overlooked. Be it a problem or an opportunity, it must be identified clearly. If the issue is perceived differently by key individuals, the search for solutions becomes confused. Start by asking the right questions, such as

1. Where are we now? What is unique about us? What should our business be?
2. What can we do that is different from and better than what our competitors do?
3. What is the driving stimulus in our organization? What determines how we make our final decisions?
4. What prevents us from moving in the direction we wish to go?
5. What kind of change is required?

This last question generates integrative thinking on the potential effect of change on the system. Organizational change involves modifications in the system's interacting components: technology, structure, and people.

The introduction of new technology necessitates changes in the structure of the organization. The physical plant will be altered if new services are added. Relationships among the people who work in the system change when the structure is changed. New units open; others close. New rules and regulations, new authority structures, and new budgeting methods may emerge. They, in turn, change staffing needs, requiring people with different skills, knowledge bases, attitudes, and motivations.

Collect Data Once the problem or opportunity has been clearly defined, the change agent collects data external and internal to the system. This step is crucial to the eventual success of the planned change. All driving and restraining forces are identified so the driving forces can be emphasized and the restraining forces reduced. It is imperative to assess the political pulse. Who will gain from this change? Who will lose? Who has more power and why? Can those power bases be altered? How?

The nurse manager can best assess the political climate by examining the reasons for the present situation. Who is in control who may be benefiting now? Egos, commitment of the involved people, and personality likes and dislikes are as important to assess as the formal organizational structures and processes. The innovator has to gauge the potential for resistance.

The costs and benefits of the proposed change are obvious focal points. The nurse manager also needs to assess resources—especially those the manager can control. A manager who has the respect and support of an excellent nursing staff has access to a powerful resource in today's climate.

Analyze Data   The kinds, amounts, and sources of data collected are important, but they are useless unless they are analyzed. The change agent should focus more energy on analyzing and summarizing the data than on just collecting it. The point is to flush out resistance, identify potential solutions and strategies, begin to identify areas of consensus, and build a case for whichever option is selected. When possible, a statistical analysis should be made; it is worth the effort, especially when the change agent will need to persuade persons in power. The case should be presented cogently and succinctly using visual aids (e.g., bar graphs and charts) if needed.

Planning

Planning the who, how, and when of the change is a key step. What will be the target system for the change? Members from this system should be active participants in the planning stage. The more involved they are at this point, the less resistance there will be later. Lewin's unfreezing imagery is relevant here. Present attitudes, habits, and ways of thinking have to soften so members of the target system will be ready for new ways of thinking and behaving. Boundaries must melt before the system can shift and restructure.

This is the time to make people uncomfortable with the status quo. Plant the seeds of discontent by introducing information that may make people feel dissatisfied with the present and interested in something new. This information comes from the data collected (e.g., research findings, quantitative data, and patient satisfaction questionnaires or staff surveys). Couch the

proposed change in comfortable terms as far as possible, and minimize anxiety about the new change.

Managers need to plan the resources required to make the change and establish feedback mechanisms to evaluate its progress and success. Establish control points with people who will provide the feedback and work with these people to set specific goals with time frames. Develop operational indicators that signal success or failure in terms of performance and satisfaction.

Implementation

The plans are put into motion (Lewin's moving stage). Interventions are designed to gain the necessary compliance. The change agent creates a supportive climate, acts as energizer, obtains and provides feedback, and overcomes resistance. Managers are the key change-process actors. Some methods are directed toward changing individuals in an organization, whereas others are directed toward changing the group.

Methods to Change Individuals   The most common method used to change individuals' perceptions, attitudes, and values is information giving (Katz & Kahn, 1978). External expert consultants or internal staff prepare and disseminate the information, usually in a top-down communication flow. Providing information is prerequisite to change implementation, but it is inadequate unless lack of information is the only obstacle to effecting change. Providing information does not address the motivation to change.

Training is often considered a method to change individuals. Training combines information giving with skill practice. Training typically shows people how they are to perform in a system, not how to change it. Therefore, it is more of a system maintenance mechanism than a change strategy.

Selecting and placing personnel or terminating key people often is used to alter the forces for or against change. When key supporters of the planned change are given the authority and accountability to make the change, their enthusiasm and legitimacy can be effective in leading others to support the change. Conversely, if those opposed to the change are transferred or leave the organization, the change is more likely to succeed.

Methods to Change Groups   Some implementation tactics use groups rather than individuals to attain compliance to change. The power of an organizational group to influence its members depends on its authority to act on an issue and the significance of the issue itself. The greatest influence is achieved when group members discuss issues that are perceived as important and make relevant, binding decisions based on those discussions. Effectiveness in implementing organizational change is most likely when groups are composed of members who occupy closely related positions in the organization.

Individual and group implementation tactics can be combined. Whatever methods are used, participants should feel their input is valued and should be rewarded for their efforts. Some people are not always persuaded before a beneficial change is implemented. Sometimes behavior changes first, and attitudes are modified later to fit the behavior. In this case, the change agent should be aware of participants' conflicts and reward the desired behaviors. It may take some time for attitudes to catch up.

Evaluation

Evaluate Effectiveness   At each control point, the operational indicators established are monitored. The change agent determines whether presumed benefits were achieved from a financial as well as a qualitative perspective, explaining the extent of success or failure. Unintended consequences and undesirable outcomes may have occurred.

Stabilize the Change   The change is extended past the pilot stage, and the target system is refrozen. The change agent terminates the helping relationship by delegating responsibilities to target system members. The energizer role is still needed to reinforce new behaviors through positive feedback.

Change Agent Strategies

Regardless of the setting or proposed change, the four-step change process should be followed. However, specific strategies can be used, depending on the amount of resistance anticipated and the degree of power the change agent possesses.

Power-Coercive Strategies

Power-coercive strategies are based on the application of power by legitimate authority, economic sanctions, or political clout. Changes are made through law, policy, or financial appropriations. Those in control enforce changes by restricting budgets or creating policies. Those who are not in power may not even be aware of what is happening. Even if they are aware, they have little power to stop it. The prospective payment system

for Medicare (DRGs) was a power-coercive strategy by the federal government. Similarly managed care has changed economic incentives in health care.

The change process continues through the seven steps, but there is little, if any, participation by the target system members. Resistance is handled by authority measures: Accept it, or leave.

Power-coercive strategies are useful when a consensus is unlikely despite efforts to stimulate participation by those involved. When much resistance is anticipated, time is short, and the change is critical for organizational survival, power-coercive strategies may be necessary.

Empirical-Rational Model

In the **empirical-rational model** of change strategies, the power ingredient is knowledge. The assumption is that people are rational and will follow their rational self-interest if that self-interest is made clear to them. It is also assumed that the change agent who has knowledge has the expert power to persuade people to accept a rationally justified change that will benefit them. The flow of influence moves from those who know to those who do not know. New ideas are invented and communicated or diffused to all participants. Once enlightened, rational people will either accept or reject the idea based on its merits and consequences. Empirical-rational strategies are often effective when little resistance to the proposed change is expected and the change is perceived as reasonable

Introduction of new technology that is easy to use, cuts nursing time, and improves quality of care would be accepted readily after in-service education and perhaps a trial use. The change agent can direct the change. There is little need for staff participation in the early steps of the change process, although input is useful for the evaluation and stabilization stages. The benefits of change for the staff and perhaps research findings regarding patient outcomes are the major driving forces. Well-researched, cost-effective technology can be implemented using these strategies.

Normative-Reeducative Strategies

In contrast to the rational-empirical model, **normative-reeducative strategies** of change rest on the assumption that people act in accordance with social norms and values. Information and rational arguments are insufficient strategies to change people's patterns of actions; the change agent must focus on noncognitive determinants of behavior as well. People's roles and relationships, perceptual orientations, attitudes, and feelings will influence their acceptance of change.

In this mode, the power ingredient is not authority or knowledge, but skill in interpersonal relationships. The change agent does not use coercion or nonreciprocal influence, but collaboration. Members of the target system are involved throughout the change process. Value conflicts from all parts of the system are brought into the open and worked through so change can progress.

Normative-reeducative strategies are well suited to the creative problem solving needed in nursing and health care today. With their firm grasp of the behavioral sciences and communication skills, nurses are comfortable with this model. Changing from a traditional nursing system to self-governance or initiating a home follow-up service for hospitalized patients are examples of changes amenable to the normative-reeducative approach. In most cases, the normative-reeducative approach to change will be effective in reducing resistance and stimulating personal and organizational creativity. The obvious drawback is the time required for group participation and conflict resolution throughout the change process. When there is adequate time or when group consensus is fundamental to successful adoption of the change, the manager is well advised to adopt this framework.

Resistance to Change

Response to change varies from ready acceptance to full-blown resistance. Rogers (1983) identified six response typologies:

- Innovators love change and thrive on it.
- Less radical, early adopters are still receptive to change.
- The early majority prefers the status quo, but eventually accept the change.
- The late majority are resistive, accepting change after most others have.
- Laggards dislike change and are openly antagonistic.
- Rejecters actively oppose and may even sabotage change.

Resistance to change is to be expected for a number of reasons: lack of trust, vested interest in the status quo, fear of failure, loss of status or income, misunderstanding, and belief that change is unnecessary or that it will not improve the situation (Yukl, 2002; Hellriegel, Jackson, & Slocum, 2002). Employees may resist change because they dislike or disapprove of the person responsible for implementing the change or they may distrust the change process. Regardless, managers continually deal with change—both the change that they themselves initiate and change initiated by the larger organization.

The change agent should anticipate and look for resistance to change. It will be lurking somewhere, perhaps where least expected. It can be recognized in such statements as

- We tried that before.
- It won't work.
- No one else does it like that.
- We've always done it this way.
- We can't afford it.
- We don't have the time.
- It will cause too much commotion.
- You'll never get it past the board.
- Let's wait awhile.
- Every new boss wants to do something different.
- Let's start a task force to look at it; put it on the agenda.

Expect resistance and listen carefully to who says what, when, and in what circumstances. Open resisters are easier to deal with than closet resisters. Look for nonverbal signs of resistance, such as poor work habits and lack of interest in the change.

Resistance has positive and negative aspects. On the one hand, resistance forces the change agent to be clear about why the change is needed. The manager must know the change inside and out because she or he must defend it against challengers. The positive part of resistance is the sharper focus and problem solving it encourages. It prevents the unexpected. It forces the manager to clarify information, keep interest level

MEDIALINK ◆ Managing Resistance to Change

KEY TERMS

Power-coercive strategies   Change agent strategies based on the application of power by legitimate authority, economic sanctions, or political clout.

Empirical-rational model   A change agent strategy based on the assumption that people are rational and follow self-interest if that self-interest is made clear.

Normative-reeducative strategy   A change agent strategy based on the assumption that people act in accordance with social norms and values.

high, and establish why change is necessary. Resistance is a stimulant as much as it is a force to be overcome. It may even motivate the group to do better what it is doing now, so that it does not have to change.

On the other hand, resistance is not always beneficial, especially if it persists beyond the planning stage and well into the implementation phase. It can wear down supporters and redirect system energy from implementing the change to dealing with resisters. Morale can suffer.

When handling resistance, the manager must first identify the need to reduce it. Resistance can be used to sharpen decision, for example, and eventually gain consensus. If it is necessary to minimize it, do not personalize the resistance. Remain rational, stick to the problem-solving change process, and proceed with the following guidelines:

1. Communicate with those who oppose the change. Get to the root of their reasons for opposition.
2. Clarify information, and provide accurate feedback.
3. Be open to revisions but clear about what must remain.
4. Present the negative consequences of resistance (e.g., threats to organizational survival, compromised patient care).

5. Emphasize the positive consequences of the change and how the individual or group will benefit. However, do not spend too much energy on rational analysis of why the change is good and why the arguments against it do not hold up. People's resistance frequently flows from feelings that are not rational.
6. Keep resisters involved in face-to-face contact with supporters. Encourage proponents to empathize with opponents, recognize valid objections, and relieve unnecessary fears.
7. Maintain a climate of trust, support, and confidence.
8. Divert attention by creating a different disturbance. Energy can shift to a more important problem inside the system, thereby redirecting resistance. Alternatively, attention can be brought to an external threat to create a bully phenomenon. When members perceive a greater environmental threat (such as competition or restrictive governmental policies), they tend to unify internally.

A nurse manager in a home health care agency used change management strategies to overcome resistance as shown in Case Study 16-1.

CASE STUDY 16-1: Change Management

Peter Beasley is nurse manager of pediatric home care for a private home health care agency. Last year the agency completed a pilot of wireless devices for use in documenting home visits. As nurses complete the documentation, charges for supplies and medical equipment are also generated. The agency director informed the nurse managers that all nurses will be required to use the wireless devices within the next 3 months.

Charlene Ramirez has been a pediatric nurse for 18 years, working for the home health care agency for the past 5 years. Charlene has been active in updating the pediatric documentation and training staff when new paper-based documentation was implemented in the past. Although she was part of the pilot, Charlene is very much opposed to using the new wireless devices. She has rarely used a computer and complains she can barely visualize text on a regular monitor. At a recent staff meeting, Charlene stated she would rather quit than learn to use the new wireless devices.

Peter empathizes with Charlene's reluctance to use the new handheld computers. He also recognizes how much

Charlene contributes in expertise and leadership to the department. However, he knows that the new performance standards require all employees to use the wireless devices. After three mandatory training sessions, Charlene repeatedly tells co-workers "We've tried things like this before, it never works. We'll be back on paper within 6 months, so why waste my time learning this stuff?" The program trainer reports that Charlene was disruptive during the class and failed her competency exam.

Peter meets privately with Charlene to discuss her resistance to the new technology. Charlene again states that she fails to see the need for wireless devices in delivering quality patient care. Peter reviews the new performance standards with Charlene, emphasizing the technology requirements. He asks Charlene if she has difficulty understanding the application or just in using the device. Charlene admits she cannot see the text on the screen and therefore cannot determine what exactly she is documenting. Peter informs Charlene that the agency's health benefits include vision exams and partial payment for corrective lenses. He suggests she talk with an optometrist to see if special glasses would help her see the screen. Peter also makes a note to speak with the technology specialist to see if there are aids to assist staff in viewing data on the device.

Manager's Checklist

The nurse manager is responsible for

- Communicating openly and honestly with employees who oppose change,
- Understanding the resistance to change,

- Maintaining support and confidence in staff even if they are resistive to change,
- Emphasizing the positive outcomes from initiating change, and
- Finding solutions to problems that are obstacles to change.

The Manager's Role in Implementing Change

Making change is not easy, but it is a mandatory skill for managers. Successful change agents demonstrate certain characteristics that can be cultivated and mastered with practice. Among these are

- The ability to combine ideas from unconnected sources.
- The ability to energize others by keeping the interest level up and demonstrating a high personal energy level.
- Skill in human relations: well-developed interpersonal communication, group management, and problem-solving skills. Knox and Irving (1997) noted that communication was the most important factor in promoting change.
- Integrative thinking: the ability to retain a big picture focus while dealing with each part of the system.
- Sufficient flexibility to modify ideas when modifications will improve the change, but enough persistence to resist nonproductive tampering with the planned change.
- Confidence and the tendency not to be easily discouraged.
- Realistic thinking.
- Trustworthiness: a track record of integrity and success with other changes.
- The ability to articulate a vision through insights and versatile thinking.
- The ability to handle resistance.

Contrary to popular opinion, change often is not initiated by top-level management (Yukl, 2002), but rather emerges as new initiatives or problems are identified. Thus, all managers must be able to initiate change and to participate in implementing change.

Energy is needed to change a system. Power is the main source of that energy. Informational power, expertise, and possibly positional power can be used to persuade others. To access optimum power, use the following strategies:

1. Analyze the organizational chart. Know the formal lines of authority. Identify informal lines as well.
2. Identify key persons who will be affected by the change. Pay attention to those immediately above and below the point of change.
3. Find out as much as possible about these key people. What are their "tickle points"? What interests them, gets them excited, turns them off? What is on their personal and organizational agendas? Who typically aligns with whom on important decisions?
4. Begin to build a coalition of support before you start the change process. Identify the key people who will most likely support your idea and those who are most likely to be persuaded easily. Talk informally with them to flush out possible objections to your idea and potential opponents. What will the costs and benefits be to them—especially in political terms? Can your idea be modified in ways that retain your objectives but appeals to more key people?

This information helps the manager develop the most sellable idea or at least pinpoint probable resistance. It is a broad beginning to the data-collection step of the change process and has to be fine-tuned once the idea is better defined. The astute manager keeps alert at all times to monitor power struggles.

Although a cardinal rule of change is: Don't try to change too much too fast, the savvy manager develops a sense of exquisite timing by pacing the change process according to the political pulse. For example, the manager unfreezes the system during a period of

MEDIALINK   Thirteen Tips for Managing Change

coalition building and high interest, while resistance is low or at least unorganized.

The manager may stall the project beyond a pilot stage if resistance solidifies or gains a powerful ally. In this case, the manager exercises mechanisms to reduce resistance. If resistance continues, two options should be considered:

- The change is not workable and should be modified to meet the strongest objections (compromise).
- The change is fine-tuned sufficiently, but change must proceed now and resistance must be overcome.

If the latter option is selected, energy is focused on overcoming resistance. Supporters are mobilized, and constant, consistent pressure is exerted to move ahead.

How the manager participates in the change process depends on whether she or he is an insider or outsider. Someone who is part of the system being changed knows that system, has a stake in the outcome, and is familiar with the people, language, and politics. However, being an insider can restrict one's ability to move freely throughout the system. The manager may be locked into certain roles, authority structures, and expectations. Perspective may be limited. However, blinders to insight can be removed. An outsider offers a fresh perspective and is independent of internal policies but is unfamiliar with the system, people's values, and personal agendas. Either insiders or outsiders can accomplish change, but change must be assessed and used differently.

What You Know Now

- In today's health care system, change is rapid, constant, persuasive, and persistent.
- Critical evaluation of planned change theory and selection of theories suitable for nursing provide guidance and direction for initiating and managing change.
- The change process is similar to the nursing process: assessment, planning, implementation, and evaluation.
- The manager will use change agent skills in initiating change and in implementing organizational change.
- Resistance to change is to be expected, and it can be a stimulant as well as a force to be overcome.
- The manager must understand resistance and develop skills to handle it.
- The manager needs to understand the politics of change and use power strategies successfully.

Tools for Initiating and Managing Change

1. Identify the problem or opportunity.
2. Collect necessary data and information.
3. Select and analyze data.
4. Develop a plan for change, including time frame and resources.
5. Identify supporters or opposers.
6. Build a coalition of supporters.
7. Help people prepare for change.
8. Prepare to handle resistance.
9. Provide a feedback mechanism to keep everyone informed of the progress of change.
10. Evaluate effectiveness of the change and, if successful, stabilize the change.

Questions to Challenge You

1. Identify a needed change in the organization where you practice. Using the change process, outline the steps you would take to initiate change.
2. Consider your school or college. What change do you think is needed? Explain how you would change it to become a better place for learning.
3. Have you had an experience with change occurring in your organization? What was your initial reaction? Did that change? How well did the change process work? Was the change successful?
4. Do you have a behavior you would like to change? Using the steps in the change process, describe how you might effect that change.
5. How do you normally react to change? Choose from the following:
    a) I love new ideas, and I'm ready to try new things.
    b) I like to know that something will work out before I try it.
    c) I try to avoid change as much as possible.
6. Did your response to the above question alter how you would like to view change? Think about this the next time change is presented to you.

Explore 🌐 MediaLink

NCLEX review questions, essay activities, group activities, and other interactive resources for this chapter can be found on the Web site at http://www.prenhall.com/sullivan-decker. Click on "Chapter 16" to select activities for this chapter.

References

Baulcomb, J. S. (2003). Management of change through force field analysis. *Journal of Nursing Management, 11*(4), 275–280.

Havelock, R. (1973). *The change agent's guide to innovation in education.* Englewood Cliffs, NJ: Educational Technology Publications.

Hawke, M. (2003). Embracing change. *Nursing Spectrum, 4* (4), 32.

Hellriegel, D., Jackson, S. E., & Slocum, Jr., J. W. (2002). *Management: A competency-based approach* (9th ed.). Eagan, MN: South-Western.

Katz, D., & Kahn, R. (1978). *The social psychology of organizations* (2nd ed.). New York: Wiley.

Knox, S., & Irving, J. A. (1997). Nurse manager perceptions of healthcare executive behaviors during organizational change. *Journal of Nursing Administration, 27*(11), 33–39.

Lewin, K. (1951). *Field theory in social science.* New York: Harper & Row.

Lippitt, R., Watson, J., & Westley, B. (1958). *The dynamics of planned change.* New York: Harcourt & Brace.

McConnell, C. R. (2002). Know when to manage less, not more. *The Health Care Manager, 20*(4), iv–vi.

Porter-O'Grady, T. (2003). A different age for leadership, Part 2: New rules, new roles. *Journal of Nursing Administration, 33*(3), 173–178.

Rogers, E. (1983). *Diffusion of innovations* (3rd ed.). New York: Free Press.

Yukl, G. (2002). *Leadership in organizations* (5th ed.). Upper Saddle River, NJ: Prentice Hall.

Managing Human Resources

CHAPTER 17

Handling Staffing and Scheduling

Staffing

Patient Classification Systems
Determining Nursing Care Hours
Determining FTEs
Determining Staffing Mix
Determining Distribution of Staff

Scheduling

Creative and Flexible Scheduling
Self-Staffing and Scheduling
Supplemental Staff

Looking Ahead

Chapter 17 introduces the human resource management section of this book: the development and management of staff, dealing with problems, and the various obligations and ways of dealing with others that go along with being a manager. The first step is to determine the number of staff needed within the health care organization. The quality of patient care is dependent on the number and competency of the staff regardless of the setting where the care is delivered (e.g., hospital, clinic, skilled nursing facility, home). Several questions must be answered: What are the workload patterns? How can staff be distributed in a way that is both efficient and effective? How are the needs of both the staff and the clients balanced? This

chapter will help you find better strategies to face these challenges.

Objectives

In this chapter, you will learn

- How to determine staffing requirements.
- What factors to consider when determining staffing requirements.
- How patient classification systems are used to determine staffing needs.
- How to use a variety of resources to plan staffing.

MediaLink www.prenhall.com/ sullivan-decker

Additional resources for this chapter can be found on the Companion Website at www.prenhall.com/sullivan-decker. Click on "Chapter 17" to select the activities for this chapter.

- NCLEX Review
- Critical Thinking Activities
- Current Events
- MediaLinks
- *Nursing Leadership & Management in Action: Self Governance: Critique of a Staff Schedule*

Staffing and scheduling is an important responsibility of the nurse manager. The higher the proportion of registered nurses with more hours of care provided by them results in higher quality care, according to a landmark study in the New England Journal of Medicine (Needleman,

Buerhaus, Mattke, Stewart, & Zelevinsky, 2002). Another study demonstrated that the number of baccalaureate-prepared nurses affected surgical patient mortality (Aiken, Clarke, Cheung, Sloane, & Silber, 2003). Mortality was higher when the organization employed nurses with less than a baccalaureate degree. In addition, Potter, Barr, McSweeney, and Sledge (2003) found that adequate staffing levels positively affected patient outcomes. Thus, staffing and scheduling adequate numbers of competent staff to meet patients' needs is the focus of this chapter.

Staffing

The goal of **staffing** is to provide the appropriate numbers and mix of nursing staff (nursing care hours) to match actual or projected patient care needs (patient care hours) that will lead to the delivery of effective and efficient nursing care. There is no single or perfect method to achieve efficient and effective staffing. There are, however, key elements that contribute to successful and satisfying staffing. Because staffing requires continuous fine-tuning, variability in patient census during the year is a big challenge for nursing managers.

In a hospital, the unit may experience a steady census during the 7 days of the week or a higher census from Monday to Friday. Its patient days may be distributed evenly during the year, or it may consistently experience peaks in occupancy in certain months (seasonality pattern) such as the months of April, July, and October. In hospitals as well as in other health care settings, staffing is one of the most pressing challenges nurse managers face.

To determine staffing requirements (number of staff), nurse managers must examine workload patterns for the designated unit, department, or clinic. For a hospital, this means determining the level of care, average daily census, and hours of care provided 24 hours a day, 7 days a week.

The Joint Commission on the Accreditation of Healthcare Organizations (JCAHO, 2002) specifies only that the right number of competent staff be provided to meet patients' needs based on organization-selected criteria. JCAHO does not identify specific levels of nursing care hours for specific patient populations or types of patient care units, or the type of patient classification system to be used.

Although they do not accredit health care organizations, the American Nurses Association (ANA, 1999) has developed principles for nurse staffing as shown in Box 17-1. ANA recommends that health care organizations shift from an industrial, technical model to a professional model and focus on the level of nurse competency required to provide quality nursing care.

Patient Classification Systems

Patient classification systems (PCSs), sometimes referred to as patient acuity systems, were developed to determine workload requirements and staffing needs objectively. To be most effective, patient classification data are collected midpoint for every shift by the unit nursing staff and analyzed before the next shift to ensure appropriate numbers and mix of nursing staff.

Initially, paper-and-pencil methods based on industrial engineering models that incorporated time and motion study data were used to estimate annual staffing needs and determine the annual personnel budget (Malloch & Conovaloff, 1999). Three methods were commonly used:

1. Descriptive
2. Checklist
3. Time standard

The descriptive system is a subjective classification of patient activities by category. Four or five categories are used to describe varying levels of care and dependence. The nurse selects the category that best represents the patient. Neither category is an actual representation of the patient's needs or the staff's time. As a result, this type of classification system is rarely used today.

The checklist format is another subjective system in which an acuity level is determined by identifying the level of activity within each category for each patient. Points ascribed for each level of activity (eating, bathing, medications, and so on) are totaled and converted to a level of acuity. For example, a new mother following a cesarean section can feed herself (1 point), has a Foley catheter in place (3 points), has an intravenous catheter (3 points), and needs minimal assistance turning (2 points). Totaled, this patient receives 9 points, which by the hospital's standards converts to an acuity of 2. The checklist format provides a more individualized

MEDIALINK   Patient Classification System

KEY TERMS

Staffing   The process of balancing the quantity of staff available with the quantity and mix of staff needed by the organization.

Patient classification systems (PCSs)   Systems developed to objectively determine workload requirements and staffing needs.

Box 17-1   American Nurses Association's Principles for Nurse Staffing

A. Patient Care Unit Related

1. Appropriate staffing levels for a patient care unit reflect analysis of individual and aggregate patient needs.

2. There is a critical need to either retire or seriously question the usefulness of the concept of nursing hours per patient day (HPPD).

3. Unit functions necessary to support delivery of quality patient care must also be considered in determining staffing levels.

B. Staff Related

1. The specific needs of various patient populations should determine the appropriate clinical competencies required of the nurse practicing in that area.

2. Registered nurses must have nursing management support and representation at both the operational level and the executive level.

3. Clinical support from experienced RNs should be readily available to those RNs with less proficiency.

C. Institution/Organization Related

1. Organizational policy should reflect an organizational climate that values registered nurses and other employees as strategic assets and exhibits a true commitment to filling budgeted positions in a timely manner.

2. All institutions should have documented competencies for nursing staff, including agency or supplemental and traveling RNs, for those activities that they have been authorized to perform.

3. Organizational policies should recognize the myriad needs of both patients and nursing staff.

From *Principles for Nurse Staffing,* copyright 1999. Retrieved from www.nursingworld.org/readroom/stffprnc.htm. American Nurses Association, Washington, DC.

representation of patients' needs but still may not adequately reflect nursing's time.

In the time standard method, work sampling techniques are used to determine time standards associated with various patient care activities. Activities required for patient care are identified; associated time standards are calculated; and, like the checklist method, patient care is totaled and converted to an acuity level. This type of PCS best represents both the patient's needs and nursing's time.

With the advent of computers, patient classification systems have become computerized and are used to determine daily staffing needs and predict monthly personnel budgets. The most common of these are Medicus, GRASP, and ARIC.

Medicus   One of the first patient classification systems developed, **Medicus,** was introduced in the late 1960s and continues to be used frequently in the United States. This instrument contains 37 indicators that determine patient dependence on nursing. The result of the applicable indicators is that the patient is placed in one of five levels of care. A patient classified as a 5 requires the greatest intensity of nursing care. Patients are clustered into categories; nursing care requirements are defined in terms of average hours of care per category. A predetermined relative value for the level of care is established by

the organization. For example, on a 22-bed acute medical unit with an average patient rating of 3.5, the hours of nursing care required might be 6.8. Total hours of care with this system reflect both direct and indirect care.

GRASP   In 1970, a patient classification system referred to as PETO was introduced. After further study and refinement, **GRASP (Grace Reynolds Application and Study of PETO)** emerged in the mid-1970s (Meyer, 1978). GRASP is probably the most commonly used PCS in the United States. GRASP identifies 40 to 50 direct care activities, as identified by a specific unit, which account for about 85 percent of the direct care activities. An example is provided in Table 17-1.

KEY TERMS

Medicus   A patient classification system that clusters patients into five categories of nursing care as predetermined by indicators.

GRASP (Grace Reynolds Application and Study of PETO)   A patient classification system that identifies direct care activities, determines total hours of care, and projects nursing interventions and required staff.

Table 17-1   Components of GRASP

Rehabilitation Example

Assessment: (Circle each shift) Patient	A	B	C	D	E	F	G	H	I	J	K	L
Assessment/update assessment	3	3	3	3	3	3	3	3	3	3	3	3
Planning: (circle each shift)												
1. Update/Revise care plan/Problem list	2	2	2	2	2	2	2	2	2	2	2	2
Knowledge deficit: (circle as applicable)												
1. Planned teaching	2	2	2	2	2	2	2	2	2	2	2	2
2. Reinforce teaching	6	6	6	6	6	6	6	6	6	6	6	6
Self-care deficit—feeding: (circle highest applicable)												
1. Feeds self independently	2	2	2	2	2	2	2	2	2	2	2	2
2. Feeds self with assistance by personnel/family	4	4	4	4	4	4	4	4	4	4	4	4
3. Total feed or self-feed with dysphagia training	24	24	24	24	24	24	24	24	24	24	24	24
4. Total feed by staff/feeds self with constant supervision	9	9	9	9	9	9	9	9	9	9	9	9
5. Tube feeding continuous/bolus	6	6	6	6	6	6	6	6	6	6	6	6
Self-care deficit—toileting: (circle highest applicable)												
1. Incontinent care—toilet/bedside commode (BSC) with constant supervision	12	12	12	12	12	12	12	12	12	12	12	12
2. Toilet with assist/BSC/bedpan/urinal	8	8	8	8	8	8	8	8	8	8	8	8
Self-care deficit—bathing/hygiene/grooming: (circle highest applicable)												
1. Total care by staff	6	6	6	6	6	6	6	6	6	6	6	6
2. Moderate care by staff	3	3	3	3	3	3	3	3	3	3	3	3
3. Minimal care by staff	2	2	2	2	2	2	2	2	2	2	2	2
Operation in safety												
1. Restraint	4	4	4	4	4	4	4	4	4	4	4	4
2. Monitor the wandering patient	10	10	10	10	10	10	10	10	10	10	10	10
Other direct: (circle as applicable)												
1. Assistive devices	4	4	4	4	4	4	4	4	4	4	4	4
2. Accucheck	3	3	3	3	3	3	3	3	3	3	3	3
3. Empty Foley/leg bags/drainage collection containers	1	1	1	1	1	1	1	1	1	1	1	1
4. Simple dressing change/remove staples/sutures/steri strips	2	2	2	2	2	2	2	2	2	2	2	2
5. Complex dressing/decubitus care	7	7	7	7	7	7	7	7	7	7	7	7
6. I & O calculation/calorie count	1	1	1	1	1	1	1	1	1	1	1	1
7. Nourishment/supplement feedings/diabetic snacks	1	1	1	1	1	1	1	1	1	1	1	1
Direct care:	10	10	10	10	10	10	10	10	10	10	10	10
Evaluation: (circle each shift)	2	2	2	2	2	2	2	2	2	2	2	2
Unit patient care hour (PCH) Total												
PCH												

Note: Time values on chart have been increased to reflect time for all unlisted activities.

Direct care activities are determined by the organization; time studies are completed to ensure that the instrument is tailored to the organization. An adjustment factor is added to account for the direct care activities that are unlisted about 15 percent of the time. Also, indirect patient care activities are added to determine the total hours of care. In the example provided, the numbers in each column correspond to the total hours of care assigned to that patient care activity. These calculations for every patient are completed every 12 hours and, based on the existing patients, can project nursing interventions and required staff for the next shift. The numbers on the form adjacent to the interventions represent the projected time it takes to complete the activity. The system incorporates interrater reliability testing to verify continued accuracy of the data.

The GRASP system operates as a multidimensional nursing management information system package and includes management reporting, staffing/scheduling, budgeting, cost identification, and quality evaluation. The patient classification portion of the system may be implemented in either a manual pen-and-paper or computerized form.

ARIC ARIC (**Allocation, Resource, Identification, and Costing**) was developed in the 1970s by the Sisters of Mercy Health Corporation. This system incorporates patient admission, discharge, and transfer information from each patient along with the classification information and recognizes the dependent activities of nurses, physicians' orders and hospital policies, and the independent activities of nurses and their professional judgments. Staffing reports are generated based on the patient classification information entered. The reports identify actual versus needed staffing, the level of productivity, and staff exceeding workload.

Computerized systems are developing that incorporate expert nurse judgments into patient assignments. They are able to classify patients' needs, match them with nurses' skills and availability, and then track and monitor results. Integrated with the clinical information systems, these programs promise the most effectiveness for the future (see Chapter 14).

Determining Nursing Care Hours

From the patient classification data, patient workload trends are analyzed for each day of the week (each hour in critical care) or for a specific patient diagnosis to determine staffing needs, known as **nursing care hours (NCHs)**. For example, if 26 patients with the following acuities required 161 nursing care hours, then an average of 6.19 nursing hours per patient per day (NHPPD) are required. NHPPD are calculated by dividing the total nursing care hours by the total census (number of patients).

Number of Patients	Acuity Level	Associated Hours of Care	Total Hours of Care
3	I	2	6
10	II	6	60
11	III	7	77
2	IV	9	18
Total 26			*161*

There are no specific standards for nursing care hours (NCHs) for any type of patient or patient care unit. NCHs may vary on the average from 5 to 7 hours of care for patients on medical and/or surgical units, to 10 to 24 hours of care for patients in critical care units, to 24 to 48 hours of care for selected patients, such as new, severely burned patients.

Determining FTEs

Positions are defined in terms of a **full-time equivalent (FTE)**. One FTE equals 40 hours of work per week for 52 weeks, or 2,080 hours per year. In a 2-week pay period, one FTE would equal 80 hours. One FTE can be filled by one person or any combination of personnel. For example, one nurse may work 24 hours per week, and two other nurses may each work 8 hours per week. Together, the three nurses fill one FTE (24+8+8=40).

Several methods are available for determining the number of FTEs required to staff a unit 24 hours a day, 7 days a week. One technique incorporates information regarding the hours of work for the staff for 2 weeks, average daily census, and hours of care. The average daily census can be determined by dividing the total patient days (obtained from daily census counts for the year) by the number of days in the year.

■ EXAMPLE

$$\text{Total patient days} = \frac{9490}{365} = 26 \text{ patients per day}$$

Data

Number of hours worked per FTE in 2 weeks = 80
Number of days of coverage in 2 weeks = 14
Average daily census = 26
Average nursing care hours (from PCS) = 6.15

Formula

$$x = \frac{\text{average nursing care hours} \times \text{days in staffing period} \times \text{average patient census}}{\text{hours of work per FTE in 2 weeks}}$$

$$x = \frac{6.15 \times 14 \times 26}{80} = \frac{2238.6}{80} = 27.98, \text{ or } 28 \text{ FTEs}$$

A second technique uses nursing care hours and annual hours of work provided by one FTE:

Data

Number of hours worked per FTE in 1 year = 2080
Total nursing care hours (from PCS) = 161

Formula

$$x = \frac{\text{Total nursing care hours} \times \text{days in a year}}{\text{Total annual hours per one FTE}}$$

$$x = \frac{161 \times 365}{2080} = \frac{58,765}{2080} = 28.25, \text{ or } 28 \text{ FTEs}$$

As previously delineated, one person working full-time usually works 80 hours (ten 8-hour shifts) in a 2-week period. However, to staff an 8-hour shift takes 1.4 FTEs, one person working ten 8-hour shifts (1.0 FTE) and another person working four 8-hour shifts (0.4 FTE) in order to provide for the full-time person's 2 days off every week. For 12-hour shifts, it takes 2.1 FTEs to staff one 12-hour shift each day, each week; two people each working three 12-hour shifts and one person working one 12-hour shift each week (0.9 FTE = 0.9 FTE = 0.3 FTE = 2.1 FTEs). Therefore, the same number of FTEs is required to staff a unit for 24 hours a day for 2 weeks, regardless of whether the staff are all on 8-hour shifts (1.4 FTEs × 33 shifts = 4.2 FTEs) or 12-hour shifts (2.1 FTEs × 32 shifts = 4.2 FTEs).

Determining Staffing Mix

The same data used to determine FTEs are used to identify **staffing mix**. For example, for patient care needs involving general hygiene care, feeding, transferring, or turning patients, unlicensed assistive personnel (UAPs) can be used. For patient care needs involving frequent assessments, patient education, or discharge planning, RNs will be needed because of the skills required. A high RN-skill mix allows for greater staffing flexibility. Again, information on typical or usual patient needs is obtained by using trends from the patient classification system.

Determining Distribution of Staff

For many patient care units, the distribution of staff varies from shift to shift and by days of the week. Patient census on a surgical unit will probably fluctuate throughout the week, with a higher census Monday through Thursday and a lower census over the weekend. In addition, some surgical units may have more complex cases earlier in the week and short-stay surgical cases later in the week. Surgical patients may have a shorter length of stay (LOS) than many medical patients. The patient census on a medical unit rarely fluctuates Monday through Friday, but may be less on weekends, when diagnostic tests are not done.

The workload on many units also varies within the 24-hour period. The care demands on a surgical unit will be heaviest early in the morning hours prior to the start of the surgical schedule; midmorning, when the unit receives patients from critical care unit(s); late in the afternoon, when patients return from the postanesthesia recovery unit; and in the evening hours, when same-day surgical patients are discharged.

Critical care units may have greater care needs in the mornings when transferring patients to medical or surgical units and in the early afternoon hours when admitting new surgical cases. Medical units usually have the heaviest care needs in the morning hours, when patients' daily care needs are being met and physicians are making rounds. On skilled nursing and rehabilitation units, care needs are greatest before and immediately after mealtimes and in the evening hours; during other times of the day, patients are often away from the unit and involved in various therapeutic activities.

KEY TERMS

ARIC (Allocation, Resource, Identification, and Costing) A patient classification system that incorporates patient and classification information with staff activities to generate staffing reports.

Nursing care hours (NCHs) The number of hours of patient care provided per unit of time.

Full-time equivalent (FTE) The percentage of time an employee works that is based on a 40-hour workweek.

Staffing mix The type of staff necessary to perform the work of the organization.

MEDIALINK American Nurses Association's Principles for Nurse Staffing

In contrast with the medical, surgical, critical care, and rehabilitation units that have definite patterns of patient care needs, labor-and-delivery and emergency department areas cannot predict when patient care needs will be most intense. Thus, labor-and-delivery and emergency department areas must rely on block staffing to ensure that adequate nursing staff are available at all times.

Block staffing involves scheduling a set staff mix for every shift. However, there may be trends in peak workload hours in emergency departments, when additional staff (RN, UAP, or secretary) beyond the block staff are necessary. Examples of peak workload hours within the emergency department may be from 6:00 P.M. to 10:00 P.M. to accommodate patient needs after physicians' offices close or from 12:00 A.M. to 3:00 A.M. to accommodate alcohol-related injuries. All these patterns of care needs must be known when staffing requirements and work schedules are established. Data reflecting peak workload times must be continuously monitored to maintain the appropriate levels and mix of staff.

Table 17-2 presents a staffing template for a 30-bed unit with fluctuating needs. This table illustrates numbers of staff and numbers of FTEs (the latter appear in brackets), as well as the staffing mix required for every shift. The direct care totals include only those nursing personnel providing direct patient care. Leadership and unit clerk positions are excluded from the direct care numbers. The decision to include or exclude these two groups of staff is a very important decision that affects the unit's productivity report. The total number of FTEs involved in direct care is based on the average NHPPD of 6.15 hours and an average patient census of 26 patients (86.7% occupancy). Average occupancy rates are determined by dividing the average patient days (obtained by

dividing total annual census by number of beds on unit) by number of days in a year.

■ EXAMPLE

Data
Annual census = 9,490
Number of beds on unit = 30

Formula

$$\text{Average patient days} = \frac{\text{Annual census}}{\text{Number of beds}}$$

$$\text{Occupancy rate} = \frac{\text{Average patient days}}{\text{Days in a year}}$$

$$\text{Average patient days} = \frac{9490}{30} = 316.33$$

$$\text{Occupancy rate} = \frac{316.33}{365} = 86.7\%$$

Scheduling

Creative and Flexible Scheduling

Nurse shortages and current restrictions in salary budgets have made creative and flexible staffing patterns necessary and probably everlasting. Combinations of 4-, 6-, 8-, 10-, and 12-hour shifts and schedules that have nurses working 6 consecutive days of 12-hour shifts with 13 days off, and staffing strategies such as weekend programs and split shifts are common. Table 17-3 presents a 2-week working schedule for RNs based on the master staffing template; four types of shifts and a weekend option are incorporated. Note that the work schedule has fewer RNs on weekends and more RNs Monday through Friday. However, the average nursing care hours

Table 17-2   Staffing Template*

Shift	Leadership Unit Manager/ Assistant Unit Manager	RNs	LPNs	UAPs	Unit Clerk	Direct Care	Total Nursing Care Hours	All Staff
Day	1 [1.0]	4 [5.6]	2 [2.8]	2 [2.8]	1 [1.4]	8 [11.2]	64	10 [13.6]
Evening	1 [1.0]	4 [5.6]	1 [1.4]	2 [2.8]	1 [1.4]	7 [9.8]	56	9 [12.2]
Night	0 [0.0]	2 [2.8]	2 [2.8]	1 [1.4]	0 [0.0]	5 [7.0]	40	5 [7.0]
Total	2 [2.0]	10 [14.0]	5 [7.0]	5 [7.0]	2 [2.8]	20 [28.0]	160	24 [32.8]

*This is a 30-bed unit, but it is staffed for an average patient census of 26 (86.7% occupancy) and an average number of hours of care of 6.15 (calculated using only direct care staff). In each column (except for "Total Nursing Care Hours"), the number on the left indicates the number of staff; the bracketed number to the right indicates the number of FTEs.

Table 17-3 Sample 2-Week Schedule for RNs on Surgical Unit Using 4-, 6-, 8-, and 12-Hour Shifts and Weekend Option (Average Patient Census of 26)

Name	Position	FTE	Week 1 S	M	T	W	T	F	S	Week 2 S	M	T	W	T	F	S
Taber	Head Nurse (HN)	1.0	-	D	D	D	D	D	-	-	D	D	D	D	D	-
Carson	Assistant HN	1.0	E	E	E	E	E	-	-	-	E	E	E	E	-	E
Lewis	RN	1.0	-	D	D	D	D	-	D	-	D	D	D	D	D	-
Cass	RN	1.0	-	D	D	D	D	D	-	-	-	D	D	D	D	D
Freeze	RN	0.9	A	A	A	-	-	-	-	-	-	-	-	A	A	A
Ritz	RN	0.9	-	-	-	-	A	A	A	A	A	A	-	-	-	-
Jakarti	RN	0.9	-	-	A	A	A	-	-	A	A	-	A	-	-	-
Chow	RN	.55	-	-	D	6	-	D	E	-	-	D	6	-	-	-
Smith	RN	0.4	-	A	-	-	-	-	-	-	-	A	-	D	-	-
Burch	RN	0.4	-	-	-	D	-	-	D	-	D	-	E	-	-	-
Jones	RN	PRN	-	-	-	5	4	-	-	-	-	-	5	-	-	A
Betz	RN	PRN	A	-	-	-	-	-	-	-	-	-	-	A	-	-
Zipp	RN	PRN	-	-	-	-	-	A	-	-	-	-	A	-	-	-
Simon	RN	PRN	-	-	-	-	D	-	-	-	-	-	-	-	A	-
Link	RN	0.9	-	E	E	E	-	E	E	-	E	E	E	E	-	-
White	RN	0.9	-	E	E	P	N	-	-	-	E	E	N	-	-	P
Turner	RN	0.9	P	P	P	-	-	-	-	P	P	P	-	-	-	-
Short	RN	0.9	P	P	P	-	-	-	-	-	P	-	-	P	P	-
Melton	RN	.75	-	-	-	P	-	P	-	-	-	P	P	P	-	-
Graham*	RN	0.6	-	-	-	-	-	P	P	-	-	-	-	-	P	P
Allen	RN	0.5	-	-	-	3	E	E	-	-	-	-	E	4	R	-
Pascheco	RN	0.5	-	E	-	-	E	-	-	-	-	-	E	-	E	E
King	RN	0.4	-	-	3	3	E	-	-	P	-	-	4	-	-	-
Boyer	RN	PRN	-	-	4	4	P	-	-	-	-	-	-	3	-	-
Lui	RN	PRN	-	-	-	-	-	-	N	-	-	-	-	N	-	-
		†7 A.M.–3 P.M.	2	4	5	5	5	4	3	2	4	5	5	5	4	3
		†3 P.M.–7 P.M.	2	5	5	5	5	4	2	2	5	5	5	5	4	2
		†7 P.M.–11 P.M.	2	5	5	5	5	4	2	2	5	5	5	5	4	2
		†11 P.M.–7 A.M.	2	2	2	2	2	2	2	2	2	2	2	2	2	2
	Daily RN Nursing Care Hours		48	88	96	96	96	80	56	48	88	96	96	96	80	56

Legend: D = 7 A.M.–3 P.M.; E = 3 P.M.–11 P.M.; N = 11 P.M.–7 A.M.; A = 7 A.M.–7 P.M.; P = 7 P.M.–7 A.M.; PRN = as needed; 1 = 7 A.M.–11 A.M.; 2 = 11 A.M.–3 P.M.; 3 = 3 P.M.–7 P.M.; 4 = 7 P.M.–11 P.M.; 5 = 7 A.M.–1 P.M.; 6 = 1 P.M.–7 P.M.

*Weekend option (works 12-hour shifts every Saturday and Sunday "A" *or* Friday and Saturday "P").
†Number of RNs scheduled to work each shift based on average patient acuity and census.

would be unchanged; more LPNs and UAPs would be included. A decrease in patient census and intensity of patient care needs on weekends (as identified from trend analysis) justify this alteration. Distribution of all staff is based on the overall data on actual patient care needs.

Flexible staffing patterns, as presented in Table 17-3, can be a major challenge for the nurse manager, and in some cases a mathematical challenge. However, once a schedule is established and agreed to by the nurse manager and the staff, it can become a cyclic schedule for an extended period of time, such as 6 to 12 months. This allows staff members to know their work schedule many months ahead of time.

KEY TERMS

Block staffing Scheduling a set staff mix for every shift so that adequate staff is available at all times.

The use of 8-hour and 12-hour shifts is fairly straightforward. Problems with combined staffing patterns may include

- The perception that nurses don't work full time when they work several days in a row and then are off for several days in a row,
- Disruption in continuity of care if split shifts are used (7:00 A.M. to 11:00 A.M.; 11:00 A.M. to 3:00 P.M.; 3:00 P.M. to 7:00 P.M.; 7:00 P.M. to 1:00 A.M.; 1:00 A.M. to 7:00 A.M. shifts), and
- Immense challenges for nurse managers to communicate with all staff in a timely manner.

Advantages of using combined staffing patterns are that it

- Better meets patient care needs during peak workload times,
- Improves staff satisfaction, and
- Maximizes the availability of nurses.

Ten-hour shifts (not included in Table 17-3) provide greater overlap between shifts to permit extra time for nurses to complete their work; for this reason, 10-hour shifts may increase salary expenditures. There are a few specialty units in which 10-hour shifts would be cost-efficient: postanesthesia recovery areas, operating departments, and emergency departments are examples.

Self-Staffing and Scheduling

Some hospitals have instituted **self-staffing and scheduling**. With this model, nurse managers and their staff completely manage staffing and schedules. This is an empowerment strategy that allows unit staff the authority to use their backup staffing options if the patient workload increases or if unscheduled staff absences occur. Likewise, staff can and must go home early if the patient workload decreases.

Hospitals can no longer arbitrarily staff patient care units on weekends or at nights with marginal numbers or levels of qualified staff. The acuity of patients in hospitals, including medical and surgical patients, mandates staffing units on the weekends by the same principles used for weekdays. Thorough trend analysis of patient classification data can provide the justification necessary to appropriately decrease the number of RNs, at least for some levels, because of differences in patient care needs throughout the day. Another creative method for staffing includes a weekend program, in which a nurse agrees to work 24 hours every weekend (usually two 12-hour shifts) for full-time benefits and full-time salary or premium salary.

Supplemental Staff

When there is a need for additional staff because of scheduled or unscheduled absences, increased workload demands, or existing staff vacancies, the nurse manager or staffing person must find additional staff. Options include using PRN staff (staff scheduled on an as-needed basis), part-time staff, or float pool staff; allowing overtime for full-time staff; scheduling nurse manager(s) for direct care assignments; using extra nurses from another unit; using outside agency nurses; or asking staff for suggestions or help.

Supplemental staff are needed when workload increases beyond that which the existing staff can manage, staff absences and resignations occur, and staff vacancies exist. Chronic staffing problems need to be addressed in a proactive manner involving the nurse manager, the chief nurse executive, and the nursing personnel on the unit having the problem. Strategies for dealing with turnover are given in Chapter 22, and strategies for managing absenteeism are discussed in Chapter 23.

Internal Pools   Acute staffing problems can be addressed by establishing internal float pools using nursing staff and unlicensed assistive personnel (UAPs). Internal float **pools** of nurses can provide supplemental staffing at a substantially lower cost than using agency nurses. Internal float pools can be centralized or decentralized. A centralized pool is the most efficient. A pool of RNs, LPNs, UAPs, and unit clerks are available for placement anywhere in the institution. However, it may be difficult to place the person with the correct skills for a particular unit at the needed time. In decentralized pools, a staff member usually works only for one nurse manager or on only one unit. The advantages of decentralized pools include better accountability, improved staffing response, and improved continuity of care. Critical care units, operating rooms, maternal–child units, and other highly specialized or technical areas tend to use a decentralized system. Other pools often used include PRN or per diem staff. PRN staff also can be centralized or decentralized. These employees, however, receive premium pay instead of benefits.

External Pools   For some institutions, agency nurses become part of the regular staff contracted to fill vacancies for a specified period of time (e.g., traveling nurses). However, most agency nurses are used as supplemental staff. All agency nurses require orientation to the facility and unit; they must work under the supervision of an experienced in-house nurse. The nurse manager must verify valid licensure, ensure that either the agency or agency nurse has current malpractice insurance, and develop a mechanism to evaluate the agency nurse's performance. Although an agency nurse may meet an urgent staffing need, continuity of care may be compromised and there may be some staff resentment because these nurses may earn two to three times the salary of in-house nurses.

Use of Existing Staff   Nurse managers also must explore opportunities to use nurse extenders, referred to as unlicensed assistive personnel (UAPs). Persons in these roles are nonprofessionals and may or may not provide direct patient care. Sometimes, UAPs complete nonnursing tasks and allow nurses time to assume direct care. Emptying trash, getting supplies, transporting patients, distributing linens, and delivering drinking water and food trays are all nonnursing tasks that take nurses away from the patient's professional care. As the demands for nursing care continue, more efficient and effective use of UAPs will remain a strong option, permitting RNs to focus exclusively on direct patient care.

What You Know Now

- The goal of staffing and scheduling is to provide an adequate mix of nursing staff to match patient care needs.
- The Joint Commission on the Accreditation of Healthcare Organizations requires that organizations determine criteria for nurse staffing and provide adequate numbers of competent staff to meet that criteria.
- Various patient classification systems exist, and they are increasingly being incorporated into computerized clinical information systems.
- Scheduling involves assigning available staff in a way that patient care needs are met. Scheduling is always a challenge.
- Flexible and creative staffing and scheduling techniques are increasingly necessary.

- Self-staffing and scheduling is an option in which nursing staff participate in designing the schedule and accepting responsibility for ensuring attendance.

Tools for Handling Staffing and Scheduling

1. Familiarize yourself with the current patient classification or acuity system in use.
2. Determine the nursing care hours needed.
3. Determine FTEs needed.
4. Create or modify a schedule that best meets your patients' needs.
5. Supplement staff as needed.
6. Consider self-staffing if appropriate.

Questions to Challenge You

1. What has been your experience with staffing? Use any work setting where you are or have been an employee. How well did it work? Was there adequate coverage to meet the needs of the organization? Explain.
2. Study Table 17-3. Where are there possible gaps in coverage? Where might there be overlap?
3. On occasion, there are more staff available than are needed. As a nurse manager, how would you handle this? How might the staff respond?
4. No one is ever completely satisfied with the schedule. How would you handle a staff member who repeatedly asks to have his schedule changed?

Explore 🌐 MediaLink

NCLEX review questions, essay activities, group activities, and other interactive resources for this chapter can be found on the Web site at http://www.prenhall.com/sullivan-decker. Click on "Chapter 17" to select activities for this chapter.

References

Aiken, L. H., Clarke, S. P., Cheung, R. B., Sloane, D. M., & Silber, J. H. (2003). Educational levels of hospital nurses and surgical patient mortality. *JAMA, 290*(12), 1617–1623.

American Nurses Association. (1999). *Principles for nurse staffing.* Washington, DC: Author.

Joint Commission on the Accreditation of Healthcare Organizations (JCAHO). (2002). *Comprehensive accreditation manual for hospitals: The official handbook.* Oakbrook Terrace, IL: Author.

Malloch, K., & Conovaloff, A. (1999). Patient classification systems, Part 1: The third generation. *Journal of Nursing Administration, 29*(7/8), 49–56.

Meyer, D. (1978). *GRASP: A patient information and workload management system.* Morganton, NC: MCS.

Needleman, J., Buerhaus, P., Mattke, S., Stewart, M., & Zelevinsky, K. (2002). Nurse-staffing levels and the quality of care in hospitals. *New England Journal of Medicine, 346*(22), 1715–1722.

Potter, P., Barr, N., McSweeney, M., & Sledge, J. (2003). Identifying nurse staffing and patient outcome relationships: A guide for change in care delivery. *Nursing Economics, 21*(4), 158–166.

Recruiting and Selecting Staff

Chapter 17 examined the process of allocating staff resources. This chapter opens the discussion with a focus on the first step, finding quality people who are suitable for a particular job and soliciting their services. This task consists of numerous components, from analyzing the job, developing a diverse recruitment strategy, and conducting interviews to comparing candidates and arriving at a consensual decision. Chapter 18 outlines these issues and helps you develop the human resource skills required of nurse managers.

Objectives

In this chapter, you will learn

- How to recruit and select staff.
- How to do a job analysis.
- How to interview prospective candidates.
- How to discriminate appropriate from inappropriate questions to ask during an interview.
- What legal issues are involved in hiring.

MediaLink www.prenhall.com/sullivan-decker

Additional resources for this chapter can be found on the Companion Website at www.prenhall.com/sullivan-decker. Click on "Chapter 18" to select the activities for this chapter.

- NCLEX Review
- Critical Thinking Activities
- Current Events
- MediaLinks
- *Nursing Leadership & Management in Action:* The Employment Interview; Selective Interviewing

In service or labor-intensive organizations such as health care organizations, the quality of personnel hired and retained determines whether an organization successfully accomplishes its objectives. The cost of improper selection can be high. The visible cost is in recruiting, selecting, and training an employee who must later be terminated because of unsatisfactory performance. The hidden costs may be even more expensive and include low quality of work performed by the unmotivated employee, disruption of harmonious working relationships, and patients' ill will and dissatisfaction, which may make patients reluctant to return to the particular clinic or hospital. The focus of this chapter is on job analysis, recruitment of applicants, and selection of personnel.

The Recruitment and Selection Process

The purpose of the selection process is to match people to jobs. It includes the following elements:

1. Job analysis
2. Methods of recruiting applicants
3. Selection technique(s) that measure applicants' skill, ability, and knowledge
4. Assurance that the selection techniques developed and used conform to legal requirements

Responsibility for selecting nursing personnel in health care organizations is usually shared by the human resources management (HRM) department and nursing management. First-line nursing managers are the most knowledgeable about job requirements and can best describe the job to applicants. HRM performs the initial screening and monitors hiring practices to be sure they adhere to legal stipulations.

Staffing responsibilities and activities can be thought of as a series of steps designed to acquire and retain personnel:

1. Planning the number and types of personnel needed according to patient care delivery systems of the organization.
2. Performing job analyses to define the duties, requirements, tasks, and qualifications of each position.
3. Developing and implementing a recruitment strategy to locate and attract enough qualified applicants to provide a pool of potential employees.
4. Interviewing, testing, and selecting needed personnel.

5. Orienting personnel to the job.
6. Enhancing employee performance through staff development and management of job performance.
7. Evaluating performance to provide feedback to the employee.
8. Managing personnel problems.
9. Developing and implementing strategies to retain staff.
10. Providing career counseling.
11. Developing exit strategies, such as preretirement counseling, exit interviews, and outplacement.

The purpose of recruitment activities is to generate a pool of qualified applicants, whereas the purpose of the selection process is to assess an applicant's ability, skills, and motivation relative to the requirements and rewards of the job so that a matching process can be carried out. To the extent that these matches are made effectively, positive outcomes such as high job satisfaction, low turnover, and high-quality performance can result.

Figure 18-1 shows a flowchart of the recruitment and selection process and suggested responsibilities. As indicated in the chart, this process is a joint effort among the nurse manager, the nursing department, and the HRM department. The recruitment and selection process begins with job analysis, which is a careful determination of job duties and requirements by nursing service, with technical assistance from HRM. Based on the job analysis and subsequent job descriptions, recruiting plans and selection systems are developed and implemented.

Once an applicant makes contact with the organization, HRM reviews the application and may conduct a preliminary interview. If the applicant does not meet the basic needs of the open position or positions, he or she should be so informed. Rejected applicants may be qualified for other positions or may refer friends to the organization and thus should be treated with utmost courtesy.

The next three stages include the selection instruments used: tests, reference checks, and managerial interviews. In most cases, the interview is last, but practices may vary. Even if an applicant does poorly on the selection test or receives poor references, it is prudent to carry out the interview so that the applicant is not aware that the test or reference checking led to the negative decision. In addition, applicants may feel they have a right to "tell their story" and may spontaneously provide information that explains poor references.

Figure 18-1 Flowchart of the typical recruitment and selection process.

The nurse manager should participate in the interview process because she or he (a) is generally in the best position to assess applicants' technical competence, potential, and overall suitability and (b) is able to answer applicants' technical, work-related questions more realistically. In some organizations, the candidate's future co-workers also participate in the interview process to assess compatibility.

After the managerial interview, the applicant is given a comprehensive medical examination to protect the organization from legal actions. For example, individuals with back problems should not be hired to work on a rehabilitation unit where a great deal of lifting of patients is required. In addition, state boards of health and other regulatory bodies require rubella, tetanus, and tuberculosis testing. The Occupational Safety and Health Administration (OSHA) requires that the hepatitis immune series be offered to health care workers who are not immune to hepatitis.

Once the medical examination has been completed, the nurse manager reviews the information available on each candidate and makes a job offer. The nurse manager must keep others involved in the selection process informed. The nurse manager is usually the first to be aware of potential resignations, requests for transfer, and maternity or family medical leaves that require personnel replacement. The manager also is aware of changes in the work area that might necessitate a redistribution of staff, such as the need for a night nurse instead of a day one. Communicating these needs to HRM promptly and accurately helps ensure effective coordination of the selection process.

Job Analysis

Before recruiting or selecting new staff, those responsible for hiring must be familiar with the job description and the skills, abilities, and knowledge required to perform the job. Duties and requirements are defined through job analysis.

Job analysis is a process that determines

1. Principal duties and responsibilities involved in a particular job,
2. Tasks inherent in those duties, and
3. Personal qualifications (skills, abilities, knowledge, and traits) needed for the job.

The outcome of a job analysis is a job description. If no job descriptions currently exist, then the nurse manager, with the assistance of HRM, should develop one for each job on the unit. All staff members (new or existing) need to have an up-to-date copy of their job description.

Job Specification   An important factor is the **job specification,** which details the knowledge, skills, and abilities needed, the tasks to be performed, and the behavior required to perform them. Although knowledge, skills, and abilities can be inferred from a description of the tasks to be performed, a description of knowledge, skills, and abilities does not necessarily explain what tasks will be done or what behaviors are expected on the job. Consequently, a job analysis that lists tasks is usually better than one that lists only knowledge, skills, and abilities.

Many tools are available for performing job analysis. They vary substantially in complexity and in applicability to different kinds of jobs. These tools include supervisory conferences, critical incidents, observation (such as work sampling and time and motion studies), interviewing, questionnaires, checklists, and logs.

Supervisory Conference   In a supervisory conference, the job analyst brings the supervisors and/or first-line managers together to identify the critical tasks or duties required in a job. Critical incidents require the managers to keep notes on subordinates' behavior that have contributed to particularly successful or unsuccessful job performance. Both methods are time consuming, and critical incident notes do not always give a complete picture of the job because they list only very positive or negative behaviors.

Work Sampling   One commonly used observational technique for collecting work activity information is work sampling. This technique can be used for jobs that consist of repetitive, short-cycle, manual operations as well as professional positions. In work sampling, data are collected at intervals of time, such as twice an hour or at randomly selected times. An inference can be made about overall work activities based on the observed activities.

Time and Motion Studies   Similar to work sampling, time and motion studies also use observations (Finkler, Knickman, Hendrickson, Lipkin, & Thompson, 1993). Time and motion studies require an observer to record exactly how much time is devoted to each skill, task, or behavior. Observation is done for extended periods. Time and motion studies are labor-intensive and expensive. A drawback to both work sampling and time and motion studies is that employees may change their behavior while being observed.

Interviewing   Interviewing, another common method, relies on staff members providing information about tasks or personal characteristics required for the job. Questionnaires and checklists also rely on staff members as a source of information on job requirements. Questionnaires may be open-ended, whereas checklists tend to be more structured and may consist of 200 or more items for the individual respondent to check off if performed. These data are analyzed to determine the tasks performed by the majority of persons currently in the job. When a checklist is used as the basis for job analysis, a large number of staff members are needed to supply enough data.

Self-Report Logs   Self-report logs may be used by staff members to report their activity at specified times. These logs are considered less reliable than other methods because staff may not record activities in a timely manner and may not be totally honest about what activities they are performing at the designated sampling times (Finkler et al., 1993).

The nurse manager often participates in developing a job analysis, usually through a supervisory conference, by interviewing, or by using questionnaires. Assuming they are free of error and distortion, job descriptions and specifications can be compared to a photograph in that they represent what the job is at the time the analysis is performed. The nurse manager can then use information regarding tasks and duties to develop selection procedures and to construct performance appraisal instruments and training programs.

Recruitment

The purpose of recruitment is to locate and attract enough qualified applicants to provide a pool from which the required number of individuals can be selected. Even though recruiting is primarily carried out by HRM staff and nurse recruiters, nurse managers and nursing staff play an important role in the process. Recruiting is easier when current employees spread the recruiting message, reducing the need for expensive advertising and bounty methods.

Box 18-1 lists ways in which your organization can attract potential employees by oft-ignored messages it sends.

To a very large extent, proper management can serve as the best recruiting tool. A nurse manager who is able to create a positive work environment through leadership style and clinical expertise will have a positive impact on efforts on recruitment because potential staff members will hear about and be attracted to that area (e.g., hospital unit, home health team). In contrast, an autocratic manager is more likely to have a higher turnover rate and is less likely to attract sufficient numbers of high-quality nurses.

Any recruiting strategy includes essentially four elements:

1. Where to look
2. How to look
3. When to look
4. How to sell the organization to potential recruits

KEY TERMS

Job analysis   A process that determines and defines the duties and requirements involved in a particular job.

Job specification   Details the knowledge, skills, and abilities needed, the tasks to be performed, and the behavior required to perform them.

Box 18-1   What Messages Does Your Organization Send?

- Does your lobby communicate a sense of inspiration?
- Do your recruitment offices convey that you are serious about developing your staff and that you will guide them through the transitions of a professional career?
- When they interview in the workplace, do they quickly get the message that the growth of staff is important?
- Do the opportunities to learn and grow clearly show?
- Are the work spaces organized and "humanized" so they are fit for human beings?
- Do the private spaces for staff areas clearly demonstrate concern about the stress levels of staff?
- Are there continual educational and inspirational offerings available for growth?
- Will the candidate have a guide/preceptor who can help with the transition to the workplace?

From "On Leadership: It's Transformation, Not Patient Care!" by K. Kerfoot, 2001, *Nursing Economics*, *19*(4), pp. 187–188.

Each of these elements may be affected by market competition, cyclic nursing shortages, reputation, visibility, and location.

Where to Look

For most health care organizations, the best place to look is in their own geographic area. During nursing shortages, however, many organizations conduct national searches. This effort is frequently futile because most nurses look for jobs in their local area. If the agency is in a major metropolitan area, a search may be relatively easy; if it is located in a rural area, however, recruitment may need to be conducted in the nearest city. Organizations tend to recruit where past efforts have been the most successful. Most organizations adopt an incremental strategy whereby they recruit locally first and then expand to larger and larger markets until a sufficient applicant pool is obtained.

Because proximity to home is a key factor in choosing a job, recruitment efforts should focus on nurses living nearby. The state board of nursing can provide the names of registered nurses by zip code to allow organizations to target recruitment efforts to surrounding areas. Also, personnel officers in large companies or other organizations in the area can be asked to assist in recruiting nurse spouses of newly hired employees.

Students in local schools of nursing are obviously an excellent potential source of employees. One way to recruit them is to serve as a clinical training site and treat students well. Nurses who work with students play a key role in recruitment. Students feel welcomed and valued when their care and contributions are acknowledged. In doing so, the staff conveys a positive impression of the work group.

Employing students as aides may provide another recruitment tool because it allows students to learn first-hand about the organization and what it has to offer. In turn, the organization can evaluate the student as a potential employee postgraduation. Some organizations provide assistance with student loan payments if the student continues to work after graduation. Baccalaureate graduates report, however, that the most critical factor they consider in seeking their first nursing position is the orientation program (Kersten & Johnson, 1992). Graduates look for an orientation that provides successful transition into professional practice. Other top factors they consider are the reputation of the agency, benefits, promotional opportunities, specialty area, and nurse–patient ratio.

How to Look

Employee referrals, advertising in newspapers and professional journals and on the Internet, attendance at professional conventions, job fairs, career days, visits to educational institutions, employment agencies (both private and public), and temporary help agencies are all recruiting sources. Most applicants are drawn to the organization by some form of advertising. During nursing shortages, some organizations offer bonuses to staff members who refer candidates, as well as bonuses to the recruits themselves.

Direct applications and employee referrals are quick and relatively inexpensive ways of recruiting people, but these methods also tend to perpetuate the current racial or social mix of the workforce. It is both legally and ethically necessary to recruit individuals without regard to their race, ethnicity, gender, or disability. In addition, organizations can benefit from the diversity of a staff composed of persons from a wide variety of social, experiential, and educational backgrounds.

Advertisements may be placed in the classified sections of local newspapers or journals and in the job listings at professional meetings. Advertising can be an effective recruiting tool, but it tends to be expensive. Nevertheless, if the organization intends to add staff, placing display ads in local newspapers reassures currently employed nurses that the organization is serious about its commitment to do so.

Another advertising medium is the Internet. Because the Internet is readily accessible, it is an attractive way to explore job opportunities anywhere in the world. There are numerous Web sites that target nurses. Ads can be purchased on some sites; others are directly available for recruiting.

In recruiting, both the **medium** and the message must be considered. The medium is the agent of contact between the organization and the potential applicant. Obviously, it is desirable to find a medium that gives the widest exposure. Unfortunately, these media tend to be inefficient and low in credibility. The more influential media tend to be the more personal ones: present employees and recruiters. Acquaintances or friends of the recruit have prior credibility and the ability to communicate more subtle aspects of the organization and the job.

Nurses referred by informal methods (e.g., employees) tend to be more productive (Breaugh & Mann, 1984). The reason is that nurses coming from informal sources of referral are likely to have more realistic information about the job and the organization and, therefore, their expectations more closely fit reality. Those who come to the job with unrealistic expectations may experience dissatisfaction as a result. In an open labor market, these individuals may leave the organization, creating high turnover. When nursing jobs are less plentiful, dissatisfied staff members tend to stay in the organization because they need the job, but they are not likely to perform as well as other employees. Consequently, even where applicants are sought may have significant consequences later on.

When to Look

The time lag in recruiting is a concern to nursing, especially during severe nursing shortages. Even when there is an excess supply of nurses, certain locations (e.g., rural areas) and specialties (e.g., critical care) may experience shortages. Careful planning is necessary to ensure that recruitment begins well in advance of anticipated needs.

How to Sell the Organization

A critical component of any recruiting effort is marketing the organization and available positions to potential employees. The nursing department and/or HRM should develop a comprehensive marketing plan. Generally, four strategies are included in marketing plans and are called the **4 Ps of marketing:**

1. Product
2. Place
3. Price
4. Promotion

The consumer is the key figure around which the four concepts are oriented, and in the recruiting process, the consumer is the potential employee.

Product is the available position(s) within the organization. Consider several aspects of the position and organization, such as

- Professionalism
- Standards of care
- Quality
- Service
- Respect

Place refers to the physical qualities and location, such as

- Accessibility
- Scheduling
- Parking
- Reputation
- Organizational culture

Price includes

- Pay and differentials
- Benefits
- Sign-on bonuses
- Insurance
- Retirement plans

Promotion includes

- Advertising
- Public relations
- Direct word of mouth
- Personal selling (e.g., job fairs, professional meetings)

Developing an effective marketing message is important. Sometimes the tendency is to use a "scatter-gun" approach, sugarcoat the message, or make it very slick. A more balanced message, which includes honest communication and personal contact, is preferable. Overselling the organization creates unrealistic expectations that may lead to later dissatisfaction and turnover.

Realistically presenting the job requirements and rewards improves job satisfaction, in that the new recruit learns what the job is actually like. Promising a nurse every other weekend off and only a 25 percent rotation to nights on a severely understaffed unit and then scheduling the nurse off only every third weekend with 75 percent night rotations is an example of unrealistic job information. It is important to represent the situation honestly and describe the steps management is taking to improve situations that the applicant might find undesirable. The candidate can then make an informed decision about the job offer.

Cross-Training as a Recruitment Strategy

In today's rapidly changing health care environment, patient census fluctuates rapidly, and staffing requirements must be adjusted appropriately. These conditions may bring about layoffs and daily cancellations and contribute to low morale. Offering cross-training to potential employees may increase the applicant pool.

Cross-training has the benefits of increasing morale and job satisfaction, improving efficiency, increasing

---

KEY TERMS

Medium   The agent of contact between the organization and the potential applicant.

4 Ps of marketing   Four strategies included in marketing plans: product, place, price, and promotion.

the flexibility of the staff, and providing a means to manage fluctuations in census. In addition, it gives nurses, such as those in obstetrics and neonatal areas, an opportunity to provide more holistic care. If cross-training is used, care should be taken to provide a didactic knowledge base in addition to clinical training. How broadly to cross-train is an important decision because training in too many areas may overload the nurse and reduce the quality of care. (See Chapter 22 on using floating to improve retention.)

Interviewing

The most common selection method, the interview, is an information-seeking mechanism between an individual applying for a position and a member of an organization doing the hiring. After the applicant's initial screening with HRM, the nurse manager usually conducts an interview.

The interview is used to clarify information gathered from the application form, evaluate the applicant's responses to questions, and determine the fit of the applicant to the position, unit, and organization. In addition, the interviewer should provide information about the job and the organization. Finally, the interview should create goodwill toward the employing organization through good customer relations.

Research suggests that decision making is improved if the interviewer postpones reviewing information not needed for the interview, such as test scores, until after the interview. Reviewing such information before the interview may lead to ignoring data that disconfirm this information (Gatewood & Feild, 1990).

An effective interviewer must learn to solicit information efficiently and to gather relevant data. Interviews typically last for 1 or $1^1/_2$ hours, and include an opening, an information-gathering and information-giving phase, and a closing. The opening is important because it is an attempt to establish rapport with the applicant so she or he will provide relevant information. Gathering information, however, is the core of the interview. Giving information also is important because it allows the interviewer to create realistic expectations in the applicant and sell the organization if that is needed. However, this portion of the interview should take place after the information has been gathered so that the applicant's answers will be as candid as possible. The interviewer should answer any direct questions the candidate poses. Box 18-2 is an example of realistic information to present to applicants. Finally, the closing is intended to provide information to the candidate on the mechanics of possible employment.

Principles for Effective Interviewing

Developing Structured Interview Guides Unstructured interviews present problems; if interviewers fail to ask the same questions of every candidate, it is often difficult to compare them. With any human skill or trait, no standard or true score exists that can serve as a basis on which to compare applicants. People can only be compared to other people. Consequently, the interview is most effective when the information on the pool of interviewees is as comparable as possible. Comparability is maximized via a structured interview supported by an interview guide. An **interview guide** is a written document containing questions, interviewer directions, and

---

Box 18-2 Staff Nurse Position, Burn Unit: Realistic Preview Information

1. Positive Information
   - Lengthy patient stays—lots of patient and family teaching
   - Presence of critical as well as recovering patients
   - Decision-making opportunities
   - Bedside nursing
   - Learning environment
   - Ability to assist with research
   - Small unit, close-knit, dedicated group
   - Burns as well as other prior difficulties or concurrent problems to work with
   - Children as well as adults
2. Negative Information
   - Patients who are sometimes difficult to deal with, that is, young children or elderly—often alcoholics, psychological difficulties
   - Emotional stress
   - Physical difficulties

Adapted from a form used by Barnes Jewish Hospital, St. Louis, MO. Used by permission.

other pertinent information so that the same process is followed and the same basic information is gathered from each applicant. The guide should be specific to the job, or job category, as shown below.

Do job analysis to determine job tasks.
↓
Use tasks to determine required personal characteristics (skills, abilities, knowledge).
↓
Write questions and develop behavioral simulations
↓
to determine
↓
whether the applicant has the required personal characteristics.
↓
Put these questions and ideas in the interview guide to direct you in the interview.

Box 18-3 lists questions you could ask in an interview, but do not copy the questions verbatim; develop your own questions based on the specific job. For example, you may want to add questions on teamwork and collaboration as they relate to position. Box 18-4 is an example of job-related questions that could be asked for an oncology unit position.

Interview guides reduce interviewer bias, provide relevant and effective questions, minimize leading questions, and facilitate comparison among applicants. Space left between the questions on the guide provides room for note taking, and the guide also provides a written record of the interview.

Preparing for the Interview   Most managers do not adequately prepare for the interview, which should be planned just like any business undertaking. All needed materials should be on hand, and the interview site should be quiet and pleasant. If others are scheduled to see the applicant, their schedules should be checked to make sure they are available at the proper time. If coffee or other refreshments are to be offered, advance arrangements need to be made. Lack of advance preparation may lead to insufficient interviewing time, interruptions, or failure to gather important information. Other problems include losing focus in the interview because of a desire to be courteous or because a particularly dominant interviewee is encountered. This typically keeps the interviewer from obtaining the needed information.

In general, when time is limited, it is better to use part of it for planning rather than squander all of it on the interview itself. This is preferable to spending more time later trying to correct the performance of a poor employee. Before the interview, the interviewer should review job requirements, the application and résumé,

> ### KEY TERMS
>
> *Interview guide*   A written document containing questions, interviewer directions, and other pertinent information so that the same process is followed and the same basic information is gathered from each applicant.

Box 18-3   Questions to Ask in an Interview

1. Tell me about yourself.
2. What do you know about our organization?
3. What are you looking for in this position?
4. Why are you looking for a new position?
5. What do you like best about being a nurse? The least?
6. How would your colleagues describe you?
7. How would your supervisor describe you?
8. How would you describe yourself?
9. What were the most significant accomplishments you made in your career so far?
10. Why do you want to work for us?
11. What other positions are you considering?
12. What continuing education have you completed recently?
13. What are your career goals?
14. How does this position fit into your long-term career goals?
15. What would you like to be doing in 5 years?
16. What are your strong points?
17. What are your weaknesses?
18. What would you like to know about the position and the area?
19. Do you have any other questions for me?

Box 18-4 Job-Related Questions for an Oncology Unit

Describe how you would intervene in the following situations:

- A patient whom you admitted with a diagnosis of lymphoma is going to begin chemotherapy, and you are preparing to hang the first dose. When you enter the room she says, "You know, I just can't believe that I have cancer. I know it is what the doctor says, but it just doesn't seem possible to me."

- The wife of a patient overhears some doctors caring for her husband say that the patient has received the incorrect dose of chemotherapy. You are caring for him.

- A young man is diagnosed with acute leukemia and expresses anger and frustration in the presence of his wife. You witness the frequent outbursts and become increasingly aware of the sense of hopelessness on the part of both him and his wife.

- A leukemia patient has been classified as a no-code. On the night shift, dyspnea develops. The patient becomes uncomfortable and anxious, and screams out periodically. The patient is on 100% oxygen already, but his wife insists that something more be done.

- A physician making rounds notices a discrepancy in your patient's intake and output record. The weights indicate that he has gained 10 pounds, but the intake records do not show how this could have happened.

- You are working nights and caring for an extremely seriously ill man receiving platelets and antibiotic therapy. The patient's blood pressure is continuing to drop. You have talked to the resident on call twice by telephone, and he tells you to continue the present orders. The man's condition continues to decline. What would you do?

Adapted from a form used by Barnes-Jewish Hospital, St. Louis, MO. Used by permission.

and note specific questions to be asked. Planning should be done on the morning of the interview or the evening before for an early morning interview. If you are sure that time will be available, planning is best done immediately before an interview or between interviews. Unfortunately, a busy manager may have to deal with unexpected minor crises between interviews and may not be able to use the time to plan the next interview.

A cardinal rule is to review the application or résumé before beginning the interview. If the interviewee arrives with the résumé or application in hand, ask him or her to wait for a few minutes while you review the material. In doing a quick review, consider four things:

1. Are there clear discrepancies between the applicant's qualifications and the job specifications? If the answer is yes, then only a brief interview may be necessary to explain why the applicant will not be considered. (If a preliminary screening is performed by the HRM, such applicants should not be referred to nurse managers.)

2. Look for specific questions to ask the applicant during the interview.

3. Look for a rapport builder (something you have in common with the applicant) to break the ice at the beginning of the interview.

4. Remember that the résumé is prepared by the applicant and is intended to market an applicant's assets to the organization. It does not give a balanced view of strengths and weaknesses. So, examine the résumé critically and make notes about areas where you need more information.

To provide a relaxed, informal atmosphere, the setting is important. Both you and the applicant should be in comfortable chairs, as close as comfortably possible. No table or desk should separate you. If an office is used, arrange chairs so that the applicant is at the side of the desk. There should be complete freedom from distracting phone calls and other interruptions. If the view is distracting, do not seat the applicant so that she or he can look out a window.

Opening the Interview The interview should start on time. Give a warm, friendly greeting, introduce yourself, and ask the applicant her or his preferred name. Try to minimize status; do not patronize or dominate. The objective is to establish an open atmosphere so applicants reveal as much as possible about themselves. Establish and maintain rapport throughout the interview by talking about yourself, discussing mutual interests such as hobbies or sports, and using nonverbal cues, such as maintaining eye contact. Finally, start the interview by outlining what will be discussed and setting the time limits for the interview.

Be careful not to form hasty first impressions and make equally hasty decisions. Interviewers tend to be influenced by first impressions of a candidate, and such judgments often lead to poor decisions. First impressions may degrade the quality of the interview by coloring the search for information to justify their first impressions, good or bad. If the first impression is negative and you decide not to hire a potentially successful candidate, you have wasted an hour or so and possibly lost a good recruit. If, because of a positive first impression, you hire an unsuccessful candidate, problems may continue for months. Conversely, your personal characteristics may influence the applicant's decisions. You create first impressions by tone of voice, eye contact, personal appearance, grooming, posture, and gestures.

Using the structured interview guide, take notes, telling the candidate that this is being done to aid recall and that you hope the candidate does not mind. There are various ways of asking questions, but only one question should be asked at a time and, where possible, open-ended questions should be used, such as, "Please tell me about your most rewarding experience as a nurse." Open-ended questions cannot be answered with a single yes, no, or one-word answer and usually elicit more information about the applicant. Closed questions (e.g., what, where, why, when, how many) should only be used to elicit specific information.

Work sample questions are used to determine an applicant's knowledge about work tasks and ability to perform the job. It is easy to ask a nurse whether she or he knows how to care for a patient who has a central intravenous line in place. An answer of yes does not necessarily prove the ability, so you might ask some very specific questions about central lines. Avoid leading questions, in which the answer is implied by the question (e.g., "We have lots of overtime. Do you mind overtime?"). You may also want to summarize what has been said, use silence to elicit more information, reflect back the applicant's feelings to clarify the issue, or indicate acceptance by urging the applicant to continue.

Giving Information Before reaching the information-giving part of the interview, consider whether the candidate is promising enough to warrant spending time in giving detailed job information. Unless the candidate is clearly unacceptable, be careful not to communicate a negative impression, because evaluation of the candidate may change when the entire packet of material is reviewed or more promising candidates decline a job offer. You also must know what information you should give and what is to be provided by others. Detailed benefit or compensation questions are usually answered by HRM. If a promising candidate's questions cannot be answered, arrange for someone to contact the candidate later with the desired information.

Closing the Interview In closing the interview, you may want to summarize the applicant's strengths. Make sure to ask the applicant whether she or he has anything to add or questions to ask related to the job and the organization. You may also want to mention the candidate's weaknesses, particularly if they are objective and clearly related to the job, such as lack of experience in a particular field. Mentioning a perception of a subjective weakness, such as poor supervisory skills, may lead to legal problems. Thanking the applicant and completing any notes made during the interview conclude the interview process.

Involving Staff in the Interview Process

Today's trend toward decentralization of decision making may lead to sharing interview responsibilities with staff. Involving staff in interviews helps to strengthen teamwork, improves work-group effectiveness, increases staff involvement in other unit activities, and increases the likelihood of selecting the best candidate for the position.

If staff are involved in interviews, several steps must be taken to protect the integrity of the interview process. An organized orientation to interviewing should be given that includes (a) federal, state, and local laws and regulations governing interviewing, as well as any collective-bargaining agreements that may affect the process; (b) tips on handling awkward interviewing situations; and (c) time for rehearsing interviewing skills. Just as the manager does, staff should follow a structured interview guide to help standardize the process.

Interview Reliability and Validity

Numerous research studies have been performed on the reliability and validity of employment interviews. In general, agreement between two interviews of the same measure by the same interviewer (**intrarater reliability**) is fairly high, agreement between two interviews of the

---

KEY TERMS

Work sample questions Used to determine an applicant's knowledge about work tasks and ability to perform the job.

Intrarater reliability Agreement between two measures by the same interviewer.

same measure by several interviewers (**interrater reliability**) is rather low, and the ability to predict job performance (**validity**) of the typical interview is very low. Research also has shown that

1. Structured interviews are more reliable and valid;
2. Interviewers who are under pressure to hire in a short time or meet a recruitment quota are less accurate than other interviewers;
3. Interviewers who have detailed information about the job for which they are interviewing exhibit higher interrater reliability and validity;
4. The interviewer's experience does not seem to be related to reliability and validity;
5. There is a decided tendency for interviewers to make quick decisions and therefore be less accurate;
6. Interviewers develop stereotypes of ideal applicants against which interviewees are evaluated, and individual interviewers may hold different stereotypes, thus decreasing interrater reliability and validity; and
7. Race and gender may influence interviewers' evaluations.

Possibly the greatest weakness in the selection interview is the tendency for the interviewer to try to assess an applicant's personality characteristics. Although it is difficult to eliminate such subjectivity, evaluations of applicants are often more subjective than they need to be, particularly when interviewers try to assess personality characteristics.

Information collected during an interview should answer three fundamental questions:

1. Can the applicant perform the job?
2. Will the applicant perform the job?
3. Will the candidate fit into the culture of the unit and the organization?

The best predictor of the applicant's future behavior in these respects is past performance. Previous work and other experience, previous education and training, and current job performance all should be considered, not personality characteristics, which even psychologists cannot measure very accurately.

Education, Experience, Licensure, and Physical Examinations

Education and experience requirements for nurses have long been important screening factors and bear a close relationship to work sample tests. Educational requirements are a type of job knowledge sample because they

tend to ensure that applicants have at least a minimal amount of knowledge necessary for the job. For nurses, educational preparation is particularly important. For example, nurses who are graduates of associate degree and diploma programs are prepared to care for individuals in structured settings and use the nursing process, decision-making process, and management skills in the care of those individuals. Baccalaureate graduates can provide nursing care for individuals, families, groups, and communities using the nursing process and decision-making process. Baccalaureate graduates also are prepared for beginning community health positions and possess the leadership and management skills needed for entry-level management positions.

Making assumptions regarding the type and number of years of experience should be avoided. Factors such as job requirements, patient acuity, autonomy, and degree of specialization vary from organization to organization. Therefore, careful interviewing is needed to determine the individual applicant's knowledge and skill level.

References and letters of recommendation also are used to assess the applicant's past job experience, but there is little evidence that these have any validity. Because few persons write unfavorable letters of recommendation, such letters do not really predict job performance. Criticisms are likely to be mild and may be reflected by the lack of positive language. Letters with any criticism should be verified with a telephone call, if possible, to avoid overreacting to an unusually honest author.

To avoid legal problems, many organizations include in letters of recommendation only employment dates, salary, and whether the applicant is eligible for rehire. Many organizations do not allow supervisors to write letters of recommendation. Negative references may be viewed as potential for slander or other legal recourse. Almost every organization will at least verify position title and dates of employment, which helps to detect the occasional applicant who counterfeits an entire work history. Unfortunately, omission of a position from the work history is more common than including a position not actually held. The only way to detect such omissions is to ask that candidates list year and month of all educational and work experiences. Caution is necessary when asking about time between jobs; be careful not to inquire about marital or family status.

In almost every selection situation, an applicant fills out an application form that requests information regarding previous experience, education, and references. Most applications also ask for the applicant's medical history and other personal data. As application forms are reviewed, the critical question to be asked is whether the applicant has distorted responses, either intentionally or unintentionally. Studies indicate that there is usually little distortion, at least not on the easily verifiable information. Applicants may stretch the truth a bit, but rarely are there complete falsehoods. Relative to other predictors, the application form may be one of the more valid predictors in a selection process.

Licensure status can be verified by asking to see the applicant's license at time of employment and by verifying the licensure information with the state board of nursing. The computerized NCLEX-RN® examination changed hiring practices for new graduates; because rapid notification (7 to 10 days) of licensure examination results are available, state boards no longer issue interim permits to new graduate nurses. Organizations generally wait for new graduates to obtain a license before starting employment.

Preemployment physical examinations can no longer be used to disqualify applicants for a job or benefits. Passage of PL 101-336, the Americans with Disabilities Act of 1990, protects individuals with physical or mental disabilities from discrimination. In fact, reasonable accommodations must be provided for an individual with disabilities. Regardless, disabled employees may be held to the same standards for employment (i.e., they must possess the necessary skills and experience to perform the job) as applicants without disabilities.

Integrating the Information

When comparing candidates, first weigh the qualities required for the job in order of importance, placing more emphasis on the most important elements.

Second, weigh the qualities desired on the basis of the reliability of the data. The more consistent the observation of behavior from different elements in the selection system, the more weight that dimension should be given. Third, weigh job dimensions by trainability—consider the amount of education, experience, and additional training the applicant can reasonably be expected to receive, and consider the likelihood that the behavior in that dimension can be improved with training. Dimensions most likely to be learned in training (e.g., using new equipment) should be given the least weight so that more weight is placed on dimensions less likely to be learned in training (e.g., being able to care for terminally ill children).

Attempt to compare data across individuals in making a decision. It is more accurate to make decisions based on a comparison of several persons than to make a decision for each individual after each interview. Analysis of the entire applicant pool requires good interview records but lessens the impact of early impressions on the hiring decision because the interviewer must consider each job element across the entire pool.

One nurse manager used the recommendations in this chapter to hire a nurse as shown in Case Study 18-1.

KEY TERMS

Interrater reliability   Agreement between two measures by several interviewers.

Validity   The ability to predict outcomes with some accuracy.

CASE STUDY 18-1: Selecting Staff

Jack Turner is nurse manager of the emergency department in a large metropolitan area hospital. He has four full-time RN positions open in his department. There are three nursing programs located in the city: a state university program, a community college program, and an RN-to-BSN completion program.

Jack recently participated in a nursing job fair hosted by his hospital. The event was well attended by nursing students, and he received several promising résumés of soon-to-be graduate nurses. Jack notes that one of the applicants, Sabrina Ashworth, will graduate next month with a BSN. She has been working for the past year as a

nursing assistant in the ER of another local hospital. In addition to her ER work, Sabrina has a high grade point average and indicates a strong interest in trauma and critical care. Jack contacts the human resource department to set up an interview with Sabrina.

Sabrina agrees to an interview for an RN position in the ER department. Jack schedules a conference room adjacent to the ER for the interview. Prior to Sabrina's arrival, he reviews her résumé and application, noting her educational background, previous work history, and recent volunteer trip to Mexico to assist with a vaccination program. Jack has assembled a packet for Sabrina,

(continued)

CASE STUDY 18-1: Selecting Staff   (Continued)

including job description and materials from human resources that outline the application process.

The interview begins promptly. Jack warmly greets Sabrina and establishes rapport. He follows the interview guide provided by the human resource department. Jack informs Sabrina that he will be taking notes during the interview process. After reviewing her educational and work history, Jack asks Sabrina several situational questions related to work in the ER. He also allows time for Sabrina to ask questions about the RN position. Jack also has two RN staff members give Sabrina a tour of the ER department. Finally, Jack outlines the next steps in the application process and indicates that he will follow up with Sabrina in 7 to 10 days.

Following the interview, Jack works with the human resource department and asks for transcript and reference checks for Sabrina. After verifying her transcript and

receiving positive references, Jack extends an offer to Sabrina, which she accepts.

Manager's Checklist

The nurse manager is responsible for

- Understanding the organization's human resource policies and procedures related to selecting staff,
- Working closely with the human resource department to facilitate the selection and hiring of qualified staff,
- Knowing state and federal regulations related to the application and interview process,
- Preparing for the interview process,
- Conducting the interview, and
- Following up with applicants in a timely manner.

Legality in Hiring

As a result of Title VII of the Civil Rights Act of 1964, the Equal Pay Act of 1963, the Age Discrimination Act of 1967, and Title I of the Americans with Disabilities Act of 1990, recruitment and selection activities are subject to considerable scrutiny regarding discrimination and equal employment opportunity. Title VII of the Civil Rights Act specifically prohibits discrimination in any **personnel decision** on the basis of race, color, sex, religion, or national origin. "Any personnel decision" includes not only selection but also entrance into training programs, performance appraisal results, termination, promotions, compensation, benefits, and other terms, conditions, and privileges of employment.

The act applies to most employers with more than 15 employees, although there are several exemptions—among them, **bona fide occupational qualification (BFOQ)**, business necessity, and validity of the procedure used to make the personnel decision (as discussed below). Discrimination is allowed on the basis of national origin (citizenship or immigration status), religion, sex, and age, for instance, if that discrimination can be shown to be a "bona fide occupational qualification reasonably necessary for the normal operation of a business." The classic example of a genuine BFOQ is a sperm donor. More realistic examples are a female part in a play, a Sunday school teacher of a certain religion, or a female correctional counselor at a women's prison. Claims of "customer

preference" for female flight attendants or gross gender characteristics such as "women cannot lift over 30 pounds" have not been supported as BFOQs.

A BFOQ allows an organization to exclude members of certain groups (such as all men or all women) if the organization can demonstrate that a selection method is a **business necessity**. Business necessity is likely to withstand legal challenge only in the unusual instances when a selection method that discriminates against a protected group is necessary to ensure the safety of workers or customers.

The Equal Employment Opportunity Commission (EEOC) is charged with enforcing and interpreting the Civil Rights Act and has issued Uniform Guidelines on Employee Selection Procedures (43 Federal Register, 1978). The guidelines specify the kinds of methods and information required to justify the job relatedness of selection procedures. These guidelines are not described in detail here; however, the methods of selection discussed in this chapter do follow their specifications. Remember that the law does not say one cannot hire the best person for the job. What it says is that race, color, sex, religion, disability, or national origin must not be used as selection criteria. As long as the decision is not made on the basis of minority status, one is complying with the Equal Employment Opportunity (EEO) law.

EEO law and succeeding court decisions have had three major impacts on selection procedures. First, organizations are more careful to use predictors and techniques that can be shown not to discriminate against protected classes. Second, organizations are reducing the use of tests, which may be difficult to defend if they screen out a large number of minority applicants. Third, organizations are relying heavily on the interview process as a selection device. Interviews also are subject to EEO and other regulations. Table 18-1 presents questions appropriate to ask in interviews. The basic rule of thumb in interviewing is when in doubt about a question's legality, ask: How is this question related to job performance? If it can be proved that only job-related questions are asked, EEO law will not be violated.

Table 18-1   Preemployment Questions

	Appropriate to Ask	Inappropriate to Ask
Name	Applicant's name. Whether applicant has school or work records under a different name.	Questions about any name or title that indicate race, color, religion, sex, national origin, or ancestry. Questions about father's surname or mother's maiden name.
Address	Questions concerning place and length of current and previous addresses.	Any specific probes into foreign addresses that would indicate national origin.
Age	Requiring proof of age by birth certificate after hiring. Can ask if applicant is over 18.	Requiring birth certificate or baptismal record *before* hiring.
Birthplace or national origin		Any question about place of birth of applicant or place of birth of parents, grandparents, or spouse.
		Any other question (direct or indirect) about applicant's national origin.
Race or color	Can request *after* employment as affirmative action data.	Any inquiry that would indicate race or color.
Sex		Any question on an application blank that would indicate sex.
Religion		Any questions to indicate applicant's religious denomination or beliefs.
		A recommendation or reference from the applicant's religious denomination.
Citizenship	Questions about whether the applicant is a U.S. citizen; if not, whether the applicant intends to become one.	Questions of whether the applicant, parents, or spouse are native born or naturalized.
	Questions regarding whether applicant's U.S. residence is legal; requiring proof of citizenship *after* being hired.	Require proof of citizenship *before* hiring.
Photographs	May require after hiring for identification purposes only.	Requesting a photograph *before* hiring.
Education	Questions concerning any academic, professional, or vocational schools attended.	Questions asking specifically the nationality, racial, or religious affiliation of any school attended.

(continued)

Table 18-1 Continued

	Inquiry into language skills, such as reading and writing of foreign languages.	Inquiries as to the applicant's mother tongue or how any foreign language ability was acquired (unless it is necessary for the job).
Relatives	Name, relationship, and address of a person to be notified in case of an emergency.	Any unlawful inquiry about a relative or residence mate(s) as specified in this list.
Children		Questions about the number and ages of the applicant's children or information on child-care arrangements.
Transportation		Inquiries about transportation to or from work (unless a car is necessary for the job).
Organization	Questions about organization memberships and any offices that might be held.	Questions about any organization an applicant belongs to that may indicate the race, age, disabilities, color, religion, sex, national origin, or ancestry of its members.
Physical condition/ disabilities	Questions about being able to meet the job requirements, with or without some accommodation.	Questions about general medical condition, state of health, specific diseases, or nature/severity of disability.
Military service	Questions about services rendered in armed forces, the rank attained, and which branch of service.	Questions about military service in any armed forces other than the United States.
	Requiring military discharge certificate *after* being hired.	Request of military service records *before* hiring.
Work schedule	Questions about the applicant's willingness to work the required work schedule.	Questions about applicant's willingness to work any particular religious holiday.
References	General and work references not relating to race, color, religion, sex, national origin or ancestry, age, or disability.	References specifically from clergymen (as specified above) or any other persons who might reflect race, age, disability, color, sex, national origin or ancestry of applicant.
Financial		Questions about banking, credit rating, outstanding loans, bankruptcy, or having wages garnished.
Other qualifications	Any question that has direct reflection on the job to be applied for.	Any non-job-related inquiry that may present information permitting unlawful discrimination. Questions about arrests or convictions (unless necessary for job, such as security clearance).

Adapted from *Americans with Disabilities Act* (EEOC Publication #M-1A), Ohio Civil Rights Commission and United States Equal Employment Opportunities Commission, 1992, Washington, DC: Government Printing Office.

The **Age Discrimination Act** prohibits discrimination against applicants and employees over the age of 40. Questions in recruitment and selection that are appropriate with respect to age are also presented in Table 18-1.

The **Americans with Disabilities Act** that took effect in July 1990 prohibits discrimination based on an individual's disability. A disability is defined as a physical or mental impairment that substantially limits one or more of the major life activities, or has a record of such impairment, or is being regarded as having such an impairment. A qualified individual is one who, with or without reasonable accommodation, can perform the essential functions of the position under consideration.

Employers with 15 or more employees are required to make accommodations to the known disability of a qualified applicant if it will not impose "undue hardship" on the operation of the business. Reasonable accommodations may include making existing facilities used by employees readily accessible to and usable by individuals with disabilities; job restructuring; part-time or modified work schedules; reassignment to a vacant position; acquiring or modifying equipment or devices; adjusting or modifying examinations, training materials, or policies; and providing qualified readers and interpreters.

Interview questions that may be asked of the disabled are also in Table 18-1. The law permits an organization to make an employment offer contingent on the applicant's passing a preemployment physical examination, but only if the examination is required of all applicants in similar jobs and is job related.

Organizations are liable for the character and actions of the employees they hire. To satisfy this requirement, the employer must check applicants' backgrounds before hiring in regard to licensure, credentials, and references. Failure to do so constitutes **negligent hiring** if that employee harms a patient, visitor, or another employee. Furthermore, an employer is expected to properly train its employees.

What You Know Now

- Job analysis, recruitment of applicants, and selection of personnel are important measures to ensure the best fit between employees and the needs of the organizations.
- The selection of staff is a critical function that requires matching people to jobs, and responsibility for hiring is often shared by HRM and nurse managers.
- Job analysis is fundamental to all selection efforts because it defines the job.
- Recruitment is the process of locating and attracting enough qualified applicants to provide a pool from which the required number of new staff members can be chosen.
- Selection processes should be job related and most often include screening application forms, résumés, medical examinations, reference checks, and interviews.

- Interviewing is a complex skill that is intended to obtain information about the applicant and give the applicant information about the organization.
- Successful interviews require planning, implementation, and follow-up in order to make the best decisions.
- Developing a structured interview guide is a critical element in interviewing.
- Selection decisions are subject to provisions in the Civil Rights Act of 1964, Equal Pay Act of 1963, the Age Discrimination Act of 1967, and the Americans with Disabilities Act of 1990.

Tools for Recruiting and Selecting Staff

1. Conduct or modify a job analysis as needed.
2. Coordinate recruitment efforts with the human resource department.
3. Ensure your area of responsibility sends the message you want (see Box 18-1).
4. Prepare adequately for interviews.
5. Conduct interviews following recommendations presented in the chapter.
6. Process the information obtained in interviews and reference checks to make a final decision.

Questions to Challenge You

1. Often organizations want to skip the job analysis step. What consequences to avoiding this step might occur? In your opinion, is it necessary to do a job analysis? Why?
2. What approach does your organization use to recruit employees? Is it effective? How could they improve?
3. Imagine that a potential candidate asks you to describe your present workplace. What would you say?
4. Cross-training has been used as a recruitment strategy. What are the pros and cons of using this strategy?
5. Consider the last interview you had for a job or school. Did the interviewer follow the principles discussed in this chapter? Explain.

Explore ⬤ MediaLink

NCLEX review questions, essay activities, group activities, and other interactive resources for this chapter can be found on the Web site at http://www.prenhall.com/sullivan-decker. Click on "Chapter 18" to select activities for this chapter.

References

Breaugh, J. A., & Mann, R. B. (1984). Recruiting source effects: A test of two alternative explanations. *Journal of Occupational Psychology, 57,* 261–262.

Finkler, S. A., Knickman, J. R., Hendrickson, G., Lipkin, M., & Thompson, W. G. (1993). A comparison of work-sampling and time-and-motion techniques for studies in health services research. *Health Services Research, 28,* 577–597.

Gatewood, R. D., & Feild, H. S. (1990). *Human resource selection.* Chicago: Dryden.

Kerston, J. W., & Johnson, J. S. (1992). Recruitment: What are new grads looking for? *Nursing management, 23*(3), 44–48.

Motivating and Developing Staff

A Model of Job Performance

> Employee Motivation
> Motivational Theories
> Employee Ability

Staff Development

> Needs Assessment
> Planning
> Implementation
> Evaluation
> Designing Staff Development
> Programs for a Multicultural
> Staff

Looking Ahead

The level of employee performance determines how successfully an organization operates. A key factor influencing performance is the manager's ability to help develop the skills and knowledge of the staff so they can perform the job better. Assessing the needs of employees, planning educational programs, and implementing those programs are important steps managers can take to improve organizational operations.

Objectives

In this chapter, you will learn

- How motivation and ability affect job performance.
- How different theories explain motivation.
- How motivational theories can help a manager.
- What factors must be considered in staff development.
- How different theories explain learning.
- What methods are used for staff development.

MediaLink www.prenhall.com/ sullivan-decker

Additional resources for this chapter can be found on the Companion Website at www.prenhall.com/ sullivan-decker. Click on "Chapter 19" to select the activities for this chapter.

- NCLEX Review
- Critical Thinking Activities
- Current Events
- MediaLinks
- *Nursing Leadership & Management in Action:* Employee Motivation; Personal Motivation: Use of Goal Setting

Acontinual and troublesome question facing nurse managers today is why some employees perform better than others. Making decisions about who performs what tasks in a particular manner without first considering individual behavior can lead to irreversible, long-term problems. Each employee is different in many respects. A manager needs to ask how such differences influence the behavior and performance of the job requirements. Ideally, the manager performs this assessment when the new employee is hired. In reality, however, many employees are placed in positions without the manager having adequate knowledge of their abilities and/or interests. This often results in problems with employee performance, as well as conflict between employees and managers.

Employee performance literature ultimately reveals two major dimensions as determinants of job performance: motivation and ability (Hersey, Blanchard, & Johnson, 2001). This chapter describes a model of job performance and presents techniques for evaluating performance.

A Model of Job Performance

Nurse managers spend considerable time making judgments about the fit among individuals, job tasks, and effectiveness. Such judgments are typically influenced by both the manager's and the employee's characteristics. For example, ability, instinct, and aspiration levels—as well as age, education, and family background—account for why some employees perform well and others poorly. Based on these factors, a model that considers motivation and ability as determinants of job performance is presented in Table 19-1.

This performance model identifies six categories likely to be viewed as important by the nurse manager:

1. Daily job performance
2. Attendance
3. Punctuality
4. Adherence to policies and procedures
5. Absence of incidents, errors, and accidents
6. Honesty and trustworthiness

Although there is conceptual overlap in these categories, separate designation of each helps emphasize their importance.

When using this model, the nurse manager should carefully consider several factors. First, the health care organization should establish and communicate clear descriptions of daily job performance so that deviations from expected behaviors can be easily identified and documented. Second, behaviors considered troublesome in one department may be acceptable in another department. Finally, some behaviors are viewed as serious only when repeated (e.g., being late to work), whereas others are classified as troublesome following only one incident (e.g., a medication error with severe consequences).

Employee Motivation

Motivation describes the factors that initiate and direct behavior. Because individuals bring to the workplace different needs and goals, the type and intensity of motivators vary among employees. Nurse managers prefer motivated employees because they strive to find the best way to perform their jobs. Motivated employees are more likely to be productive than are nonmotivated workers. This is one reason that motivation is an important aspect of enhancing employee performance.

Motivational Theories

Historically, motivational theories were concerned with three things:

1. What mobilizes or energizes human behavior
2. What directs behavior toward the accomplishment of some objective
3. How such behavior is sustained over time

Table 19-1   A Simplified Model of Job Performance

Motivation	and	Ability	=	Employee Performance
Compensation		Responsibilities		Daily job performance
Benefits		Education—basic/advanced		Attendance
Job design		Continuing education		Punctuality
Leadership style		Skills/abilities		Adherence to policies and procedures
Recruitment and selection				Absence of incidents/errors/accidents
Employee needs/goals/abilities				Honesty and trustworthiness

The usefulness of motivational theories depends on their ability to explain motivation adequately, to predict with some degree of accuracy what people will actually do, and, finally, to suggest practical ways of influencing employees to accomplish organizational objectives. Motivational theories can be classified into at least two distinct groups: content theories and process theories.

Content Theories In general, **content theories** emphasize individual needs or the rewards that may satisfy those needs. There are two types of content theories: instinct and need. Instinct theorists characterized instincts as inherited or innate tendencies that predisposed individuals to behave in certain ways. These theories were attacked for their difficulty in pinpointing the specific motivating behaviors and the acute awareness of the variability in the strengths of instincts across individuals. In addition, the development of need theories supported the concept that motives were learned behaviors. Perhaps the most noted of the need theorists were Abraham Maslow, Clayton Alderfer, and Frederick Herzberg.

Maslow (1943, 1954) identified five hierarchical needs. A lower-level need controls behavior until it is satisfied, and then the next higher need energizes and directs behavior. Maslow's theory is frequently used in nursing to provide an explanation of human behavior. This hierarchy, from the lowest to the highest level, is as follows:

1. Physiological needs, such as hunger and thirst
2. Safety needs, that is, bodily safety
3. Belongingness or social needs, such as friendship, affection, and love

---

> **KEY TERMS**
>
> **Motivation** The factors that initiate and direct behavior.
>
> **Content theories** Motivational theories that emphasize individual needs or the rewards that may satisfy those needs.

---

4. Esteem needs, such as recognition, appreciation, and self-respect
5. Self-actualization, that is, developing one's whole potential

The three content theorists are compared in Figure 19-1.

Alderfer (1972) suggested three, rather than five, need levels in his existence–relatedness–growth theory:

1. Existence needs, which include both physiological and safety needs
2. Relatedness needs (Maslow's belongingness or social needs)
3. Growth needs, which include the needs for self-esteem and self-actualization

This theory is similar to Maslow's in that it assumes that the satisfaction of needs on one level activates a need at the next higher level (Figure 19-1). An example is that staff who have a sense of job security will strive for a means of feeling related or connected to the organization or unit. Today's employees want to have a voice in how things are done; they want to make a difference and feel that they are valued by the organization.

Maslow	Alderfer	Herzberg
Self-actualization	Growth needs	Motivating factors
Esteem needs		
Belongingness (social needs)	Relatedness needs	Hygiene factors
Safety needs	Existence needs	
Physiological needs		

Figure 19-1 **Comparison of content theories.**

Empowerment, self-managing teams, and continuous quality improvement programs are built on recognition of these needs.

Alderfer suggests, however, that frustrated higher-level needs cause a regression to and reemphasis of the next lower-level need in the hierarchy. In addition, Alderfer's model suggests that more than one need may operate at any point in time. Although it is somewhat less rigid than Maslow's hierarchy, it presents little that is new or substantially different from Maslow's.

Herzberg's two-factor theory explains motivation as a function of job satisfaction (Herzberg, 1966; Herzberg, Mausner, & Snyderman, 1959). Herzberg states that job satisfaction and job dissatisfaction are not opposite ends of the same continuum; rather, they are two different phenomena. The factors that lead to no job satisfaction are quite different from those that lead to no job *dissatisfaction*, and the resulting behaviors from these two states are also quite different.

Based on this concept, Herzberg proposed that hygiene factors and motivating factors, respectively, affect dissatisfaction and satisfaction. Hygiene factors are extrinsic to the job itself; they include pay, supervision, organizational policies, relationships with co-workers, working conditions, personal life, status, and job security. Unsatisfactory hygiene factors lead to dissatisfaction, which, in turn, leads to increased absences, grievances, or resignations. Herzberg likens hygiene factors to a water filtration plant. Not having one will likely result in illness, but drinking purified water will not necessarily keep one from becoming sick.

Satisfaction and motivation then result from factors intrinsic to the job, such as a sense of achievement for performing a task successfully, recognition and praise, responsibility for one's own or another's work, growth, and advancement or changing status through promotion. To the extent that these intrinsic, or motivating, factors are present, an employee is assumed to experience job satisfaction and hence will be highly motivated to perform the job effectively.

Process Theories   Whereas content theories attempt to explain why a person behaves in a particular manner, **process theories** emphasize how the motivation process works to direct an individual's effort into performance. These theories add another dimension to the manager's understanding of motivation and help to predict employee behavior in certain circumstances. Examples of process theories are reinforcement theory, expectancy theory, equity theory, and goal-setting theory.

Reinforcement theory, also known as behavior modification, views motivation as learning (Skinner, 1953).

According to this theory, behavior is learned through a process called **operant conditioning**, in which a behavior becomes associated with a particular consequence. In operant conditioning, the response–consequence connection is strengthened over time—that is, it is learned.

Consequences may be positive, as with praise or recognition, or negative. Positive reinforcers are used for the express purpose of increasing a desired behavior.

Kyle, a staff nurse, offered a creative idea to redesign work flow on the unit. His manager supported the idea and helped Kyle implement the new process. In addition, the manager praised Kyle for the extra effort and publicly recognized him for the idea. Kyle was encouraged by the outcome and sought other solutions to work-flow problems.

Negative reinforcers are used to inhibit an undesired behavior. **Punishment** is a common technique.

To get Rose to chart adequately, the manager required her to come to his office daily with her patient charts until she achieved an acceptable level of charting. Rose found the task laborious and humiliating. As a result, Rose soon was charting appropriately.

Because punishment is negative in character, an employee may fail to improve and also may avoid the manager and the job, as well. Research has shown that the effects of punishment are generally temporary. Undesirable behavior will be suppressed only as long as the manager monitors the situation and the threat of punishment is present. Conversely, research has demonstrated that positive reinforcement is the best way to change behavior.

Extinction is another technique used to eliminate negative behavior. By removing a positive reinforcer, undesired behavior is extinguished.

Consider the case of Jasmine, a chronic complainer. To curb this behavior, her manager chose to ignore her many complaints and not try to resolve them. Initially Jasmine complained more, but eventually she realized her behavior was not getting the desired response and stopped complaining.

A problem with operant conditioning (behavior modification) is that there is no sure way to elicit the desired behavior so that it can be reinforced. In addition, staff and the manager may view consequences differently.

Take Thad, for example. As a new employee, Thad conscientiously completed critical paths for his assigned patients. When the manager recognized Thad for his good work, his peers began to exclude him from the group. Although the manager was attempting positive reinforcement, Thad quit completing critical paths because he felt the manager had alienated him from his co-workers.

Another procedure is **shaping.** Shaping involves selectively reinforcing behaviors that are successively closer approximations to the desired behavior. The principles of positive reinforcement may take some time, especially when shaping procedures must be implemented. Each successively closer approximation to the desired behavior is reinforced and well established before progressive reinforcement is given to closer approximations of the desired behavior. When people become clearly aware that desirable rewards are contingent on a specific behavior, their behavior will eventually change.

Behavior modification works quite well, provided that rewards can be found that, in fact, employees see as positive reinforcers and provided that supervisory personnel can control such rewards or make them contingent on performance. This does not mean that all rewards work equally well or that the same rewards will continue to function effectively over a long time. If a nursing manager praised someone four or five times a day every day, the praise would soon begin to wear thin; it would cease to be a positive reinforcer. Care must be taken not to overdo a good thing.

Figure 19-2 illustrates the use of various schedules of reinforcement. *Partial schedules* of reinforcement, reinforcing behavior with every second or third occurrence, is more effective in changing behavior.

KEY TERMS

Process theories   Motivational theories that emphasize how the motivation process works to direct an individual's effort into performance.

Reinforcement theory (behavior modification) The motivational theory that views motivation as learning and proposes that behavior is learned through a process called operant conditioning.

Operant conditioning   Process by which a behavior becomes associated with a particular consequence.

Punishment   A process used to inhibit an undesired behavior by applying a negative reinforcer.

Extinction   The technique used to eliminate negative behavior, in which a positive reinforcer is removed and the undesired behavior is extinguished.

Shaping   The selective reinforcement of behaviors that are successively closer approximations to the desired behavior.

	Interval	Ratio
Fixed	**Fixed interval** Reinforcer given after a given time Weekly or monthly paychecks Regularly scheduled exams	**Fixed ratio** Reinforcer given after a given number of behavior occurrences Piece rate pay Commissioned salespeople; certain amount is given for each dollar of sales
Variable	**Variable interval** Reinforcer given at random times Occasional praise by boss on unscheduled visits Unspecified number of pop quizzes to students	**Variable ratio** Reinforcer given after a random number of behavior occurrences Random quality checks with praise for zero defects Commissioned salespeople; a varying number of calls is required to obtain a given sale
	Time based	Behavior occurrence based

Figure 19-2   Four types of intermittent reinforcement schedules. From *Organizational Behavior*, 8th ed. (p. 107), by J. R. Schermerhorn, J. G. Hunt, and R. N. Osborn, 2003, Hoboken, NJ: Wiley.

This *fixed-ratio schedule* of reinforcement requires very close monitoring to reinforce every *n*th response and is obviously not very practical. Reinforcing on a fairly regular basis is known as a fixed-interval schedule of reinforcement; an example is the distribution of weekly or monthly paychecks.

Some rather interesting research findings have emerged over the years on continuous and partial schedules of reinforcement. On the one hand, for example, we know that a continuous schedule of reinforcement is the fastest method of establishing or learning a new behavior, whereas any kind of partial schedule of reinforcement is much slower. On the other hand, behaviors learned under a continuous schedule also extinguish very quickly once reinforcement stops. Behavior learned on a partial schedule continues for a much longer time without being reinforced. In addition, continuous schedules of reinforcement are probably better when money is used rather than other reinforcers, such as praise.

Like reinforcement theory, **expectancy theory** (Vroom, 1964) emphasizes the role of rewards and their relationship to the performance of desired behaviors. Expectancy theory regards people as reacting consciously and actively to their environment.

Vroom asserts that individuals are motivated by their expectancies (beliefs) about future outcomes (consequences of behavior) and by the value they place on those outcomes. Three components are important in predicting what and how much effort a person will exert:

1. **Expectancy** is the perceived probability that effort will lead to a specific performance level or behavior, that is, the degree to which people expect they "can do" something.
2. **Instrumentality** is the belief that a given performance level or behavior will lead to some outcome (reward or punishment).
3. **Valence** is the perceived value (attractiveness or unattractiveness) of an outcome.

Thus, a manager must determine an individual's beliefs regarding the expectancy that will achieve the desired result (expectancy), that the achievement will yield rewards (instrumentality), and how the rewards are valued (valence).

In an effort to improve the amount of delegation by the nurses on her unit, Andrea approached the situation from an expectancy theory perspective. She identified that the nurses wanted to assign more duties to assistive personnel but were reluctant because of concerns about liability. Once Andrea was able to clarify liability issues, the nurses were eager to delegate nonprofessional tasks in order to be able to devote more time to their professional responsibilities.

The net effect of these three components is the amount of effort an individual will exert. Thus, when any one component is drastically reduced, so is motivation (effort). If staff members do not believe that they are capable of performing a task (expectancy), or if they believe there is little chance of reward for their work (instrumentality), or if the value of the outcome (valence) is low, motivation is reduced.

Expectancy theory also considers multiple outcomes. Consider the possibility of a promotion to nurse manager. Even though a staff nurse believes such a promotion is positive and is a desirable reward for competent performance in patient care, the nurse also realizes that there are possibly some negative outcomes (e.g., working longer hours, losing the close camaraderie enjoyed with other staff members). These multiple outcomes will influence the staff nurse's decision.

Expectancy theory is useful because of its clear managerial implications. First, managers can maximize expectancies by assigning to employees tasks that they are capable of performing or by providing them with the necessary training. In addition, removing obstacles (inadequate resources, lack of information or cooperation from others) increases employees' expectancies. Second, instrumentalities can be maximized by making certain that rewards (and punishment) are made contingent on performance. Finally, rewards must be perceived as desirable enough to make the effort toward high performance worthwhile. Similarly, to act as a successful deterrent to inappropriate job behavior, punishment must be regarded as sufficiently undesirable.

Similarly, **equity theory** suggests that effort and job satisfaction depend on the degree of equity, or perceived fairness, in the work situation (Adams, 1963, 1965). **Equity** simply means that a person perceives that one's contribution to the job is rewarded in the same proportion that another person's contribution is rewarded. Job contributions include such things as ability, education, experience, and effort, whereas rewards include job satisfaction, pay, prestige, and any other outcomes an employee regards as valuable.

Thus, equity theory is concerned with the conditions under which employees perceive their contributions to the job and the rewards obtained as fair and equitable. Equity does not in any way imply equality; rather, it suggests that employees who bring more to the job will receive greater rewards. Inequity occurs when an employee's effort and rewards are perceived to be disproportional to that of another person, whether a co-worker or a person doing a similar job for a different employer. Inequity, then, motivates a change in behavior that may either increase or decrease actual effort and job performance. However, reducing inequity may or may not change performance.

Employees can try to restore what they perceive as equity in a variety of ways. First, they can increase or decrease effort. Nurses can attempt to increase their status by assuming more patient care assignments, spending more time on charting, or exhibiting other behaviors reflecting additional effort. Second, they may attempt to persuade the person(s) to whom they are comparing themselves to increase or decrease their inputs—persuading nursing assistants to work less, for instance. Third, they may attempt to persuade the organization to change either their own rewards or those of the comparison persons (e.g., salary changes or perquisites). Fourth, they may psychologically distort the perceived importance and value of their own contributions and rewards ("How could they run this unit without me?"). Fifth, they may distort the perceived importance and value of the comparison persons' contributions or rewards ("What can you expect of assistants?").

Psychologically distorting the perceptions of a comparison person's outcomes or inputs is probably the easiest way to restore equity without actually changing one's effort. Alternatively, the staff member may select a different comparison person, someone who is seen as more relevant for the comparison being made, such as the nurse manager. Finally, the individual may actually leave the organization.

The important point is that perceived fairness of rewards affects the manner in which individuals view their jobs and the organization, and it can affect the amount of effort they expend in accomplishing tasks. Moreover, evidence indicates that inequitable rewards, especially underpayment inequity, lead to increased psychological tension, lower job satisfaction, and poor job performance. In times of economic retrenchment, when no one in the organization receives a salary increase, employees, for example, may perceive the situation as equitable if they believed it to be equitable prior to the retrenchment; thus, job satisfaction may not be adversely affected. However, simply distributing rewards equitably does not necessarily improve an otherwise poor motivational environment. In today's economic environment, with organizations being redesigned and reengineered and positions reduced, problems with perceived equity can be anticipated.

Unlike expectancy theory and equity theory, **goal-setting theory** suggests that it is not the rewards or

outcomes of task performance per se that cause a person to expend effort, but rather the goal itself.

There are three basic propositions in goal setting (Locke, 1968):

1. Specific goals lead to higher performance than do such general goals as "Do your best."
2. Specific, difficult goals lead to higher performance than specific, easy goals, provided that those involved accept the goals.
3. Incentives such as money, knowledge of results, praise and reproof, participation, competition, and time limits affect behavior only if they cause individuals to change their goals or to accept goals that have been assigned to them.

Timothy, for example, was new to a home care hospice program. An important skill in care with the terminally ill is therapeutic communication. Timothy and his manager recognized that he needed help to improve his skills in communicating with these patients and their families. His manager asked him to write two goals related to communication. Timothy expressed a desire to attend a communications workshop and also indicated he would try at least one new communication technique each week. Within a month, Timothy's therapeutic communication skills had already improved. As a result, Timothy was more satisfied with his position, his patients

---

KEY TERMS

Expectancy theory The motivational theory that emphasizes the role of rewards and their relationship to the performance of desired behaviors.

Expectancy The perceived probability that effort will lead to a specific performance level or behavior.

Instrumentality The belief that a given performance level or behavior will lead to some outcome.

Valence The perceived value of an outcome.

Equity theory The motivational theory that suggests effort and job satisfaction depend on the degree of equity or perceived fairness in the work situation.

Equity The perception that one's work contribution is rewarded in the same proportion that another person's contribution is rewarded.

Goal-setting theory The motivational theory that suggests that the goal itself is the motivating force.

received more compassionate care, and Timothy found his work more rewarding.

According to goal-setting theory, the function of rewards is to help ensure that the individual will accept an assigned goal or to set a more specific, difficult personal goal. The specificity and difficulty of the goal mobilize energy and direct behavior toward goal accomplishment. If the person sees tasks and duties as reasonable and specific, difficult goals are likely to produce higher performance as long as such performance is rewarded and the individual is held accountable for the task.

Obviously there is no single approach to motivating staff members. Some methods work better than others with different people or in different settings. However, each theory of work motivation contributes something to our understanding of, and ultimately our ability to influence, employee motivation.

Figure 19-3 illustrates a simple model of how the various motivational theories are related. First, there is a task to be accomplished. If this task is expressed in terms of a specific, difficult goal that is accepted by the staff member, a relatively high degree of performance may realistically be expected in most situations. How does this happen? Goals, perceived ability, and perceived situational constraints all combine to form the perceived likelihood that effort will lead to a given level of performance or goal accomplishment. This expectancy, when combined with the belief that valued rewards will follow from goal attainment (instrumentality), prompts the expenditure of effort (motivation). Thus, goal-setting and expectancy theory suggest not only that staff members should know exactly what they should be doing, but also that they should perceive rewards as contingent on performance of their assigned tasks.

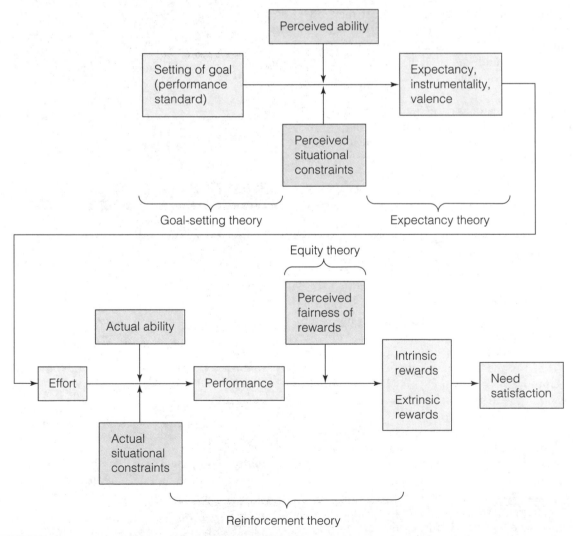

Figure 19-3   Integrated model of the motivational process.

Managers who are effective leaders draw from their knowledge of various motivational theories to create the environment in which their staff derive needs satisfaction from the work itself. No motivation theory provides a complete description of the motivational process; each theory or technique brings a different perspective and contribution to understanding and influencing motivation. Effective staff motivation is best accomplished by judiciously combining theories and techniques so that their effects are complementary.

Case Study 19-1 illustrates how one nurse manager used her ingenuity to motivate staff.

CASE STUDY 19-1: Motivating Staff

Jamie Edgar is nurse manager of the mental health outpatient clinic for a large county health department. Her staff includes nurses, licensed clinical social workers, licensed mental health technicians, and clerical support staff. State funding for mental health services has been drastically cut. Jamie had a difficult decision to make regarding who on the staff would receive pay increases and who would not. Compounding her problem is the shortage of qualified psychiatric nurses and two vacant nursing positions she has been unable to fill due to the low starting salary.

Jamie decides that the nursing staff will receive a 4 percent raise and the licensed clinical social workers will receive a 3 percent raise. The mental health technicians and clerical staff will not receive a wage increase this year. The mental health technicians and clerical staff members are upset when Jamie tells them there will not be any pay increases this year. Kevin Adams, a licensed mental health technician, and Charlotte DuBois, an administrative assistant, have both expressed frustration about the disparity in pay increases. Over the past 2 workweeks, Kevin has been clocking in 10 minutes late each work day and taking longer lunch periods than scheduled. The quality of Charlotte's work has decreased, and she is using more business time for personal telephone calls and personal business.

Jamie is concerned that Kevin's and Charlotte's negative attitudes will continue to affect their work, as well as the morale of the staff. Initially, she tried more frequent praise of Kevin's and Charlotte's work, but after 3 weeks, noted no improvement in their attitude or performance. She counseled each employee individually about performance expectations; however, neither employee made an effort to improve their behavior. After receiving a final budget for her clinic, Jamie allocated $800 for training of clerical staff and mental health technicians. She met with Kevin, Charlotte, and two other staff members. Jamie asked the group to assist her in determining how to best spend the $800 training budget. The group agreed that time-management skills could be improved among many of the staff. After reviewing the cost associated with several time-management training programs, the group was surprised at the expense. Jamie challenged her group to think of alternative ideas other than sending staff members to a seminar and offered a restaurant gift certificate for the most creative ideas.

At their next meeting, Kevin produced reviews of several interactive CD-ROM training programs. Kevin had searched the Internet for the best price for the programs and brought in several demonstration CDs of the top two time-management programs. Charlotte proposed purchasing planners for those staff members who didn't already have a planner or personal digital assistant. Charlotte had spoken to the supplier who had the contract for county office supplies. They had agreed to a price of $12 per planner for a complete year of time-planning supplies. The group agreed that both Kevin and Charlotte's ideas were excellent, as well as coming in under the $800 limit.

Kevin and Charlotte were responsible for implementing their ideas with staff who requested training in time management. Although neither employee received a raise in base salary, Jamie was able to secure approval for both to work extra hours to complete training for the clinic staff. Jamie continued to praise both employees for their commitment to the clinic and their co-workers. Kevin began to arrive promptly for each work shift and kept his lunch periods to 30 minutes. Charlotte was eager to demonstrate to co-workers how her new planner helped her prioritize work and personal tasks. Her use of work time for personal business greatly decreased.

Manager's Checklist

The nurse manager is responsible for

- Understanding motivating factors for employees and how motivation affects job performance,
- Using motivational techniques to enhance employee performance,
- Utilizing creative techniques to motivate staff when traditional rewards such as pay or benefit increases are unavailable, and
- Empowering staff to use creativity to enhance job performance.

Employee Ability

Managers can arrange for staff to participate in development programs that upgrade the knowledge and skills of employees as job requirements change and in special programs, such as intensive workshops and continuing education. The nurse manager plays a crucial role in ongoing assessment and evaluation of employees, providing opportunities and encouragement for their advancement and maintenance of abilities. In addition, the nurse manager is in the best position to communicate the department's educational needs to the administration so that adequate resources are allocated for this function.

Staff Development

Every individual is unique and, therefore, will vary in education, skills, and ability. There are a few common denominators; for example, all new staff nurses will have passed state board examinations. Yet educational preparation will vary, and some people will not have developed all of the skills and knowledge necessary to perform at the expected level. Furthermore, new nursing practice and technology call for ongoing staff education. One of the nurse manager's major responsibilities is to enhance staff performance, an activity usually referred to as **staff development**.

Most early educational theories were based on the belief that the fundamental purpose of education was the transmission of the totality of human knowledge from one generation to the next. This is a workable assumption, provided that the quantity of knowledge is small enough to be managed collectively by the educational system and that the rate of change is small enough to allow the increase of knowledge to be packaged and delivered.

Today, however, these conditions do not exist. Instead, we live in a period of knowledge explosion in which cultural and technological change is rapid. For example, from the time a student enters nursing school to a few years after completing the educational program some of the early learning already is out of date. The implications of this are twofold. First, education must be viewed as a lifelong continuous process. Second, education must become a partnership between the learner and experts so that it occurs every day in an unstructured manner.

The process of education operates constantly during conscious human activity. How people learn, the content of what they need to learn, the processes of learning, and how to teach all are important to education.

People even need to be taught how to learn so they can do their learning efficiently and are prepared to learn new information as it becomes available.

Every health care organization has specific goals, and their attainment requires trained personnel. Therefore, most organizations have specialized educational personnel, either assigned directly to nursing service or as part of an education department. Such departments administer ongoing employee development and orientation programs; nonetheless, the nurse manager remains extensively involved in the instructional process. A new employee, for example, must be taught specific work rules and tasks as well as new nursing or medical practices at the unit level. Trained personnel are the key to success in a work group and in the organization itself. Properly educating employees usually results in higher productivity, fewer accidents or mistakes, better morale, greater pride in work, and better nursing care.

Needs Assessment

The first step in staff development is a **needs assessment** for an educational program. Too often, staff development programs are initiated simply because they have been advertised and marketed, because they have been done in the past, or because other organizations have offered them. Because only educational institutions can legitimately view education as an end in itself, health care organizations must justify how an educational activity can achieve an organizational goal, such as better patient care, reduced operating costs, or more efficient or satisfied personnel. Systematic determination of educational needs based on organizational goals can be used as a basis for developing specific content. In this way, staff development programs are used in the most cost-effective and efficient manner.

The decision to offer educational programs should be based on teaching behaviors that

1. Can be made more effective and efficient by educational efforts (e.g., a streamlined dressing technique),
2. Need maintenance (e.g., cardiopulmonary resuscitation, infection control),
3. New employees need to learn (e.g., required documentation),
4. Employees who are transferred or promoted need to learn (e.g., a nurse who transfers to intensive care and needs education about thermodilution catheters), and
5. Are needed as a result of new knowledge or new technology (e.g., a new chemotherapeutic agent).

Staff development specialists and managers can identify learning needs through a variety of strategies: checklists, advisory groups, quality improvement data, professional standards, and group brainstorming.

Some educational programs are dictated by federal, state, or local regulations. Among these mandatory classes are the following:

- Infection control
- Employee fire and patient safety
- Quality assurance/quality improvement (QA/QI)
- Cardiopulmonary resuscitation (CPR)
- Handling of hazardous materials

Additional requirements may be established through professional organization standards. The Joint Commission on the Accreditation of Healthcare Organizations (JCAHO, 2002) requires organizations to provide education and training necessary to maintain a knowledgeable and skilled staff.

Planning

After needs have been determined, the next step is to plan staff development programs. **Planning** entails identifying learner objectives and matching them with educational methods. Learner objectives, like client outcomes, should be specific, measurable statements about desired behaviors, skills, or knowledge to be acquired within a specific time frame. The strategy used to affect the desired outcome should be based on learning needs, the employee, and available resources.

Nurse managers have a variety of resources at their disposal. The staff development or education department may use a variety of media, such as closed-circuit television, online computer instruction, satellite programs, competency-based programs, self-study, and traditional didactic programs. Other alternatives are using experienced staff members as teachers, preceptors, or mentors; unit-based educators; or off-site continuing education programs.

Three main questions should be considered in assessment and planning: Can the learner do what is required? How should the staff development program be arranged to facilitate learning? What can be done to ensure that what is learned will be transferred to the job? Educators must rely on principles of learning and basic knowledge about educational materials to develop instructional interventions. Also, theories of motivation can be applied to build the individual's desire to learn and to apply skills and concepts learned. Three learning theories help guide what we know

about staff development. They are social learning theory, relapse prevention, and adult education theory.

Social Learning Theory Bandura described **social learning theory** in 1977. It is a behavioral theory based on reinforcement. Bandura believed people learn new behaviors through direct experience or by observing other people performing the behaviors, which result in positive and negative outcomes. The observer learns that successful behaviors should be retained and behavior that is punished or not rewarded should be abandoned.

According to social learning theory, the anticipation of reinforcement influences what the person does or does not observe. This response suggests that observational learning is more effective when the observer is informed in advance about the benefits of adopting a certain behavior than when the observer is rewarded for imitative behavior. Knowing the benefits in advance also increases the observer's attentiveness to the model's actions.

After observing the model, the observer formulates how and in what sequence certain response components must be combined to produce the desired, new behavior. In other words, behavior is learned through cognitive processes before it is performed. Information is commonly conveyed by physical demonstrations, pictorial representations, verbal or written descriptions, and different media sources. Figure 19-4 illustrates this theory.

Relapse Prevention **Relapse prevention** emphasizes learning a set of self-control and coping strategies to

KEY TERMS

Staff development The process of enhancing staff performance with specific learning activities.

Needs assessment An evaluation of learning needs in a select population.

Planning The preparation for learning including obtaining materials and matching learner needs with educational methods.

Social learning theory A behavioral theory based on reinforcement theory that proposes new behaviors are learned through direct experience or observation that can result in positive or negative outcomes.

Relapse prevention A model that emphasizes learning a set of self-control and coping strategies to increase the retention of newly learned behavior.

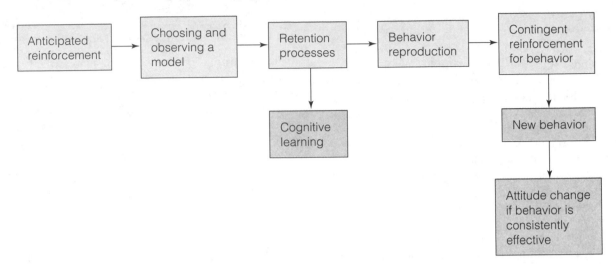

Figure 19-4 **Social learning theory.**

increase retention of newly learned behaviors. The premise behind this model is that learners are

1. Taught to anticipate high-risk situations,
2. Taught coping strategies for avoiding high-risk situations, and
3. Taught that slight slips or relapses are predictable and need not become failures.

As a result, learner self-efficacy increases because the learner anticipates potential problems and is confident in using coping strategies. In addition, this model minimizes the possibility of small relapses turning into absolute failure due to a violation of abstinence. Based on this model, learners should be encouraged to identify possible failure situations and ways to cope with them and practice such situations using new skills in the neutral environment of education.

Adult Education Theory Knowles proposed the **adult education theory**, which described differences in the learning styles of adults and children; it was assumed that the same teaching principles could be used for both children and adults. Knowles suggests four basic conceptual differences between adult and child education: self-concept, experience, readiness to learn, and time perspective. These characteristics are described in Table 19-2.

Implementation

Implementation involves bringing together educators, learners, and the materials and methods needed for education. Although most staff development is carried out by the staff development or education department,

staff development is also a unit responsibility. Two areas, orientation and on-the-job training, involve the nurse manager.

Orientation Getting an employee started in the right way is very important. Among other things, a well-planned **orientation** reduces the anxiety that new employees feel when beginning the job. In addition, socializing the employee into the workplace contributes to unit effectiveness by reducing dissatisfaction, absenteeism, and turnover.

Orientation is a joint responsibility of both the organization's staff development personnel and the nursing manager. In most organizations, the new staff nurse completes the orientation program, whereupon the nurse manager (or someone appointed to do this) provides an on-site orientation. Staff development personnel and unit staff should have a clear understanding of their respective, specific responsibilities so that nothing is left to chance. The development staff

---

KEY TERMS

Adult education theory A theory, described by Knowles, that children and adults learn differently.

Implementation Bringing together materials, methods, speakers, and learners for education.

Orientation A process by which staff development personnel and managers ease a new employee into the organization by providing relevant information.

| Table 19-2 | Characteristics of Adult Learners and Educational Implications |

Adult Learner Characteristics	Implications for Adult Learning
1. *The need to know.*	Adults need to know why they need to learn something before undertaking to learn it. The first task of the facilitator of learning is to help the learners become aware of the "need to know." At the very least, facilitators can make an intellectual case for the value of the learning in improving the effectiveness of the learners' performance or the quality of their lives. Even more potent tools for raising the level of awareness of the need to know are real or simulated experiences in which the learners discover for themselves the gaps between where they are now and where they want to be. Personnel appraisal systems, job rotation, exposure to role models, and diagnostic performance assessments are examples of such tools.
2. *The learners' self-concept.*	Adults have a self-concept of being responsible for their own decisions, for their own lives. Once they have arrived at that self-concept they develop a deep psychological need to be seen by others and treated by others as being capable of self-direction. They resent and resist situations in which they feel others are imposing their wills on them. This presents a serious problem in adult education: the minute adults walk into an activity labeled "education," "training," or anything synonymous, they hark back to their conditioning in their previous school experience, put on their dunce hats of dependency, fold their arms, sit back, and say "teach me."
3. *The role of the learners' experiences.*	Adults come into an educational activity with both a greater volume and a different quality of experience from youths. The emphasis in adult education is on experiential techniques—techniques that tap into the experience of the learners, such as group discussion, simulation exercises, problem-solving activities, case method, and laboratory methods instead of transmittal techniques. Also, greater emphasis is placed on peer-helping activities.
4. *Readiness to learn.*	Adults become ready to learn those things they need to know and be able to do in order to cope effectively with their real-life situations. An especially rich source of "readiness to learn" is the developmental tasks associated with moving from one developmental stage to the next. The critical implication of this assumption is the importance of timing learning experiences to coincide with those developmental tasks.
5. *Orientation to learning.*	There are ways to induce readiness through exposure to models of superior performance, career counseling, simulation exercises, and other techniques. In contrast to children's and youths' subject-centered orientation to learning (at least in school), adults are life-centered (or task-centered or problem-centered) in their orientation to learning. Adults are motivated to learn to the extent that they perceive that learning will help them perform tasks or deal with problems that they confront in their life situations. Furthermore, they learn new knowledge, understandings, skills, values, and attitudes most effectively when they are presented in the context of application to real-life situations.
6. *Motivation.*	While adults are responsive to some external motivators (better jobs, promotions, higher salaries, and the like), the most potent motivators are internal pressures (the desire for increased job satisfaction, self-esteem, quality of life, and the like), but this motivation is frequently blocked by such barriers as negative self-concept as a student, inaccessibility of opportunities or resources, time constraints, and programs that violate principles of adult learning.

From: The Adult Learner, 5th ed. (pp. 64-69), by M.S. Knowles, E. F. Holton III, and R. A. Swanson, 1998, Woburn, MA: Butterfield-Heinemann. Reprinted with permission from Elsevier.

should provide information involving matters that are organization-wide in nature and relevant to all new employees, such as benefits, mission, governance, general policies and procedures, safety, quality improvement, infection control, and common equipment. The nurse manager should concentrate on those items unique to the employee's specific job.

New employees often have unrealistically high expectations about the amount of challenge and responsibility they will find in their first job. If they are assigned fairly undemanding, entry-level tasks, they feel discouraged and disillusioned. The result is job dissatisfaction, turnover, and low productivity. So one function of orientation is to correct any unrealistic expectations.

The nurse manager needs to outline very specifically what is expected of new employees and assure them that they will eventually be able to progress to more challenging tasks. Such realistic job previews should cover the informal aspects of the job, about which an employee could possibly have more unrealistic expectations than about such concrete areas as the pay scale or hours.

Socializing new employees can sometimes be difficult because of the anxiety people feel when they first come on the job. They simply do not hear all of the information they are given. They spend a lot of energy attempting to integrate and interpret the information presented, and consequently they miss some of it. So repetition may be necessary the first few days or weeks on the job.

Because nurse managers are an extremely important part of the socialization process, they should discuss everything that they expect of the new employee openly and specifically. The new employee adapts more rapidly if this is done. The manager should address everything from standards of performance, attendance, and treatment of patients to the feedback the employee should expect in performance appraisals.

One method of orientation is the **preceptor** model, which can be used to assist new employees and to reward experienced staff nurses. The preceptor model provides a means for orienting and socializing the new nurse as well as providing a mechanism to recognize exceptionally competent staff nurses. Staff nurses who serve as preceptors are selected based on their clinical competence, organizational skills, ability to guide and direct others, and concern for the effective orientation of new nurses. The primary goal is for preceptors to assist new nurses to acquire the necessary knowledge and skills so that they can function effectively on the job.

Preceptorships offer new nurses the advantage of an on-the-job instruction program tailored specifically to their needs. Staff nurses (preceptors) benefit by having an opportunity to sharpen their clinical skills and increasing their personal and professional satisfaction. The new nurse works closely with the preceptor for approximately 3 weeks, although the duration of the preceptorship may vary according to the nurse's individual learning needs or the organization's policies.

The primary function of the preceptor is to orient the new nurse to the unit. This includes proper socialization of the new nurse within the group as well as familiarizing her or him with unit functions. The preceptor teaches any unfamiliar procedures and helps the new nurse develop any necessary skills. The preceptor acts as a resource person on matters of unit functions as well as policies and procedures.

New nurses may need to use their preceptors as counselors as they make their transition to the unit. If new nurses experience discrepancy between their educational preparation or their expectations and the realities of working in the unit, the preceptor's role as counselor can prove invaluable in helping them cope with "reality shock."

The preceptor also serves as a staff nurse role model demonstrating work-related tasks, how to set priorities, solve problems and make decisions, manage time, delegate tasks, and interact with others. In addition, the preceptor evaluates the new nurse's performance and provides both verbal and written feedback to encourage development. The staff development department plays an integral role in the preceptor arrangement by providing the initial orientation, familiarizing the new employee with the organization and general policies and procedures before he or she begins work with the preceptor. The staff development department's function is to teach the experienced nurse the role of a preceptor, principles of adult education applicable to learning needs, how to teach necessary skills, how to plan teaching, how to evaluate teaching and learning objectives, and how to provide both formal and informal feedback.

Staff Development Methods   Staff development can be divided into internal (on the unit) and external (off the unit) sources. Internal sources include on-the-job instruction, workshops for staff, and in-service programs. External sources are formal workshops presented by an education department within the hospital and educational activities outside the hospital, including college courses, conferences, and continuing education workshops.

For effective adult education, the student needs, at a minimum,

1. Material to be presented,
2. Practice using the new knowledge and/or skill, and
3. Feedback about performance.

There must be opportunity for practice of the desired behaviors and feedback about it. For instance, if an individual is shown how to perform CPR, practices it, and is given feedback on his or her success, the person could be expected to be able to perform CPR. Reading about or listening to a lecture about how to do cardiopulmonary resuscitation provides no assurance that the recipient actually could resuscitate an individual in an emergency.

The most widely used educational method is **on-the-job instruction**. This often involves assigning new employees to experienced nurses, preceptors, or the nurse manager. The learner is expected to learn the job by observing the experienced employee and by performing the actual tasks under supervision.

On-the-job instruction has several positive features, one of which is its cost-effectiveness. Learners learn effectively at the same time they are providing necessary nursing services. Moreover, this method reduces the need for outside instructional facilities and reliance on professional educators. Transfer of learning is not an issue because the learning occurs on the actual job. However, on-the-job instruction often fails because there is no assurance that accurate and complete information is presented, and the on-the-job instructor may not know learning principles. As a result, presentation, practice, or feedback may be inadequate or omitted.

On-the-job instruction fulfills an important function; however, staff members involved may not view it as having equal value to more standardized and formal classroom instruction.

To implement effective on-the-job instruction, the following are suggested:

1. Employees who function as educators must be convinced that educating new employees in no way jeopardizes their own job security, pay level, seniority, or status.
2. Individuals serving as educators should realize that this added responsibility will be instrumental in attaining other rewards for them.
3. The manager should carefully pair teachers and learners to minimize any differences in background, language, personality, attitudes, or age that may inhibit communication and understanding.

4. The manager should select teachers on the basis of their ability to teach and their desire to take on this added responsibility.
5. Staff nurses chosen as teachers should be carefully educated in the proper methods of instruction.
6. The manager should formalize assignments so that nurses do not view on-the-job instruction as happenstance or second-class instruction.
7. The manager should rotate learners to expose each learner to the specific know-how of various staff nurses or education department teachers.
8. The manager must make it clear to employees serving as teachers that their new assignment is by no means a chance to get away from their own jobs but that they must build instructional time into their workload.
9. The nurse manager must realize that the efficiency of the unit may be reduced when on-the-job instruction occurs.
10. The teacher and nurse manager must supervise the learner closely to prevent him or her from making any major mistakes and carrying out procedures incorrectly.

Other Educational Techniques   As technology continues to advance rapidly and the number of people requiring instruction increases, teaching is becoming more efficient and the learning process accelerating. Many organizations are using self-learning modules, such as online computer classes, closed-circuit television, computerized clinical simulations, interactive video instruction, satellite broadcasts (some of which are interactive), audiotapes, videotapes, and long-distance learning via cable television. These methods allow an instructor to convey information in a uniform manner on several occasions or at several locations at one time; many lessons can be repeated. These methods can enhance the instructor's presentation as well as reduce the need for an instructor to present every detail in person.

KEY TERMS

Preceptor   An experienced individual who assists new employees in acquiring the necessary knowledge and skills to function effectively in a new environment.

On-the-job instruction   An educational method using observation and practice that involves the employees learning new skills after being employed.

MEDIALINK ● Job Satisfaction in the Registered Nurse

Evaluation

Few issues in education create as much controversy or discussion as evaluation. **Evaluation** is an investigative process to determine whether the education was cost-effective, the objective was achieved, and learning was applied to the job. Educators usually agree on the need for sound appraisal of educational programs, but they seldom agree on the best method to do evaluation and rarely do empirical evaluation. Typically, a program is initially reviewed at the corporate level before its implementation. The same program is used over and over until someone in authority decides the program is no longer useful or no longer effective, or, more commonly, until attendance decreases.

The purpose of evaluation is to determine whether the educational program has a positive effect on day-to-day operating problems and to identify elements of the program that need improvement. Designing sound evaluation tools is difficult and costly, though necessary.

Four evaluation criteria should be used:

1. Learner reaction
2. Learning acquired
3. Behavior change
4. Organizational impact

Learner reaction is usually ascertained through a questionnaire completed at the end of a program. The questionnaire may ask about the program's content, the educator, the educator's objectives, the methods used, physical facilities, and meals. Only required questions should be asked; irrelevant data should not be gathered.

Learner reactions are important because

1. Positive reactions ensure organizational support for a program,
2. Reactions can be used to assess the program, and
3. Reactions indicate whether the learners liked the program.

Learning criteria assess the knowledge—the facts and figures—learned in the educational program. Knowledge is typically measured by paper-and-pencil tests that can include true–false, multiple-choice, fill-in-the-blank, matching, and essay questions.

But the acquisition of knowledge is not enough. Was that knowledge converted into behavioral change? One of the biggest problems in education is that instruction does not necessarily transfer from the classroom to the job—often because learners are taught the theory and the technique but never learn how to translate these into behavior on the job. There is a big difference between learning and doing; if behavior is not measured after the program (or on the job), it cannot be determined whether the instructional program has affected behavior or helped the employee transfer the new behavior to the job. Transfer from the classroom to the job is critical to the success of the educational program.

The objective of many staff development programs can be expressed in terms of organizational impact, such as reduced turnover, fewer grievances, reduced absenteeism, improved quality of care, and fewer accidents. These are usually expressed in quantified data and can be easily tied to dollars.

It is often difficult to determine whether changes in such areas can be unequivocally attributed to the staff development program or to other variables in the organization, such as changes in management, increased pay, new equipment, better selection, or changes of some other kind. To rule out the effect of these variables, those who establish the program must take particular care in deciding the length of time for data collection, the unit of analysis, randomization, and other experimental design issues. The most important criteria for measuring results are those that are closely related to the key training behaviors. Despite all of the difficulties in collecting and analyzing such data, cost-related data should be collected because they can provide evidence to higher administration that educational efforts do affect organizational effectiveness.

Designing Staff Development Programs for a Multicultural Staff

Addressing cultural differences, particularly those of the foreign-born nurse, is an important consideration in planning staff development programs. Some cultures outside the United States are more group-oriented than Americans are and often place group needs over individual needs in an attempt to promote harmony and solidarity. In addition, some cultures avoid confrontation and emphasize group cooperation.

The goal of designing culturally sensitive programs is to eliminate stereotypes, remove barriers, prevent misinterpretations, and promote functioning. Common social barriers are language and cultural expectations. In some countries, nurses defer to physicians for all decision making, whereas in the United States such behavior would be viewed as inappropriate and inefficient. Therefore it is important to include during the orientation period information about the role of the nurse, including interdependent and independent functions, management expectations, and effective communication skills.

KEY TERMS

Evaluation   The investigative process to determine whether outcomes were achieved and to what extent.

Cultural barriers also may exist. In many developing countries, needles and other disposable items are reused, families provide personal care, certain types of technology may not be available, or views on using technology to sustain life may differ. In addition, many foreign nursing programs do not incorporate psychosocial skills into their educational programs. Therefore, special programs may need to be developed to ensure a level of competence in this area. Basic nursing skills may need to be reviewed as well as safety procedures. Several such programs have been described in the literature. Common components include

1. Socialization into the nursing role,
2. How to understand and be understood,
3. The development of social skills, and
4. The use of preceptors.

The manager must consider other cultural aspects of employees, especially religious beliefs and practices and family roles and obligations because these vary among and within cultures. To meet the goal of helping staff to provide culturally sensitive care to patients, the manager must ensure that the staff also are treated in a culturally sensitive manner.

What You Know Now

- Motivational theories are classified as content theories or process theories. Content theories emphasize individual needs or the rewards that may satisfy those needs.

- Process theories emphasize how the motivation process itself directs individual performance.

- Job performance is determined by motivation and ability.

- Staff development is used to enhance employee performance through development of specific job skills using orientation, formalized education, and on-the-job instruction.

- The functions of staff development include assessment of educational needs, planning and implementation based on principles of learning and cultural needs, and evaluation.

- The most important aspect of staff development programs is transferring knowledge in order to change work behavior.

- Educational programs should enhance the organization's effectiveness.

- Cultural sensitivity is important in dealing with staff and providing for patients.

Tools for Motivating and Developing Staff

1. Become familiar with various theories of motivation and use the information to help you understand others' motivations.

2. Recognize that an employee's job performance includes both ability to do the job and motivation.

3. Identify staff and department educational needs and communicate those to the appropriate decision makers.

4. Participate in in-service and/or staff development activities as appropriate.

5. Evaluate staff members' abilities to transfer learning to the job.

6. Become sensitive to the needs of a multicultural staff and design programs and activities to meet those needs.

Questions to Challenge You

1. What motivational theory appeals to your sense of how you learn? Why?

2. You are a new nurse manager:
   a) How would you discover what motivates the individuals on your staff?
   b) What would you do first to identify your staff's learning needs?
   c) What are the next steps you would take to meet those needs?

3. What has been your experience working with individuals from other cultures? Describe any problems that emerged and how they were handled.

4. What recommendations would you make to a new nurse manager regarding motivating staff? Have you seen any of these work? Explain.

Explore 🌐 MediaLink

NCLEX review questions, essay activities, group activities, and other interactive resources for this chapter can be found on the Web site at http://www.prenhall.com/

sullivan-decker. Click on "Chapter 19" to select activities for this chapter.

References

Adams, J. S. (1963). Toward an understanding of inequity. *Journal of Abnormal and Social Psychology, 67*, 422.

Adams, J. S. (1965). Injustice in social exchange. In L. Berkowitz (Ed.), *Advances in experimental social psychology* (Vol. 2). New York: Academic Press.

Alderfer, C. P. (1972). *Existence, relatedness, and growth.* New York: Free Press.

Bandura, A. (1977). *Social learning theory.* Englewood Cliffs, NJ: Prentice Hall.

Hersey, P., Blanchard, K., & Johnson, D. E. (2001). *Management of organizational behavior: Utilizing human resources* (8th ed.). Upper Saddle River, NJ: Prentice-Hall.

Herzberg, F. (1966). *Work and the nature of man.* Cleveland, OH: World.

Herzberg, F., Mausner, B., & Snyderman, B. (1959). *The motivation to work.* New York: Wiley.

Joint Commission on the Accreditation of Healthcare Organizations (JCAHO). (2002). *Comprehensive accreditation manual for hospitals: The official handbook.* Oakbrook Terrace, IL: Author.

Locke, E. A. (1968). Toward a theory of task motives and incentives. *Organizational Behavior and Human Performance, 3*, 157.

Maslow, A. H. (1943). A theory of human motivation. *Psychological Review, 50*, 370.

Maslow, A. H. (1954). *Motivation and personality.* New York: Harper.

Skinner, B. F. (1953). *Science and human behavior.* New York: Free Press.

Vroom, V. H. (1964). *Work and motivation.* New York: Wiley.

Evaluating Staff Performance

The Performance Appraisal

Evaluation Philosophy
Components to Be Evaluated
Specific Evaluation Methods
Potential Appraisal Problems

The Appraiser

Documenting Performance
Diagnosing Performance Problems
The Performance Appraisal
    Interview

Improving Appraisal Accuracy

Appraiser Ability
Appraiser Motivation

Rules of Thumb

Looking Ahead

Evaluating job performance by determining the strengths and weaknesses of individual employees within the organization and the motivation of those employees is a vital function of managers. It helps determine and develop the future role of an employee and provides a basis for administrative decisions.

This chapter explains the importance of this process and provides methods of evaluation, criteria to take into consideration, and the accuracy and problems of performance appraisal.

Objectives

In this chapter, you will learn

- What criteria are used to evaluate staff performance.
- How different methods are used to evaluate performance.
- What problems to expect when evaluating performance.
- How to conduct a performance evaluation.

MediaLink www.prenhall.com/sullivan-decker

Additional resources for this chapter can be found on the Companion Website at www.prenhall.com/sullivan-decker. Click on "Chapter 20" to select the activities for this chapter.

- NCLEX Review
- Critical Thinking Activities
- Current Events
- MediaLinks
- *Nursing Leadership & Management in Action:* Assuring Accurate Appraisals; Management of Human Resources

A desired result of any employee's behavior is effective job performance. An important part of the manager's job is to define performance in advance and to state desired results. Performance-related behaviors are directly associated with job tasks and need to be accomplished to achieve a job's objectives.

Enhancing performance includes such actions as

- Identifying performance problems;
- Integrating, facilitating, and coordinating the work of employees; and
- Creating a motivational climate.

Managers also may enhance an employee's performance by removing situational constraints, such as rotating shifts or providing assistance in overcoming constraints. Recognition also enhances performance. Careful management of these factors helps ensure that a staff member's effort or motivation is actively translated into effective job performance.

The Performance Appraisal

The **performance appraisal** process includes

- Day-to-day manager–employee interactions (coaching, counseling, dealing with policy/procedure violations, and disciplining discussed in Chapter 21),
- Making notes about an employee's behavior,
- Completing the performance appraisal form,
- The formal appraisal interview, and
- Follow-up sessions that may involve coaching and/or discipline when needed.

Performance appraisals are conducted for a number of reasons. The primary reason is to give constructive feedback. A good appraisal system ensures that staff know what they are to do and how well they are doing it.

Performance appraisals often serve as the basis on which administrative decisions, such as the size of a salary increase or who gets promoted, are made. Ideally, accurate appraisal information allows the organization to tie rewards to performance. However, accuracy is a skill developed only with experience.

A final reason for doing performance reviews concerns fair employment practice law (see Chapter 18 for information about employment law). Performance appraisals and the decisions based on those appraisals, such as layoffs, are covered by several federal and state laws. In the past two decades, many employees have successfully sued their organizations over employment decisions that were based on questionable performance appraisal results.

Although you can never be certain that your appraisal system is legally defensible, there are several steps to help ensure that an appraisal system is nondiscriminatory (also see Chapter 5).

1. The appraisal should be in writing and carried out at least once a year.
2. The performance appraisal information should be shared with the employee.
3. The employee should have the opportunity to respond in writing to the appraisal.
4. Employees should have a mechanism to appeal the results of the performance appraisal.
5. The manager should have adequate opportunity to observe the employee's job performance during the course of the evaluation period. If adequate contact is lacking (e.g., the appraiser and the appraisee work different shifts), then appraisal information should be gathered from other sources.
6. Anecdotal notes on the employee's performance should be kept during the entire evaluation period (e.g., 3 months, 1 year). These notes, called critical incidents and discussed later, should be shared with the employee during the course of the evaluation period.
7. Evaluators should be trained to carry out the performance appraisal process, including
   a. What is reasonable job performance,
   b. How to complete the form, and
   c. How to carry out the feedback interview.
8. As far as possible, the performance appraisal should focus on employee behavior and results rather than on personal traits or characteristics, such as
   a. Initiative,
   b. Attitude, and
   c. Personality.

Regardless of how an organization uses performance appraisals, they must accurately reflect the employee's actual job performance. If performance ratings are inaccurate, an inferior employee may be promoted, another employee may not receive needed training, or there may not be a tie between performance and rewards (thus lessening employee motivation). For appraisal to be successful, the needs of the staff and requirements of the organization must be bridged (Wilson & Smith-Bodden, 1999).

Evaluation Philosophy

Although nurse managers may not have formal input into the type of appraisal instrument used in their organization, an understanding of the philosophy that underlies the appraisal system as well as the general focus of the system is important.

First, one needs to consider whether evaluations are absolute or comparative. Most evaluation systems are based on **absolute judgment**: In appraising staff, the nurse manager evaluates performance against an internal standard. This internal standard reflects what the manager perceives as reasonable and acceptable performance for the employee. When evaluations are absolute in nature, it is possible for all employees to be evaluated as exceeding the standard for acceptable performance. Alternatively, it is possible that all employees are seen as barely meeting or as falling below the standard. In other words, the ratings received depend entirely on the judgment of the nurse manager.

In contrast, evaluations based on **comparative judgment** require the nurse manager to rate employees by comparing them with one another: An employee's evaluation depends on the level of performance of his or her peers. A teacher who grades on a curve is making evaluations based on comparative judgment. Thus, comparative judgments are based on the relative standing among employees.

Because comparative judgment evaluation systems call for the nurse manager to differentiate among those rated and because not all staff can receive high ratings, it is not surprising that most nurse managers prefer to make ratings based on absolute judgment. Examples of rating scales based on absolute judgment and comparative judgment are presented in Figure 20-1.

Components to Be Evaluated

Nurses engage in a variety of job-related activities. To reflect the multidimensional nature of the job, the performance appraisal form usually requires a nurse manager to rate several different performance dimensions, such as use of the nursing process, professionalism, safety, continuing education, and initiative. In developing an appraisal device, an organization can focus on employee traits, results, behaviors, and/or some combination thereof (Bernardin & Beatty, 1984). The specific focus of the form affects the whole appraisal process.

Traits and Personal Characteristics Many appraisal systems focus on personal traits and characteristics, such as stability or ability to handle stress, because trait-oriented instruments are inexpensive to develop

and can be used for a wide variety of positions. In recent years, however, there has been a gradual shift away from trait-oriented systems, primarily because of charges that they discriminate against some groups. To satisfy legal requirements, the organization should be able to demonstrate the validity (job-relatedness) of the appraisal ratings. In most court cases, trait ratings have not been found to be job-related, and many organizations have been found guilty of discrimination (Bernardin & Beatty, 1984).

Organizations have also moved away from relying exclusively on trait ratings because they are not useful in helping to develop employees. In most health care organizations, a major reason for doing performance appraisals is to help employees improve. However, because most trait-rating dimensions are somewhat ambiguous (for example, what precisely is meant by "initiative"?), trait-oriented systems do not tell a staff nurse what to do differently in the future.

Results-Oriented System All organizations, even non-profit health care organizations, need to be concerned with the bottom line. If a hospital has a 35 percent occupancy rate or a 20 percent employee absenteeism rate, its future is in jeopardy. In recent years, therefore, top management has turned to appraising some employees at least partly on results. There are pros and cons to evaluating health care personnel on such a basis.

In theory, a results-oriented appraisal system is ideal. Employees know in advance what is expected. Objectives are quantifiable, objective, and easily measured. Unfortunately, in most health care jobs, it is not easy to identify measured, concrete objectives. For example, some aspects of a staff nurse's job, such as providing quality patient care, are not easily quantified.

Other aspects, such as the average number of minutes before answering a patient's call button, may be

---

KEY TERMS

Performance appraisal The process of interaction, written documentation, formal interview, and follow-up that occurs between managers and their employees to give feedback, make decisions, and cover fair employment practice law.

Absolute judgment An evaluation method based on reasonable and acceptable standards set by the organization.

Comparative judgment An evaluation method in which employees are compared with one another.

MEDIALINK ● Evaluating Staff Employees

Absolute judgment items "Rate each staff nurse based on what you consider satisfactory performance."	Fails to meet performance standard (1)	Does not quite meet performance standard (2)	Meets performance standard (3)	Exceeds performance standard (4)	Far exceeds performance standard (5)
1. Initiative					
2. Dependability					
3. Job knowledge					
4. Adherence to hospital policies					

Comparative judgment items "Rate each staff nurse you supervise by comparing him/her with others you supervise."	Bottom 10% of all staff nurses	Next 20%	Middle 40% of all staff nurses	Next 20%	Top 10% of all staff nurses
1. Initiative					
2. Dependability					
3. Appearance					
4. Proper utilization of time					

Figure 20-1   Sample items based on absolute and comparative judgment.

counted, but they are not worth the cost of measuring them. In addition, a results-oriented system is of little use for staff development; telling someone that he or she did not accomplish a goal does not tell the person how to accomplish it in the future. Although a results-oriented appraisal system has a number of positive attributes, total reliance on such a system for most health care jobs is often impractical.

Behavioral Criteria   In recent years, many health care organizations have adopted behavior-oriented performance appraisal systems rather than focusing on difficult-to-measure results or on vague traits that may cause legal problems. Behavior-oriented systems focus on what the employee actually does, as exemplified in Figure 20-2.

Such a system gives new employees specific information on how they are expected to behave and is less likely to lead to legal problems. The behavioral focus facilitates employee development. The major drawbacks of a behavior-oriented appraisal system are that it is relatively time consuming to develop and is tied to only one job or a narrow range of jobs. For example, the behavioral items presented in Figure 20-2 would be applicable only to staff nurses.

Combining Different Types of Criteria   As health care organizations have become more concerned with

	Outstanding (5)	Above average (4)	Average (3)	Needs improvement (2)	Unacceptable (1)
1. Performs and documents physical assessment according to unit standard.					
2. Completes patient plan of care according to unit standard on each assigned patient within 24 hours of admission.					
3. Administers medications in a safe and timely manner.					
4. Participates in all mandatory in-service programs.					
5. Dresses according to unit dress code.					
6. Adheres to universal precautions with each patient.					

Figure 20-2   **Behavior-oriented performance appraisal items for the job of staff nurse.**

employee productivity in the last few years, some have developed appraisal systems that combine various types of criteria. In such a system, each employee may have a few major objectives he or she is expected to accomplish. In addition to being evaluated on whether these results were attained, individuals are also evaluated in terms of both general personal characteristics and behaviorally specific criteria.

Specific Evaluation Methods

Traditional Rating Scales   Many organizations use a **traditional rating scale** for all employees in a class (e.g., staff nurse, clinical nurse specialist), regardless of their specific job setting (e.g., outpatient surgery, ambulatory clinic).

A traditional rating scale includes

- General performance dimensions not necessarily based on a job analysis,
- Equally weighted dimensions,
- Absolute judgment standards, and
- Judgments based on the supervisor's idea of satisfactory performance.

In filling out a traditional rating scale, the appraiser is required to reflect on the appraisee's performance over

the entire evaluation period (usually 12 months) and rate the individual against the rater's internal standard of performance. Individuals using trait-rating scales commonly complain either that the performance dimension (e.g., leadership) is irrelevant to the job in question or that they do not know exactly what is meant by the dimension. Such complaints arise because one appraisal form is being used across a variety of jobs and because the performance dimensions are not tied to concrete behaviors.

Essay Evaluation   With the **essay evaluation** technique, the nurse manager is required to describe the employee's performance over the entire evaluation period by writing a narrative detailing the strengths and weaknesses of the appraisee. If done correctly, this approach can provide a good deal of valuable data for

---

KEY TERMS

Traditional rating scale   An evaluation method that uses performance dimensions to rate employees.

Essay evaluation   An evaluation method in which an employee's performance is described through a detailed written narrative.

discussion in the appraisal interview. If used alone, however, an essay evaluation is subject to a number of constraints that can limit its effectiveness. For example, essay evaluations can be time consuming to write, they depend on appraisers' abilities to express themselves in prose, and they can be difficult to defend in court because comments made by the manager may not be closely tied to actual job performance. Most organizations have found that essay evaluations are more useful when they are used in combination with other evaluation formats and when they are based on notes taken by the manager during the course of the evaluation period.

Forced Distribution Evaluation   The **forced distribution evaluation** is similar to grading on a curve. The manager is required to rate employees in a fixed manner (see the comparative judgment items in Figure 20-1). If the rating scale has five categories, the manager may be required to spread employees' ratings equally over the five categories.

Because this technique is constraining, most evaluators do not like it. One hears such complaints as:

"I have two exceptional employees, but this system only allows me to put one of them in the highest category."

"I don't have an employee who deserves to be rated in the lowest category."

Because of the general dislike of forced distribution systems, they are not commonly used. In those instances where they are used, forced distribution systems were generally implemented because managers were giving all of their employees high ratings.

Behavior-Oriented Rating Scales   As noted earlier, focusing on specific behaviors in appraising performance has tremendous advantages. For example, new employees have specific information on how they should behave. Although there are several varieties of **behavior-oriented rating scales**, they all share a number of things in common:

1. Groups of workers who are very familiar with the target job (generally, individuals doing the job and their immediate supervisors) provide written examples (*critical incidents*) of superior and inferior job behaviors.
2. These critical incidents are stated as measurable/ quantifiable behaviors. (Examples are given in Figure 20-2.)
3. Critical incidents that are similar in theme are grouped together. These behavioral groupings

(*performance dimensions*) are labeled, for example, nursing process or communication.

4. Statistical procedures are used to arrive at a subset of the original pool of critical incidents. These procedures eliminate items that do not clearly reflect the performance dimension into which they were grouped, overlap other critical incidents, or are poorly worded.

In view of the way that behavior-oriented rating scales are developed, it is apparent that such behavior-oriented appraisal measures can be used only for one job or a cluster of very similar jobs and that these scales are time consuming and therefore expensive to develop. For these reasons, behavior-oriented systems are generally developed when a large number of individuals are doing the same job, such as staff nurses. Because employees and their managers actually develop the appraisal instrument, they have faith in the system and are motivated to use it.

Focus on Results   Whereas the other approaches to performance evaluation focus on an employee's personal characteristics (traits) or behavior, a focus on results requires setting objectives for what the employee is to accomplish. Although this technique has many variations, basically it involves two steps.

First, a set of work objectives is established at the start of the evaluation period for the employee to accomplish during some future time frame. These objectives can be developed by the employee's supervisor and given to the employee; however, it is better if the manager and employee work together to develop a set of objectives for the employee.

Each performance objective should be defined in concrete, quantifiable terms and have a specific time frame. For example, one objective may need to be accomplished in 1 month (e.g., "Revise the unit orientation manual to reflect the new JCAHO standards"); another objective may not have to be met for 12 months (e.g., "Take and pass the CCRN examination within the next year"). In setting objectives, it is important that the employee perceive them as challenging yet attainable.

The second step involves the actual evaluation of the employee's performance. At this time, the supervisor and employee meet and focus on how well the employee has accomplished his or her objectives.

Although this system can be excellent for evaluating some jobs, such a system has not met with much success in health care, primarily because it is difficult to set challenging, clear, quantifiable goals for health care jobs, where tasks are based on variable patient needs. With increasing emphasis on outcomes, however, results-oriented assessments are becoming more commonly used in health care settings.

Potential Appraisal Problems

No matter what type of appraisal device is used, problems that lessen the accuracy of the performance rating can arise, such as leniency, recency, and halo errors; ambiguous evaluation standards; and written comments problems. These, in turn, limit the usefulness of the performance review. For example, if a performance rating can be shown to be inaccurate, it will be difficult to defend in court.

Leniency Error   Many nurse managers tend to overrate their staff's performance. This is called **leniency error**. For example, a manager may rate everyone on her or his staff as "above average." Although numerous reasons are given for inflated ratings (e.g., "I want my nurses to like me," "It's difficult to justify giving someone a low rating"), these reasons do not lessen the problems that leniency error can create for both the manager and the organization. For example, if you give a mediocre nurse lenient ratings, it is difficult to turn around and take some corrective action, such as demoting the person.

Leniency error can also be demoralizing to the best staff nurses, because they would have received high ratings without leniency. However, with leniency error, these outstanding nurses look less superior compared to their co-workers. Thus, leniency error tends to be welcomed by poorer performers and disliked by better ones.

Recency Error   Another difficulty with most appraisal systems is the length of time over which behavior is evaluated. In most organizations, employees are formally evaluated every 12 months. Evaluating employee performance over such an extended period of time, particularly if one supervises more than two or three individuals, is a difficult task. Typically, the evaluator recalls recent performance and tends to forget more distant events. Thus, the performance rating reflects what the employee has contributed lately rather than over the entire evaluation period. This tendency is called **recency error**; it too can create both legal and motivational problems.

Legally, if a disgruntled employee can demonstrate that an evaluation that supposedly reflects 12 months actually reflects performance over the last 2 or 3 months, an organization will have difficulty defending the validity of its appraisal system. In terms of motivation, recency error demonstrates to all employees that they only need to perform at a high level near the time of their performance review. In such situations, an employee is highly motivated (e.g., asking the supervisor for more work) just prior to appraisal but considerably less motivated as soon as it is completed.

As with leniency error, recency error benefits the poorly performing individual. Nurses who perform well year round may receive ratings similar to those mediocre nurses who spurt as their evaluation time approaches. Fortunately, a simple procedure (recording critical incidents, discussed later in the chapter) greatly lessens the impact of recency error.

Halo Error   Sometimes an appraiser fails to differentiate among the various performance dimensions (e.g., nursing process, communication skills) when evaluating an employee and assigns ratings on the basis of an overall impression, positive or negative, of the employee. Thus, some employees are rated above average across dimensions, others are rated average, and a few are rated below average on all dimensions. This is referred to as **halo error**.

If a nurse is excellent, average, or poor on all performance dimensions, she or he deserves to be rated accordingly, but in most instances, employees have uneven strengths and weaknesses. Thus, it should be relatively uncommon for an employee to receive the same rating on all performance dimensions. Although

---

KEY TERMS

Forced distribution evaluation   An evaluation method in which employees are rated in a fixed method, similar to grading on a curve.

Behavior-oriented rating scales   A type of scale used in evaluation that focuses on specific behaviors and uses critical incidents grouped into performance dimensions.

Leniency error   The tendency of a manager to overrate staff performance.

Recency error   The tendency of a manager to rate an employee based on recent events, rather than over the entire evaluation period.

Halo error   The failure to differentiate among the various performance dimensions when evaluating.

halo error is less common and troublesome than leniency and recency error, it still is not an accurate assessment of performance.

Ambiguous Evaluation Standards   Most appraisal forms use rating scales that include words such as "outstanding," "above average," "satisfactory," or "needs improvement"; but different managers attach different meanings to these words, giving rise to what has been labeled the **ambiguous evaluation standards** problem. Organizations have attempted to address this problem in two ways. One approach is to have a group of nurse managers meet and discuss what each of them sees as outstanding performance, above-average performance, and poor performance on each dimension. The goal is to arrive at a consensus on what level of performance is expected on each dimension. Thus, the group of nurse managers may decide that to be rated excellent on the dimension of self-development, a nurse must attend at least 10 inservice meetings in a year. When agreement is reached on the behavior that reflects each level of a dimension, this information should be communicated to those being evaluated.

A more formal approach to dealing with the ambiguous evaluation standards problem is to develop rating forms that have each gradation along the performance continuum (e.g., excellent, satisfactory) anchored by examples of behavior that is representative of that level of performance. Although a detailed discussion of the process an organization would use for developing such performance standards is too complex to go into here (usually, a consulting firm works with the organization), it involves groups of knowledgeable employees (e.g., job incumbents and their managers) meeting to discuss the important performance dimensions (e.g., nursing process) of a job. Then examples of different levels of performance are developed for each performance standard. For example, a rating of excellent on the performance standard of nursing process/assessment might be anchored by "assessment documented on 95 percent of charts reviewed," whereas a rating of poor on the same standard might be anchored by "assessment completed on 75 percent of charts reviewed."

Written Comments Problem   Almost all performance appraisal forms provide space for written comments by the appraiser. The wise manager uses this space to justify in detail the basis for the ratings, to discuss developmental activities for the employee in the coming year, to put the ratings in context (e.g., although

the evaluation period is 12 months, the appraiser notes on the form that he or she has only been the nurse's manager for the past 3 months), or to discuss the employee's promotion potential. Unfortunately, few nurse managers use this valuable space appropriately; in fact, the spaces for written comments are often left blank. When there are comments, they tend to be few and general (e.g., "Joan is conscientious"), focus totally on what the individual did wrong, or reflect only recent performance.

The existence of the **written comments problem** should not be surprising. Most nurse managers wait until the end of the evaluation period to make written comments; thus, the manager is faced with a difficult, time-consuming task. Small wonder, then, that the few comments tend to be vague, negative in tone, and reflect recent events. Fortunately, regular note taking can lessen the problems associated with written comments (see Documenting Performance).

The Appraiser

In most organizations, an employee's immediate manager is in charge of evaluating her or his performance. In many situations, this makes sense. The manager is familiar with the employee's work and thus is best able to evaluate it. If the immediate supervisor does not have enough information to evaluate an employee's performance accurately, alternatives are necessary. The manager can informally seek out performance-related information from other sources, such as the employee's co-workers, patients, or other managers who are familiar with the person being evaluated. The manager weighs this additional information, integrates it with his or her own judgment, and completes the evaluation.

Another alternative involves a formal use of other sources. Peer review or ratings are growing in use and are appropriate for professionals. **Peer review** is a process by which registered nurses assess and judge the performance of professional peers against predetermined standards. Peer review is designed to make performance appraisal more objective because multiple ratings give a more objective appraisal. It is used frequently in clinical ladder programs, self-governance models, and evaluation of advanced practice nurses.

The steps for peer review are as follows:

1. The employee selects peers to conduct the evaluation. Usually, two to four peers are identified through a predetermined process.

2. The employee submits a self-evaluation portfolio. The portfolio might describe how he or she met objectives and/or predetermined standards during the past evaluation cycle. Supporting materials are included.

3. The peers evaluate the employee. This may be done individually or in a group. The individuals or group then submit a written evaluation to the manager.

4. The manager and employee meet to discuss the evaluation. The manager's evaluation is included, and objectives for the coming evaluation cycle are finalized.

Implementing a peer review involves several considerations. First, it is best to avoid selecting personal best friends for the review. Friends can provide poor ratings as well as inflated ratings, resulting in a negative experience. Second, consider how often to evaluate expert practitioners, for example, those nurses who have reached the top of a clinical ladder. The usual annual evaluations may not be necessary. Third, monitor the time needed for portfolio preparation. The object is to improve professionalism and quality of patient care, not to create more paperwork.

Another technique is **group evaluation**. In group evaluation, several managers are asked to rank employee performance based on job descriptions and performance standards. Usually, one manager facilitates the process. In addition to evaluating individual performance, performance of groups of nurses can also be evaluated in this way and group variances can be benchmarked and evaluated. Using group evaluation reduces personal bias, is timely, and can be effective (Huddleston, 1999).

Documenting Performance

Appraising an employee's performance can be a difficult job. A nurse manager is required to reflect on a staff member's performance over an extended period of time (usually 12 months) and then accurately evaluate it. Given that many nurse managers have several employees to evaluate, it is not surprising that they frequently forget what an individual did several months ago or that they may actually confuse what one employee did with what another worker did.

A useful mechanism for fighting such memory problems is the use of **critical incidents**, which are reports of employee behaviors that are out of the ordinary, in either a positive or a negative direction. These critical incidents are recorded on a form or an index card with space for four items: name of

employee, date and time of incident, a brief description of what occurred, and the nurse manager's comments on what transpired (Figure 20-3). Index cards are usually preferred to a page-size form because cards are more easily carried and are less likely to get torn.

Recording critical incidents as they occur is bound to increase the accuracy of the year-end performance appraisal ratings. Although this type of note taking may sound simple and straightforward, a manager can still run into problems; for instance, some managers feel sheepish about this kind of record keeping. Many managers are uncomfortable about recording behaviors; they see themselves as spies lurking around the work area attempting to catch someone. What they need to remember is that this note taking will enable them to evaluate the employee more accurately and makes recency error much less likely.

The best time to write critical incidents is just after the behavior occurred. The note should focus specifically on what took place, not on an interpretation of what happened. For example, instead of writing, "Ms. Hudson was rude," write, "Ms. Hudson referred to the patient as a slob." The nurse manager is responsible for deciding what are critical incidents. In some departments, coming to work on time may be noteworthy; in other departments, coming to work late is. Once a critical incident has been recorded, the manager should share it with the employee in private. If the behavior is positive, this

---

KEY TERMS

Ambiguous evaluation standards problem The tendency of evaluators to place differing connotations on rating scale words.

Written comments problem The tendency of evaluators not to include written comments on appraisal forms.

Peer review A process by which other employees assess and judge the performance of professional peers against predetermined standards.

Group evaluation An evaluation process whereby a group of managers compare individual and group performance to organizational standards.

Critical incidents Reports of employee behaviors that are out of the ordinary, either positive or negative.

1. Name of employee: ___Cindy Siegler___

2. Date and time of incident: ___March 22, 8:22 A.M.___

3. Description: ___Ms. Siegler came to work late. This was the third time in the___
   ___past 2 weeks.___

4. Comments: ___Ms. Siegler has only worked for the clinic for 4 months and her___
   ___repeatedly late attendance is having an effect on the other clinic staff. I___
   ___spoke with her privately and conveyed the above concerns on March 22___
   ___at 10:35 A.M. She acknowledged the problem she has had with baby___
   ___sitters but reassured me that she has enrolled her child in preschool and___
   ___that she should be on time from now on. We agreed to meet again in 2___
   ___weeks to evaluate her attendance.___

Figure 20-3   Example of a critical incident.

provides a good opportunity for the nurse manager to praise the employee; if the behavior is considered in some way undesirable, the manager may need to coach the employee (see Chapter 21).

Because most nurse managers are extremely busy, they sometimes question whether note taking is a good use of their time. In fact, keeping notes is not a time-consuming process. The average note takes less than 2 minutes to write. If one writes notes during the gaps in the day (e.g., while waiting for a meeting to start), little, if any, productive time is used. In the long run, such note taking saves time. For example, keeping and sharing notes forces a manager to deal with problems when they are small and thus are more quickly addressed. In addition, completing the appraisal form at the end of the evaluation period takes less time when one has notes for reference.

A key factor in effectively using this note-taking approach is how nurse managers introduce the technique to their staff. To get maximum value out of note taking, nurse managers need to keep in mind two important facts:

1. The primary reason for taking notes is to improve the accuracy of the performance review.
2. When something new is introduced, people tend to react negatively to it.

Managers should be open and candid about the first fact, admitting that they cannot remember every event associated with every employee and telling employees that these notes will make more accurate evaluations possible. Even then, employees will still be suspicious about this new procedure. One way to get this note-taking procedure off to a good start is for managers to make the first note they record on an employee a positive one, even if they have to stretch a bit to find one. By doing this, each employee's first contact with critical incidents is positive.

Based on the experience of organizations that have formally introduced the use of critical incidents, nurse managers tend to make three types of mistakes in using notes.

1. Some managers fail to make them specific and behavior oriented; rather, they record that a nurse was "careless" or "difficult to supervise."
2. Some managers record only undesirable behavior.
3. Some managers fail to give performance feedback to the employee at the time that a note was written.

Each of these errors can undermine the effectiveness of the note-taking process. If the notes are vague, the employee may not know specifically what was done wrong and therefore does not know how to improve. If only poor performance is documented, employees will resent the system and the nurse manager. If the nurse manager does not share notes as they are written, the employee will often react defensively when confronted with them at the end of the evaluation period. In sum, any nurse manager who is considering using this powerful note-taking procedure needs to take the process seriously and to use it as it is designed.

By increasing the accuracy of the performance review, written notes also diminish the legal liability of lawsuits. If a lawsuit is brought, written notes are very persuasive evidence in court. Sharing the notes with employees throughout the evaluation period also improves the communication flow between the manager and the employee. Having written notes also gives the manager considerable confidence when it comes time to complete the evaluation form and to carry out the appraisal interview.

The nurse manager will be less prone to leniency and recency error and will feel confident that the appraisal ratings are accurate. Not only does the nurse manager feel professional, but also the staff nurse shares that perception. In fact, it is typically found that with the use of notes, the performance appraisal interview focuses mainly on how the employee can improve next year rather than on how he or she was rated last year. Thus, the tone of the interview is constructive rather than argumentative.

One final issue needs to be addressed. Different employees react differently to the use of notes. Good employees react positively. Although the nurse manager records both what is done well and what is done poorly, good employees will have many more positive than negative notes and therefore will benefit from notes being taken. In contrast, poorer employees do not react well to notes being taken.

Whereas once they could rely on the poor memory of the nurse manager as well as on a leniency tendency to produce inflated ratings, note taking is likely to result in more accurate (i.e., lower) ratings for poor employees. The negative reaction of poor employees, however, tends not to be a lasting one. Generally, the poor performers either leave the organization, or when they discover that they no longer can get away with mediocre performance, their performance actually improves.

Diagnosing Performance Problems

If the manager notes poor or inconsistent performance during the appraisal process, the manager must investigate and remedy the situation. Certain questions should be asked:

"Is the performance deficiency a problem?"
"Will it go away if ignored?"
"Is the deficiency due to a lack of skill or motivation? How do I know?"

The first step is to begin with accepted standards of performance and an accurate assessment of the current performance of the staff member. This means job descriptions must be current and performance appraisal tools must be written in behavioral terms. It also implies that employee evaluations are regularly carried out and implemented according to recognized guidelines. Also, the employee must know what behavior is expected.

Next decide whether the problem demands immediate attention and whether it is a skill-related or motivation-related problem. Skill-related problems can be solved through informal training, such as demonstration and coaching, whereas complex skills require formal training (e.g., in-service sessions or workshops). If there is a limit to the time an employee has to reach the desired level of skill, the manager must determine whether the job could be simplified or whether the better decision would be to terminate or transfer the employee.

In any deliberations, the manager must include budgetary considerations in the decision-making process. For example, would it be more cost-effective to hire an experienced nurse at a higher salary rather than to provide the necessary staff development to have the current employee reach a satisfactory performance level? Often, the resources of the organization determine which option the manager is able to exercise.

If the performance problem is due to motivation rather than ability, the manager must address a different set of questions. Specifically, the manager must determine whether the employee believes that there are obstacles to the expected behavior or that the behavior leads to punishment, reward, or inaction. For example, if the reward for conscientiously coming to work on holidays (rather than calling in sick) leads to always being scheduled for holiday work, then good performance is associated with punishment.

Only when the employee sees a strong link between valued outcomes and meeting performance expectations will motivation strategies succeed. The manager plays a role in tailoring motivational efforts to meet the individual needs of the employee. Unfortunately, creating a performance–reward climate does not eliminate all problem behaviors. When the use of rewards proves ineffective, other strategies, such as coaching and discipline, are warranted (see Chapter 21).

To differentiate between lack of ability and lack of motivation, the manager can analyze past performance. If past performance has been acceptable and little change in standards of performance has taken place, then the problem results from a lack of motivation. In contrast, if the nurse has never performed at an acceptable level, then the problem may be primarily skill related. Different intervention strategies should be used, depending on the source of the problem. The objective should be to enhance performance rather than to punish the employee. Figure 20-4 summarizes the steps to take.

The Performance Appraisal Interview

Once the manager completes an accurate evaluation of performance, he or she should arrange an appraisal interview. The appraisal interview is the first step in employee development.

Preparing for the Interview   The nurse manager must keep in mind what needs to be accomplished during the interview. If the appraisal ratings are accurate, they are more likely to be perceived as so by the employee. This perception should, in turn, make the employee more likely to accept them as a basis for both rewards as well as developmental activities. More specifically,

to motivate employees, rewards need to be seen as linked to performance.

The performance appraisal interview is the key to this linkage. In the interview, the nurse manager needs to establish that performance has been carefully assessed and that, when merited, rewards will be forthcoming. Developmental activities also need to be derived from an accurate evaluation. If an employee is rated as "needs immediate improvement" on delegation skills, for example, any effort to remedy this deficiency must stem from the employee's acceptance of the need for improvement in delegation.

Even though they have tried to fill out the appraisal form accurately, nurse managers should still anticipate disagreement with some of their ratings. Most employees tend to see themselves as above-average performers. This tendency to exaggerate our own performance results from the fact that we tend to forget our mistakes and recall our accomplishments; we often rationalize away those instances where our performance was substandard (e.g., "I forgot, but with this heavy workload, what do you expect?"). Given this tendency to overevaluate one's own performance and the fact that most staff previously have had poor experiences with the evaluation process, nurse managers

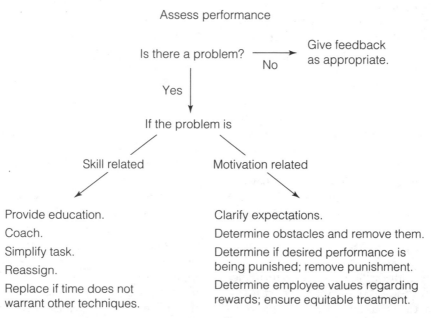

Figure 20-4   Decision tree for evaluating performance.

should expect that staff will lack confidence in the whole appraisal process.

A key step for making the appraisal interview go well is proper planning. The manager should set up the performance appraisal interview in advance, preferably giving at least 2 days' notice. The manager should schedule enough time: Most interviews last 20 to 30 minutes, although the time needed will vary considerably depending on the degree to which the nurse manager and the staff nurse have talked regularly during the year.

In preparing for the appraisal interview, the nurse manager should have specific examples of behavior to support the ratings. Such documentation is particularly important for performance areas in which an employee receives low ratings. In addition, the manager should try to anticipate how the staff member will react to the appraisal. For example, will the individual challenge the manager's ratings as being too low? Anticipating such a reaction, one can respond by saying, "Before I made my ratings, I talked with two other unit managers to make sure my standards were reasonable."

The setting also should be considered in planning the meeting. It is critical that the interview take place in a setting that is private and relatively free from interruptions. This allows a frank, in-depth conversation with the employee. Although it is difficult to limit interruptions in a health care setting, choosing the meeting time carefully will help. A nurse manager may be able to schedule the meeting when another manager can cover, or at a time when interruptions are least likely to occur. The most important point to remember is that a poor setting limits the usefulness of the interview. No one wants weaknesses discussed in public. Similarly, interruptions destroy the flow of the feedback session.

The Interview   The appraisal interview is most likely to go well if the nurse manager has written and shared critical incidents throughout the evaluation period. If such feedback has occurred, staff members go into the interview with a good idea of how they are likely to be rated, as well as what behaviors led to the rating. If the nurse manager has not kept notes throughout the year, it is very important to recall numerous, specific examples of behavior, both positive and negative, to support the ratings given.

The major focus of the feedback interview should be on how the nurse manager and the staff member can work together to improve performance in the coming year. However, establishing such an improvement-oriented climate is easier said than done. In giving feedback, a manager needs to be aware that every employee has a tolerance level for criticism beyond which defensiveness sets in. Thus, in reviewing an employee's performance, a manager should emphasize only a few areas—preferably, no more than two—that need immediate improvement.

Unfortunately, evaluators often exceed an employee's tolerance level, particularly if performance has been mediocre. Typically, the manager will come up with an extensive list of areas needing improvement. Confronted with such a list, the staff member gradually moves from a constructive frame of mind ("I need to work on that") after one or two criticisms are raised to a destructive perspective ("She doesn't like me," "He's nitpicking," "How can I get even?") as the list of criticisms continues.

Following are recommendations for conducting an appraisal interview:

1. *Put the employee at ease.* Many subordinates are nervous at the start of the appraisal interview, especially new employees who are facing their first evaluation or those who have not received frequent performance feedback from their manager over the course of the evaluation period. To facilitate two-way communication during the interview, some managers rely on small talk; others begin the interview by giving an overview of the type of information that was used in making the performance ratings, such as, "In preparing for this review, I relied heavily on the notes I have taken and shared with you throughout the year." Rather than trying to reduce the tension an employee may have at the start of the interview, it is better for a manager to ignore it. In many cases, if the manager has given the employee feedback throughout the evaluation period, the employee will not be unduly nervous at the start of the session.

2. *Clearly state the purpose of the appraisal interview.* This improvement-oriented theme should be conveyed at the beginning of the interview and will help the employee do the best possible job in the coming year.

3. *Go through the ratings one by one with the employee.* Provide a number of specific examples of behavior that led to each rating. Some nurse managers use only negative examples to support ratings, and this can cause problems. Employees are more likely to become defensive because the entire focus is on problem areas. If the manager

pays no attention to good performance in certain areas, the employee will pay less attention to these behaviors in the future.

In reviewing the ratings, the nurse manager should be careful not to rush. By systematically going through the ratings and providing behavioral examples, the nurse manager projects an image of being prepared and of being a professional. This is important for getting the staff nurse to accept the ratings and act on them.

4. *Draw out the employee's reactions to the ratings.* More specifically, the nurse manager needs to ask for the employee's reaction to the ratings and then listen, accept, and respond to them. Of the seven key behaviors for doing performance reviews, nurse managers have the most difficulty with this one. To carry out this phase of the interview effectively, the nurse manager must have confidence in the accuracy of the ratings.

When asked to express their reactions, individuals who have received low ratings will frequently question the rater's judgment ("Don't you think your standards are a little high?"). Not surprisingly, the manager whose judgment has been questioned then tends to get defensive, cutting off the employee's remarks and arguing for the rating in question. Being cut off sends a contradictory message to the employee. The individual was asked for reactions, but when given, the supervisor did not want to hear them. The nurse manager should anticipate that the ratings will be challenged and must truly want to hear the staff nurse's reaction to them.

After having listened to the employee's reactions, the nurse manager should accept and respond to them in a manner that conveys the manager has heard what the employee said (e.g., paraphrase some of the comments) and accepts the individual's opinion ("I understand your view"). In addition, the manager may want to clarify what has been said ("I do not understand why you feel your initiative rating is too low. Could you cite specific behavior to justify a higher rating?"). The nurse manager strives for a candid, two-way conversation and wants to know exactly how the employee feels.

5. *Decide on specific ways in which performance areas can be strengthened.* The focus of the interview should now shift to the future. If a thorough review of an employee's performance reveals deficiencies, the manager and employee may jointly develop action plans to help the individual improve. An action plan describes mutually agreed-on activities for improving performance. Such developmental activities may include formal training, academic course work, or on-the-job coaching. Together, the nurse manager and the staff nurse should write down the resulting plans.

Because of the possibility of defensiveness, only one or two performance areas needing improvement should be addressed. The nurse manager should choose the area(s) that (is) are most troublesome and focus attention on this (these). In arriving at plans for improving performance, the nurse manager should begin by asking the staff member for ideas on how to enhance personal performance. After the individual has offered suggestions, the nurse manager can offer additional suggestions. It is critical that such performance plans refer to specific behavior. In some cases, not only will the staff member be expected to do things in a different manner (e.g., "I will refer to a patient as Mr., Mrs., or Ms. unless specifically told otherwise"), but the manager may also be expected to change behavior ("I will post changes in hospital policy before enforcing them").

6. *Set a follow-up date.* After having agreed on specific ways to strengthen performance in problem areas, the nurse manager should schedule a subsequent meeting, usually 4 to 6 weeks after the appraisal interview. At this later meeting, the manager provides specific feedback on the nurse's recent performance. This meeting also gives the manager and the nurse an opportunity to discuss any problems they have encountered in attempting to carry out their agreed-on performance/improvement plans. In most cases, this follow-up session is quite positive. With only one or two areas to work on and a specific date on which feedback will be given, the nurse's performance usually improves dramatically. Thus, the follow-up meeting is one in which the nurse manager has the opportunity to praise the employee.

7. *Express confidence in the employee.* The final key behavior is simple but often overlooked. It is nevertheless important that the manager indicate confidence that improvement will be forthcoming.

Since no more than two problem areas should be addressed in the appraisal interview, other problem areas may be considered later in the year. If the targeted performance areas continue to improve significantly, then 1 or 2 weeks after this follow-up session, the manager should meet again with the staff member, this time raising an additional area that needs attention. As before, specific ways to improve the performance deficiency are developed and written down, and another follow-up meeting is scheduled. In short, performance deficiencies are not ignored, they are merely temporarily overlooked.

Improving Appraisal Accuracy

For the manager and employee to get maximum benefit from an appraisal, it needs to encompass all facets of job performance and be free from rater error. Although attempting to get totally accurate evaluations is much like the search for the Holy Grail, there are ways to greatly improve the accuracy of appraisals.

Appraiser Ability

Accurately evaluating an employee's performance involves using the job description to identify behaviors required, observing the worker's performance over the course of the evaluation period and recalling it, and knowing how to use the appraisal form accurately (e.g., understanding what is meant by performance dimensions such as "initiative"). To the extent that any of these things are lacking, a manager's ability to rate accurately is limited.

Fortunately, a manager's ability to rate employees can be improved. An organization can develop detailed job descriptions and share them with the rater. Steps can be taken to give the rater greater opportunity to directly or indirectly observe an employee's behavior. For example, other supervisors can provide information on an employee's performance when the immediate supervisor is not present. Managers can be taught to take notes on an employee's behavior to facilitate recall. Also, managers can learn to use the appraisal form better through formal training.

Formal training programs help to increase appraiser ability by making raters aware of the various types of rating errors (the assumption being that awareness may reduce the error tendency), by improving raters' observational skills, and by improving raters' skill in carrying out the performance appraisal interview.

Appraiser Motivation

Although it is often assumed that managers are motivated to accurately appraise their employees, such an assumption is often fallacious. Nurse managers have a multitude of tasks to perform, often immediately. Not surprisingly, then, they often view performance appraisals as something that can be done later. Furthermore, many managers do not see doing appraisals as a particularly important task, and some question the need for doing them at all. This is especially true if all employees receive the same percentage salary increase. Thus, if nurse managers are to be motivated to do appraisals well, they need to be rewarded for their efforts.

A nurse manager may spend little time on appraisals for several reasons:

- The organization does not reward the person for doing a good job.
- The manager's superior spends little time on the nurse manager's own appraisal (thus sending the message that doing appraisals is not important).
- If a nurse manager gives low ratings to a poor employee, a superior may overrule and raise the ratings.

In short, in many health care organizations, the environment may actually dampen appraiser motivation rather than stimulate it. Given these reasons for not spending time on appraisals, it is fairly obvious how an organization can enhance appraiser motivation:

- The nurse manager needs to be rewarded for conscientiously doing performance reviews.
- The nurse manager's superior needs to present a good model of how an appraisal should be carried out.
- As far as possible, the nurse manager should be able to reward the highly rated staff.

This becomes more likely as outcomes are used as the basis for reimbursement to the organization and, subsequently, the organization bases rewards on productivity. For the organization and its employees to benefit from the performance appraisal system, pay increases should not be across the board, layoffs should not be based on seniority, and promotions should be tied to superior performance.

Learn how one manager used a performance evaluation to help a staff member and benefit the organization at the same time (see Case Study 20-1).

CASE STUDY 20-1: Evaluating Staff

Brenda Tice has been nurse manager for the medical intensive care unit (MICU) in a large urban hospital for 6 months. The MICU rarely has staff openings and the average nurse has 12 years of experience on the unit. Brenda herself was a nurse on the unit for 10 years prior to her promotion to nurse manager.

Lori Cook has been an RN on the MICU day shift for the past 18 months. Lori is pleasant and tries hard to please her patients and co-workers. However, she consistently stays late to complete her charting, relies heavily on co-workers to help her throughout the shift, and has little confidence in her own ability to handle complex patients. Often Lori will break down and cry during a patient code and is seemingly overwhelmed by the code process. Although the other nurses are supportive of Lori, they are aware of her limitations. Several nurses have complained when they have been assigned two high acuity patients and Lori is assigned one lower acuity patient.

Brenda has arranged for Lori to attend several training programs designed specifically for ICU nurses, provided opportunities for experienced nurses to mentor Lori on more complex patients, and provided her with reference materials to reinforce Lori's skill set. Brenda also reviewed Lori's personnel records for the past 18 months. While Lori is rated high for attendance and her interpersonal skills, her clinical skills are rated as fair. Brenda notices three separate performance counseling documents dated within the past 12 months, with little improvement noted in her clinical performance.

Following another code incident in which Lori started crying and was asked to leave by a physician, Brenda determines that while Lori is a nice person and has many positive qualities, she does not have the clinical skills necessary to function independently in the MICU. After contacting the human resources department to discuss the transfer process, she schedules a meeting with Lori to discuss her performance issues. Brenda reviews the performance concerns with Lori and informs her that she has 30 days to accept reassignment within the hospital to a unit that more closely matches her clinical abilities. Lori decides to interview for positions in the geriatric psychiatric unit and the psychiatric day treatment program.

Manager's Checklist

The nurse manager is responsible for

- Understanding the performance appraisal process and appraisal tools used by the organization,
- Providing honest and timely feedback to all employees,
- Communicating as needed with the human resources department when performance issues arise,
- Accurately and thoroughly documenting all performance-related issues,
- Identifying the impact of poor performers on the morale and productivity of staff, and
- Making staffing decisions in a timely manner.

Rules of Thumb

For approximately 5 percent of employees, the prescriptions given in this chapter will not work, for reasons yet unknown. Additional suggestions or "rules of thumb" derived from practical experience include the following.

- *Go beyond the form.* Too often, people doing evaluations cite an inadequate form as an excuse for doing a poor job of evaluating their employees. No matter how inadequate an appraisal form is, managers can go beyond it. They can focus on behavior even if the form does not require it. They can set goals even if other supervisors do not. They can use critical incidents. In short, nurse managers should do the best job of

managing that they can and not let the form handicap them.

- *Postpone the appraisal interview if necessary.* Once the appraisal interview begins, there appears to be some natural law of management that the session must be completed in the time allotted, whether the session is going well or has degenerated into name calling. Managers forget the goal of the appraisal interview is not merely to get an employee's signature on the form but also to get the employee to improve performance in the coming year. Therefore, if the interview is not going well, a manager should discontinue it until a later time. Such a postponement allows both the manager and the employee some time to reflect on what has transpired as well as some time to calm down.

In postponing the meeting, the manager should not assign blame ("If you're going to act like a child, let's postpone the meeting"), but should adopt a more positive approach ("This meeting isn't going as I hoped it would; I'd like to postpone it to give us some time to collect our thoughts"). Most managers who have used this technique find the second session, which generally takes place 1 to 2 days later, goes much better.

- *Don't be afraid to change an inaccurate rating.* New managers often ask whether they should change a rating if an employee challenges it. They fear that by changing a rating, they will be admitting an error. They also fear that changing a rating will lead to other ratings being challenged. A practical rule of thumb for this situation is if the rating is inaccurate, change it, but never change it during the appraisal interview. Rather, if an employee challenges a rating and the manager believes the employee has a case, the manager should tell the person that some time is needed to think about the rating before getting back to the employee.

The logic behind this rule of thumb is as follows: If a manager does a careful job of evaluating performance, few inaccurate ratings will be made. But no one is perfect, and on occasion, managers will err. When such an error occurs, the manager should correct it. Most employees respect a manager who admits a mistake and corrects it. By allowing for time to reflect on the ratings, a manager eliminates the pressure to make a snap judgment.

Karlene Kerfoot (2000) states that "Performance management systems are a way to hold a mirror up to employees and let them see their performance through the eyes of others" (p. 305). An effective performance evaluation contributes to the employee's development, improves job satisfaction, and enhances employee morale. Learning how to evaluate employees is one of the nurse manager's useful activities.

What You Know Now

- Doing performance appraisals is one of the most difficult and most important management activities.
- Accurate appraisals provide a sound basis for both administrative decisions (e.g., salary increases) and employee development.
- Absolute judgment or comparative judgment may be used to evaluate employees.

- Criteria to be evaluated may include individual traits, outcome results, behavioral criteria, or a combination.
- Evaluation methods include rating scales, essays, forced distribution categories, behavior rating scales, and evaluation of results.
- To enhance the accuracy of the performance appraisal, the manager should record critical incidents throughout the evaluation period.
- Problems with employee appraisal include leniency error, recency error, halo error, ambiguous standards, and the inadequate use of written comments.
- To improve the value of the appraisal interview, the manager should follow the key behaviors for conducting an appraisal interview.

Tools for Evaluating Staff Performance

1. Become familiar with the evaluation process adopted by your organization.
2. Familiarize yourself with the appraisal instrument used for staff evaluation.
3. Learn to use critical incidents and include positive behaviors as well as those needing improvement.
4. Be alert to the chances for error in the appraisal process.
5. Prepare for an appraisal interview using the strategies suggested in the chapter.
6. Follow the key behaviors for conducting an appraisal interview.

Questions to Challenge You

1. What is the evaluation philosophy at your workplace or clinical site? If you do not know, find out and share it with a colleague or class.
2. What components of your job (or clinical placement) are evaluated? Are they the appropriate ones?
3. What types of evaluation methods have been used to evaluate you? Were they the best ones to evaluate your performance? What would you suggest?
4. What has been your experience with being evaluated as an employee? What did you learn from the experience?
5. Have you ever evaluated someone else's performance at work? How closely did your actions follow the suggestions in the chapter?

Explore 🌐 MediaLink

NCLEX review questions, essay activities, group activities, and other interactive resources for this chapter can be found on the Web site at http://www.prenhall.com/sullivan-decker. Click on "Chapter 20" to select activities for this chapter.

References

Bernardin, H. J., & Beatty, R. W. (1984). *Performance appraisal: Assessing human behavior at work*. Boston: Kent-Wadsworth.

Huddleston, D. (1999). Empowerment of nursing staff for optimal performance. *Journal of Nursing Administration, 29*(12), 5, 16.

Kerfoot, K. (2000). On leadership: Leading from the inside out. *Nursing Economics, 18*(6), 7.

Wilson, P., & Smith-Bodden, J. (1999). Does your appraisal system measure up? *Nursing Management, 6*(1), 27–30.

Coaching, Disciplining, and Terminating Staff

Day-to-Day Coaching

Dealing with a Policy or Procedure Violation

Disciplining Staff

Terminating Employees

Looking Ahead

This chapter provides an overview of day-to-day and long-term actions that can be used to develop and maintain employees as well as steps to discipline employees and, when necessary, to terminate staff.

Objectives

In this chapter, you will learn

- What techniques can be used to coach employees.
- How to conduct day-to-day coaching.

- How to confront an employee about a violation.
- How to discipline an employee.
- How to terminate an employee.

MediaLink **www.prenhall.com/ sullivan-decker**

Additional resources for this chapter can be found on the Companion Website at www.prenhall.com/ sullivan-decker. Click on "Chapter 21" to select the activities for this chapter.

- NCLEX Review
- Critical Thinking Activities
- Current Events
- MediaLinks
- *Nursing Leadership & Management in Action*: Key Behaviors in Coaching; A Coaching Experience— Alternative 1: Acting as Team Leader; A Coaching Experience—Alternative 2

Some of the most challenging problems for managers is what to do when employees fail to perform to expectations. Managers often want to ignore the problems, hoping they'll disappear, but that seldom happens. Instead the manager can learn how to handle these problems. This chapter provides an overview of day-to-day coaching, disciplining, and terminating employees when necessary. Chapter 22 covers reducing turnover and retaining staff, and Chapter 23 focuses on absenteeism and other staff problems in more detail.

Day-to-Day Coaching

Coaching, the day-to-day process of helping employees improve their performance, is an important tool for effective nurse managers. Yet coaching is probably the most difficult task in management and often is neglected. In one short interaction, it encompasses needs analysis, staff development, interviewing, decision making, problem solving, analytical thinking, active listening, motivation, mentoring, and communication skills. Intervening immediately in performance problems on a day-to-day basis usually eliminates small problems before they become larger ones and the subject of discussion in performance appraisal interviews or disciplinary actions. Coaching also should be used when performance meets the standard but improvement can still be obtained.

Before entering into a coaching session, the nurse manager (coach) should prepare for the interaction. The goal of the meeting is to eliminate or improve performance problems such as incorrect flow sheet documentation, excessive absenteeism, or frequent personal phone calls. The manager should try to anticipate how the employee will react ("Everybody gets personal phone calls") in order to formulate an appropriate response ("I am here to talk about the number of personal phone calls you receive"). In general, coaching sessions should last no more than 5 to 10 minutes. The steps in successful coaching are as follows:

1. *State the targeted performance in behavioral terms.* "For the past 2 days, the physical assessment portions of your flow sheets have not been filled out."
2. *Tie the problem to consequences for patient care, the functioning of the organization, or the person's self-interest.* "It's difficult for other nurses and physicians to know whether the patient's status is changing, and therefore it's hard to know how to treat the patient. Physical assessments are

a standard of practice in our unit. Failure to document assessments could lead to legal problems should the patient's record go before a court of law." This is an important but often overlooked step because it cannot be taken for granted that the employee knows why the behavior is a problem. If employees are expected to act in a certain way, they need to understand why the behavior is important and be rewarded when it has improved. Also, avoid threatening language, such as "if you want to stay in this unit, you had better complete your documentation." This puts the employee on the defensive and makes the person less receptive to change.

3. *Having stated the problem behavior, avoid jumping to conclusions but instead explore reasons for the problem with the employee.* Listen openly as the employee describes the problem and the reasons for it. If the problem was caused by ignorance—for instance, lack of familiarity with the standard of care on performing and documenting assessments—simply inform the nurse of the appropriate behavior and end the coaching session.
4. *Ask the employee for his or her suggestions and discuss ideas on how to solve the problem.* In many cases, the employee knows best how to solve the problem and is more likely to be committed to the solution if it is his or her own. It is better to encourage employees to solve their own problems, but this does not mean that managers cannot add suggestions for improvement. It is essential to listen openly to understand the employee's perspectives.
5. *How formal should the coaching session be?* If the problem is minor and a first-time occurrence, you may simply state what actions will be taken to solve the problem and end the meeting. In most cases, however, you and the employee should agree on specific behavioral steps each will take to solve the problem; write down these steps for later reference.
6. *Arrange for a follow-up meeting, at which time the employee will receive performance feedback.* It is possible that an employee may bring up personal problems as a cause for the work problems. The coaching session then verges on becoming a counseling session. When the employee brings up personal problems, nurse managers should convey their concern and willingness to work with the employee to get help for the problems. In most cases, nurse managers will not be the direct source of the help but rather will help the employee seek out other, more appropriate, sources. Nurse managers should not

delve into potential personal problems ("Are there problems at home that I should know about?") unless staff raise them. The employee's personal life is not the manager's business.

Dealing with a Policy or Procedure Violation

As with day-to-day coaching, the nurse manager should prepare to **confront** an employee about a policy or procedure violation. The leadership style of the manager is important in determining whether the employee perceives he or she is being told what to do versus being sold on the idea that she or he is an important contributor to the staff. The steps involved in confrontation are similar to coaching. These steps are outlined in Box 21-1.

The first key behavior is to determine whether the employee is aware of the policy. The employee should have received policy information at orientation, and an updated policy manual should be readily accessible to all employees. It is also important to know whether the policy has been enforced consistently. If policies regarding tardiness are not applied to everyone on a daily basis, efforts to change this behavior in one individual predictably will be unsuccessful. It is better to identify policies and procedures that the majority of staff accept and to determine which employee(s) need direction in compliance.

Second, the nurse manager should describe the behavior that violated the policy in a manner that conveys concern to the employee regarding the outcome. By focusing on the employee's behavior, the manager avoids making the interaction a personal issue.

After stating that the policy has been violated, the nurse manager should have documents stating the policy so that interpretation issues can be clarified. For example, if the policy being violated is the requirement that nurses report to a peer about their patients when leaving the unit, the nurse manager should have a copy of the policy in hand.

The next step is to solicit the employee's reason for the behavior (e.g., what is preventing the person from informing a peer about patients when leaving the unit).

KEY TERMS

Coaching   The day-to-day process of helping employees improve their performance.

Confrontation   A communication technique used to address specific issues.

Box 21-1   Steps in Confrontation

1. Prepare before the meeting.	Is the employee aware of the policy and procedure? Desired behavior? Has the policy/procedure been consistently enforced? How will the employee react?
2. Without attacking the person, describe the undesired behavior. Tie that behavior to its consequences for the patients, organization, or employee.	Jane, were you aware that it is clinic policy to notify *both* the clinic manager and the hospital supervisor when you will be absent from work? Not only were we worried about you, but we had to reschedule patient procedures because we did not have the staff to attend to both clinic appointments and special procedures.
3. Solicit and openly listen with empathy to the employee's reasons for the behavior.	Why didn't you notify someone about your absence?
4. Explain why the behavior cannot continue, and ask for suggestions in solving the problem. If none are offered, suggest solutions. Agree on steps each will take to solve the problem.	In the future, you will need to notify both the clinic manager and the hospital supervisor if you cannot come in. How do you suppose you might do this since you do not have a phone?
5. Set and record a specific follow-up date.	Can we meet again in 1 month to review this plan?

Allow sufficient time for the employee to respond while at the same time guarding against the pursuit of extraneous, unrelated issues. In the latter event, redirect the employee's attention to the policy violation and suggest dealing with other issues at another time.

The nurse manager also must convey to the employee that she or he cannot continue breaking an established policy. In the previous example, the manager could discuss the effects of the behavior, such as medications not given, IVs running dry, and patients being left unattended, as reasons for the policy.

Next, the manager should explore alternative solutions so that negative outcomes will be avoided. Ask the employee for suggestions for solving the problem, and discuss each of the suggestions. Offer help if it is appropriate. Decide and agree on a course of action. The last step in the process is to set up a reasonable date to follow up with the employee on adherence to the established policy.

Although dealing with policy or procedure violations in a distinct step-by-step sequence is not always possible, the nurse manager should proceed in an orderly manner. Many policy violations require early and decisive interventions, and these must be handled in an immediate, forthright manner. Positive results will emerge when the manager addresses policy violations within the context of a formalized plan of action.

Disciplining Staff

Most managers, including those in nursing, dread having to **discipline** an employee for many reasons. Nevertheless, there will be occasions where discipline is necessary (e.g., when a regulation has been violated, jeopardizing patient safety). Lack of management support or training, letting past inappropriate behavior go by without mention, rationalization to avoid disciplining, and fear that the employee will respond negatively are a few of the reasons managers hesitate to discipline employees (Anderson & Pulich, 2001). Learning how to discipline effectively can reduce the manager's concerns and improve morale for all employees.

The nurse manager must never lose sight of the reason for discipline. The primary function of discipline is not to punish the guilty party, but to teach new skills and encourage that person and others to behave appropriately in the future.

When faced with a disciplinary situation, the nurse manager should maintain close contact with the organization's human resource department and administration. Before taking any disciplinary action, the manager should discuss the action he or she intends to take and seek approval for it. This close coordination between the nurse manager and administration is essential to guarantee that any disciplinary action is administered in a fair and legally defensible manner.

To further ensure fairness, rules and regulations must be clearly communicated, a system of progressive penalties must be established, and an appeals process must be available. To enforce rules or regulations, managers must inform employees of them ahead of time, preferably in writing.

If a rule is violated, penalties should be progressive. For minor violations (e.g., smoking in an unauthorized area), penalties may progress from an oral warning, to a written warning placed in the employee's personnel folder, to a suspension, and ultimately to termination. For major rule violations (e.g., theft of property), initial penalties should be more severe (e.g., immediate suspension). An appeals process should be built into an organization's disciplinary procedures to ensure that discipline is carried out in a fair, consistent manner. Guidelines for effective discipline can be found in Box 21-2.

Box 21-2 Guidelines for Effective Discipline

1. Get the facts before acting.
2. Do not act while you are angry.
3. Do not suddenly tighten your enforcement of rules.
4. Do not apply penalties inconsistently.
5. Discipline in private.
6. Make the offense clear. Specify what is appropriate behavior.
7. Get the other side of the story.
8. Do not let the disciplining become personal.
9. Do not back down when you are right.
10. Inform the human resource department and administration of the outcome and other pertinent details.

Terminating Employees

Unfortunately, some employees do not respond to techniques to enhance performance, and nurse managers will face the day when they must **terminate**, or fire, an employee. As with a disciplinary action, the nurse manager should maintain close contact with the organization's human resource department and nursing administration. Again, the manager must discuss the termination and seek approval for it.

Preparation before terminating an employee is essential. To prepare, answer the following questions:

1. Did you set your expectations clearly from the beginning? Did you review the job description, performance appraisal criteria, and pertinent policies and procedures with the employee? These expectations should have been in writing.
2. Did you document the employee's performance on a continuing basis using the critical incident or a similar method?
3. Did you keep the employee informed about his or her performance on a regular basis?
4. Did you conduct coaching sessions or deal with policy or procedure violations in a timely manner? Were the sessions and the agreed-on actions in these meetings documented?
5. Were you honest with the employee about the poor performance or the policy that was violated? Were you specific about behaviors that failed to meet expected standards? Was the expected performance stated in behavioral terms?
6. Were you consistent among employees in how you dealt with performance issues and policy or procedure violations?
7. Did you follow up? Did you deliver the actions you agreed to in the coaching sessions?
8. Did you document everything in writing? The importance of this cannot be overstated.

This checklist applies to almost every instance of termination. The few exceptions might be theft or physical abuse of a patient. Even in the latter instances, observation and documentation are crucial to avoid legal challenges.

The steps in terminating an employee are similar to those for disciplining, except there are no plans to correct the behavior and no follow-up. See how one manager handled terminating an employee in Case Study 21-1.

KEY TERMS

Discipline   The action taken when a regulation has been violated.

Terminate   To fire an employee.

CASE STUDY 21-1: Terminating Staff

Carrie Lyle is nurse manager of a 20-bed medical–surgical unit in a suburban hospital. Six months ago, Margaret Johnson, LPN, transferred to the unit from the skilled nursing unit. Carrie noted that although Margaret had been an employee of the hospital for 12 years, her personnel record included several entries regarding substandard performance. Carrie also found gaps in her performance appraisals from other units. Carrie discussed these issues with Margaret prior to her transfer and clearly indicated performance expectations. However, Margaret often arrives late to work and leaves before report is finished for the day shift.

Claire Kindred, RN and night shift charge nurse, has worked with Margaret for the past 6 months. Claire requested a meeting with Carrie to discuss patient care concerns. Claire indicated that during most shifts, Margaret takes extended meal and break times. She has been found sleeping during her shift in empty patient rooms. Recently, Claire assisted one of Margaret's patients to the bathroom. When recording the patient's output, she noted that Margaret had charted the patient's IV intake for the entire shift even though it was only 3 hours into the night shift. When confronted, Margaret laughed and told Claire she was "just saving time." Claire had documented the dates of the incidents and provided them to Carrie. Carrie met that evening with Margaret to discuss her performance and informed her that she will be on probation for the next 30 days. The next morning, Robert Adams, RN, brought one of his patient's charts to Carrie's office. The patient had been assigned to Margaret on the night shift. In addition to diabetes, the patient has bilateral below-the-knee amputations. On the patient's physical assessment, Margaret had charted positive pedal pulses. She also charted she had changed the patient's IV tubing and IV dressing. On closer inspection, Robert found that the date stickers had been covered over by new stickers and no IV tubing charges were noted on the patient's chart. Carrie immediately contacts the human

(continued)

CASE STUDY 21-1: Terminating Staff   Continued

resource department. She tells them that Margaret has falsified patient documentation, in direct violation of her probation and hospital policy. The human resource department reviews Margaret's file and concurs that immediate termination is appropriate. Exit paperwork is initiated by the human resource department and forwarded to Carrie.

Carrie meets Margaret as she arrives for her scheduled shift. She asks Margaret to come into her office to discuss her immediate termination of employment. Margaret is visibly shaken. Carrie calmly outlines the performance problems and compliance issues that support Margaret's termination. She has a security officer escort Margaret to her locker to gather her personal items. Carrie documents the meeting outcome in Margaret's personnel file.

Manager's Checklist

The nurse manager is responsible for

- Understanding the organization's discipline and termination policies and procedures,
- Reviewing personnel files and identifying past performance problems that may affect current or future performance,
- Addressing employee performance issues in a timely manner,
- Verifying performance problems rather than personality problems, and
- Working with the human resources department when employee termination is indicated.

Even with careful documentation and the most conscientious adherence to organizational policies regarding termination, firing an employee may be followed by legal action, grievance procedures, and stressful and time-consuming hearings. A preferable alternative is that the employee voluntarily resign. Careful documentation may allow the manager to suggest that the employee voluntarily leave the organization. This allows the employee to leave without a record of termination.

What You Know Now

- Coaching is the day-to-day process of helping employees improve their performance or eliminate a performance problem.
- When a policy or procedure violation occurs, confrontation is necessary.
- To confront an employee, the manager should make the employee aware of the violation and its consequences, elicit reasons for the behavior, and agree on steps to prevent future recurrence.
- When rule violations occur, disciplinary action is needed. Penalties should be progressive.
- When staff members do not respond to discipline, managers must terminate their employment.
- If an employee must be terminated, the manager must stay in close contact with the human resources department and administration when planning and carrying out the termination.

Tools for Coaching, Disciplining, and Terminating Staff

1. To prepare and conduct a coaching session,
   a. Note the behavior and why it is unacceptable,
   b. Explore reasons for the behavior with the employee,
   c. Ask the employee for suggestions to solve the problem, and
   d. Arrange for follow-up.
2. To conduct a discipline session,
   a. Be certain you are calm before beginning,
   b. Assure privacy before beginning,
   c. Apply rules consistently,
   d. Get both sides of a story,
   e. Keep the focus on the problem, not the person,
   f. Arrange for follow-up, and
   g. Inform the human resources department and administration.
3. To prepare to terminate a staff member,
   a. Inform the human resources department and administration beforehand,
   b. State the offending behavior and the reason for termination,
   c. Explain the termination process,
   d. Remain calm,
   e. Arrange for employee to be escorted out, and
   f. Report back to the human resources department and administration.

Questions to Challenge You

1. Have you ever been coached, confronted, or disciplined in your workplace or clinical site? How well was it handled? How well did you handle it? Did you learn from it?

2. Have you ever had to coach, confront, or discipline someone? How did the person respond? How well did you do? What did you learn?

3. Do you think you could terminate a staff member? If not, how would you prepare yourself?

4. Select a colleague or classmate and role play four situations:

   a. A coaching session

   b. A confrontation

   c. A discipline session

   d. A termination

After you have completed these sessions, reverse positions and play the opposite role.

5. Critique each other's performance.

Explore MediaLink

NCLEX review questions, essay activities, group activities, and other interactive resources for this chapter can be found on the Web site at http://www.prenhall.com/sullivan-decker. Click on "Chapter 21" to select activities for this chapter.

References

Anderson, P., & Pulich, M. (2001). A positive look at progressive discipline. *Health Care Manager, 20*(1), 1–9.

Reducing Turnover, Retaining Staff

Turnover

> Measurement Issues
> Consequences of Turnover
> Voluntary Turnover
> Strategies for Controlling Turnover
> A Systems Perspective

Retaining Staff

> Financial Considerations
> Pay for Performance
> Magnet Hospital Recognition
>   Program
> Floating
> Mentoring

Looking Ahead

In the last chapter we looked at coaching, disciplining, and terminating staff. In this chapter we examine the opposite—how to reduce the number of staff who leave and better retain the most productive employees. Reducing turnover and retaining motivated, competent staff is a priority for managers to be effective.

Objectives

In this chapter, you will learn

- What causes turnover.
- What happens when turnover occurs.
- How to manage turnover.
- Why retention is an issue in health care.
- What factors influence job satisfaction.
- How to retain valuable employees.

MediaLink 🌐 www.prenhall.com/sullivan-decker

Additional resources for this chapter can be found on the Companion Website at www.prenhall.com/sullivan-decker. Click on "Chapter 22" to select the activities for this chapter.

- NCLEX Review
- Critical Thinking Activities
- Current Events
- MediaLinks
- *Nursing Leadership & Management in Action*: Planning Strategies for Staff Retention; What Do Nurses Want?

Turnover

Where nurses practice and what mix of nursing staff is required to adequately care for tomorrow's patients continue to shift (e.g., ambulatory care, home care). Regardless of the setting, reducing **turnover,** the number of staff members who vacate a position, is essential for the health care organization to thrive.

The actual dollar cost of nursing turnover is difficult to estimate. However, given the numerous expenses incurred in hiring a new nurse (e.g., recruiting, selection, orientation, on-the-job training) and temporarily replacing a nurse who quits or is fired (e.g., paying other nurses to work overtime or filling the vacancy with a temporary replacement), the costs are certainly sizable.

Given its cost, nursing turnover clearly needs to be understood better and controlled more effectively. Turnover has been thought of in simplistic terms and seen as universally negative. Such a primitive view of turnover is not helpful to managers as they attempt to deal with this costly problem. Rather, varieties of turnover need to be differentiated:

- Did the employee leave of her or his own accord, or was the person asked to leave?
- Was the departed individual's performance exceptional or mediocre?
- Did the employee leave for career development (e.g., return to school) or because of dissatisfaction with the organization?
- Will the departed nurse be easy or difficult to replace?

Questions such as these have only recently been asked by health care organizations. Yet until they are answered, it is difficult to establish whether the organization truly has a turnover problem and, if so, what can be done about it.

The discussion in this chapter focuses on **voluntary turnover** (i.e., employees choose to leave). If an organization finds a significant amount of **involuntary turnover** (i.e., employees being terminated), then it needs to carefully examine the way it recruits, selects, trains, and motivates employees. These topics are addressed in detail in other chapters in this book.

Measurement Issues

Before a supervisor can hope to manage turnover, its causes must be understood. Traditionally, organizations have attempted to determine the reason(s) for voluntary turnover through two sources: The exiting employee's supervisor is asked why the employee is leaving, and an exit interview with the departing employee is conducted by someone in the human resources department.

Such an approach for determining the cause of voluntary turnover is certainly straightforward, but its validity has been questioned. Hinrichs (1975) has shown that the reasons that departing employees give in their exit interviews differ greatly from their responses to surveys completed several months after leaving the organization. Hinrichs argues that because future employers often ask for reference information from prior employers, exiting employees provide safe responses (e.g., "a better opportunity came along") during an exit interview. In summarizing his results, Hinrichs found it was rare that departing employees would say anything negative about an organization they were leaving or about their immediate supervisor.

Although this tendency for departing employees to make safe responses is understandable, it makes it difficult to determine why turnover is occurring. Surveys sent to former employees several weeks after they have resigned may be more useful. Former employees need to be assured that their responses will not influence any future reference information furnished about them, but rather will be used only to help the organization identify the reasons why nurses are leaving. Another way to attempt to discover the cause of nurse turnover is to conduct interviews with the former employee's co-workers, who often know why an employee left.

Turnover is either functional or dysfunctional (Dalton, Krackhardt, & Porter, 1981). Losing a nurse who is an excellent performer is a greater loss than losing a mediocre performer. Similarly, if a nurse can be replaced easily, the loss to the organization is less than if she or he is hard to replace.

Thus, a nurse manager needs to be particularly concerned about turnover when the nurses who are leaving are of high quality and difficult to replace

KEY TERMS

Turnover   The number of staff members who vacate a position.

Voluntary turnover   The employee chooses to leave the organization.

Involuntary turnover   The employee is terminated by the employers.

(i.e., **dysfunctional turnover**). In contrast, if poorly performing nurses who can be easily replaced resign, the organization actually may benefit from the turnover (i.e., **functional turnover**). Managers need to disregard the myth that all turnover is bad and replace it with an appreciation of the numerous factors that should be involved in determining whether turnover is a problem meriting attention.

Consequences of Turnover

Although turnover obviously involves real costs to the organization, turnover also can have undesirable effects on patients, co-workers, and others. And, as discussed earlier, voluntary turnover is not always undesirable. Anyone with work experience can remember some individual (e.g., a co-worker, a supervisor) whose departure would have improved the organization's functioning significantly. In evaluating the consequences of turnover, a nurse manager (and the organization) must remember that voluntary turnover can have costs and/or benefits. What may be seen as a desirable departure by some (e.g., the nurse manager) may be viewed as a loss by others (e.g., a subset of co-workers).

However, turnover has consequences that go far beyond direct dollar costs. Turnover can have a number of repercussions among other nurses who worked with the departed nurse. Steers and Stone (1982) suggest that turnover can be interpreted by co-workers as a rejection of the job and a recognition that better job opportunities exist elsewhere.

For those who remain, ways must be found to reconcile their decision to stay in light of evidence from others that the job may not be good. As a result, those who remain may reevaluate their present position in the organization and develop more negative job attitudes. In addition, nurses who remain may have to work longer hours (overtime) or simply work harder to cover for a departed nurse; this can cause both physical and mental strain and may result in additional departures. Thus, one often finds a turnover spiral.

If temporary replacements are used, problems still can result as the workflow of the unit is disturbed and communication patterns within the unit are disrupted. Turnover, and the resultant decrease in the number of nurses, also may cause the organization to postpone, cancel, or not pursue potentially profitable new ventures. An organization may delay opening new clinics or services or even close existing units.

As suggested earlier, turnover also can have several desirable consequences, especially if the departed nurse was a poor performer. Steers and Stone (1982) state that among these are the possibility that performance may improve in the following ways:

- Recently trained employees may be more enthusiastic.
- Long-running conflicts between people will be reduced or eliminated through attrition.
- Opportunities for promotion and transfer will increase for those who remain.
- Innovation and adaptation brought about by the introduction of fresh ideas may be enhanced.

To this list of desirable consequences could be added three additional outcomes:

- Opportunity for overtime will increase (some nurses desire voluntary overtime as a way to increase wages).
- Organization may be stimulated to change a troublesome policy (as a result of losing a "star performer").
- Layoffs may be avoided (natural attrition may lessen or eliminate the need for forced reduction of staff during tight labor markets).

Although a detailed discussion of the consequences of turnover is beyond the scope of this chapter, the abbreviated discussion provided should make clear the numerous issues that need to be considered in attempting to determine whether a given turnover rate actually is a "turnover problem."

If the nurse manager decides that she or he has a turnover problem, then action should be initiated. The turnover model introduced in the next section should be a useful vehicle for helping the manager diagnose the cause of voluntary turnover and actively manage it (e.g., attempt to reduce the overall turnover rate, influence who is resigning).

Voluntary Turnover

Voluntary turnover is a direct function of a nurse's perceptions of both the ease and the desirability of leaving the organization.

Perceived ease of movement depends on

- The nurse's personal characteristics
  - Education
  - Area of specialization

- Age
- Geographic mobility
- Contacts at other hospitals
- Transportation
- Market forces
  - Number of job openings at other organizations
  - Non–health care organizations hiring nurses for nursing or nonnursing positions

As with ease of movement, perceptions of the desirability of movement can be affected by several factors:

- Job alternatives within the health care organization
- Work characteristics
- Organizational characteristics

The more a nurse perceives that other work opportunities (positions) exist within the organization, the less voluntary turnover there should be; that is, a nurse may be able to leave her or his current position by means of a lateral transfer, promotion, or demotion. Thus, a nurse who is having problems with a co-worker may be able to transfer to a new unit rather than leave the organization.

To some degree, a nurse manager may be able to facilitate alternative job opportunities (e.g., helping a nurse transfer) as a way to reduce voluntary turnover by

- Work characteristics
  - Autonomy
  - Communication
  - Group cohesion
  - Job stress
  - Job satisfaction
  - Organizational commitment
- Organizational characteristics
  - Unit structure
  - Distributive justice

A number of studies have shown that the greater an employee's satisfaction level or level of organizational commitment, the lower the probability of the individual's quitting.

Job satisfaction is affected by various facets of the work environment, including

- Relationships with the nurse manager, other staff nurses and unit employees, patients, and physicians;
- Shift worked (e.g., day versus evening, rotating versus fixed);
- Compensation level; and
- Equal and fair distribution of rewards and punishments.

In dealing with turnover, managers need to be aware of three important considerations:

1. Voluntary turnover can be caused by several factors, only some of which the nurse manager can influence.
2. The manager needs to assess why nurses are leaving; this may be done in cooperation with the human resources department.
3. Any action taken to reduce voluntary turnover may have other unintended ramifications.

Typically, an organization determines the reasons for turnover by means of exit interviews. However, as noted earlier, the use of exit questionnaires (mailed several weeks after a resignation) and interviews with remaining co-workers often provide more accurate data on turnover causes. The nurse manager should carefully think through a strategy for dealing with turnover prior to implementing it.

Strategies for Controlling Turnover

The nurse manager's goal should be to reduce dysfunctional voluntary turnover. The manager's first opportunity to reduce turnover is when the decision to hire is made. An individual's length of stay at past employers is an indication of how long the person could be expected to stay on a new job (Breaugh & Dosset, 1989).

To retain a valued employee in the organization, the manager can facilitate movement within the organization. Thus, if a staff nurse is "burned out" from working on an oncology floor, one option is to allow a transfer to another service area in the organization (e.g., home care). Unfortunately, many nurse managers hinder or even prohibit such a transfer (particularly if the potential transferee is an excellent performer), not wanting to lose a good nurse. However, this perspective is shortsighted. If the staff nurse cannot transfer to another area (intraorganizational mobility), she or he may leave the organization entirely (interorganizational mobility).

Work characteristics (e.g., job satisfaction, group cohesion, job stress) and organizational characteristics

KEY TERMS

Dysfunctional turnover When nurses who are high quality and are difficult to replace leave the organization.

Functional turnover When poorly performing nurses leave the organization.

(e.g., unit structure) also can be influenced by the nurse manager both directly and indirectly by

- Providing a realistic job preview,
- Enriching or redesigning the staff nurse's job,
- Facilitating upward and downward communication,
- Linking rewards with performance (see next section on pay for performance),
- Developing group cohesiveness,
- Helping resolve interpersonal conflicts, and
- Providing training and educational opportunities.

A Systems Perspective

Employee absenteeism (see Chapter 23) and turnover have been referred to as withdrawal behaviors because they allow an employee to leave the workplace, in one case temporarily and, in the other, permanently. In many cases, these withdrawal behaviors share a common cause: job dissatisfaction. Some effective strategies for reducing absenteeism include

- Providing child care,
- Improving supervisory behavior,
- Coordinating car pools,
- Offering stress management workshops, and
- Creating a cohesive work group.

The nurse manager must avoid the temptation to look for a quick fix in dealing with turnover. In addition, the manager must recognize that what appears to be a simple change (e.g., trying to enrich the job of a high-performing nurse) may not be. For example, providing additional duties to enrich a nurse's job may lead to complaints of favoritism from other nurses or the human resources department may worry about assigning duties that are not included in the job description.

Such potential difficulties should not cause a nurse manager to revert back to status quo behavior. Rather, the manager needs to anticipate such potential problems and deal with them (e.g., be able to justify the differential treatment through the use of performance appraisal data, have the affected nurse agree to the additional duties in writing).

An environment that rewards good performance is the goal. Obviously, this calls for careful attention to the performance appraisal process (see Chapter 20). Such a performance-oriented climate increases the likelihood of functional turnover (i.e., the departure of poorly performing nurses) and decreases the probability of dysfunctional turnover.

Work scheduling (self-scheduling, fixed versus rotating shifts, flexible work hours, job sharing) is a particu-

larly important area not only because of its relationship to voluntary turnover but also because of its frequent linkage to unionization attempts. It should not be surprising that working conditions that lead to turnover also can motivate interest in unionization. Two key causes of turnover-related unionization are staff shortages and rotating work schedules.

Innovative work schedules have had positive impacts on both nurse recruitment and retention. Although changing to work schedules that staff nurses see as more advantageous (e.g., fixed shifts, flexible hours, job sharing) obviously involves costs (e.g., coordination time, paperwork), it also provides benefits. Most nurses prefer fixed shifts. If possible, nurses also prefer flexible hours. For many nurses with child care responsibility, job sharing provides a perfect means for remaining in health care and, at the same time, fulfilling parental responsibilities.

Before implementing such innovative work schedules, considerable planning (e.g., cost–benefit analysis) clearly needs to take place. Unfortunately, many health care organizations, even those that are having trouble recruiting and retaining nurses, simply dismiss such schedules. As with a number of the strategies for reducing turnover, a single nurse manager is unlikely to be able to change an organization's policy concerning work schedules. However, if several managers coordinate their efforts, change is more likely to occur. To increase their likelihood of a successful attempt, the group of managers may need to build a persuasive case for the program they are suggesting (e.g., document the success of job sharing at other hospitals, cost out the possible financial gain—often, part-time nurses are paid at a lower rate and do not receive pension benefits).

Sometimes a nurse manager may simply need to adapt to a high turnover rate. Even if this is the case, the manager may be able to lessen potential problems by doing two things:

1. The nurse manager may want to "manage" beliefs about why a nurse left. Sometimes, the reason is unclear, and the grapevine often will provide an inaccurate and less attractive reason from the organization's perspective (e.g., "she left for $1.05 more an hour at a competitor institution").

2. The nurse manager may be able to provide human resources with a preferred list of replacement workers. One health care organization keeps an up-to-date list of former nurses who will fill in on an occasional basis. Such former employees are more familiar with organizational procedures and thus can handle things more efficiently.

A nurse manager wants to do everything possible to lessen the problem of turnover. Sometimes this involves coordinating efforts with other managers to change organizational policy. The strategies outlined in this chapter have been shown to be effective in reducing turnover. However, not all are equally applicable to all situations.

As a manager, the nurse must be able to analyze situational factors and determine what is appropriate for the set of circumstances. For example, flexible work hours may be suitable for a clinic but not for an around-the-clock operation. By being creative, nurse managers not only can reduce the overall turnover rate but also can have an influence on which nurses leave by providing incentives for the exceptional nurse to stay and by doing less to retain mediocre nurses.

Retaining Staff

Retention begins with recruitment and selection (see Chapter 18). The shortage of nurses makes staff retention a more pressing problem, and the shortage is expected to worsen (AACN, 2003; JCAHO, 2003). An aging workforce coupled with an aging population and the spiraling cost of health care exacerbate the problem of too few nurses to care for many more patients. It behooves the nurse manager to make every effort to enhance the environment so that the best nurses remain.

Financial Considerations

As the largest group of health care professionals, nurses' wages account for the majority of an organization's salary budget. It is reasonable (although not cost effective) that organizations imagine they can reduce expenses by constraining nurses' salaries or allowing open positions to go unfilled. Thus, nurses employed for many years find their salaries only slightly greater than (or even less than) nurses with only a few years of experience.

Salary compression is an ever-present problem in nurses' compensation (Greipp, 2003). **Salary compression** is the effect of higher starting pay of new nurses or rewarding those with fewer years of experience with higher increases that results in the salaries of long-term employees being at or below those of less-experienced nurses. Sign-on bonuses and loan-forgiveness programs are strategies used to attract new graduates. They are, however, only quick fixes that serve to disadvantage already-employed nurses whose salary ceilings remain fixed. One union negotiated for the largest percentage of wage increase to be given to those nurses with the shortest employment time (Greipp, 2003).

Pay scales must be reconfigured to reflect achievement and accomplishment. One institution has done just that.

Pay for Performance

At the Methodist Hospital in Houston, Texas, a performance-driven clinical ladder program was developed and implemented (Triolo, 2003). The purpose was to integrate "organizational values, evidence-based practice, relationship-centered care" with pay for performance (Perry, 2003, p. 1). The American Nurses Credentialing Center magnet hospital criteria were used along with a differentiated practice model.

The **performance-driven clinical ladder** program uses a system of using performance indicators to advance an employee within the organization. An analysis of current salaries was conducted, using years of experience and performance ratings (Triolo, 2003). Then pay for performance replaced across-the-board increases. Three key concepts guided decision making:

1. Horizontal promotion
2. Clinical ladder
3. Clinical mentor

Horizontal promotion rewarded the excellent clinical nurse without promoting the nurse to management. A clinical ladder, based on Benner's (2001) novice-to-expert concepts, was designed. The five designations are:

1. Clinical apprentice—new nurse or nurse new to the area
2. Clinical colleague—a full partner in care
3. Clinical mentor—demonstrates preceptor ability

KEY TERMS

Salary compression The effect of higher starting pay of new nurses or rewarding those with fewer years of experience with higher increases that results in the salaries of long-term employees being at or below those of less-experienced nurses.

Performance-driven clinical ladder A system of using performance indicators to advance an employee within the organization.

Horizontal promotion A program to reward a high-performing employee without promoting the employee to a management position.

4. Clinical leader—demonstrates leadership in practice
5. Clinical expert—combines teaching and research with practice

The strength of the system is that superb, clinical nurses can remain at the bedside, clinical excellence can be rewarded, and nurses can move back and forth among the levels based on their personal and professional goals and needs.

Financial considerations, however, are not the only reason for difficulty in retaining nurses in one organization or retaining them in the nursing profession for that matter. Today's young nurses want to have challenging careers that offer opportunities for growth and advancement. They do not define challenge as working longer hours with fewer staff (Greipp, 2003).

Magnet Hospital Recognition Program

Magnet hospitals are those institutions that have met the stringent guidelines for nurses and are credentialed by the American Nurses Credentialing Center. Two studies of magnet hospitals revealed that these hospitals were more successful in attracting and retaining nurses (Buchan, 1999; Aiken, Havens, & Sloane 2000). A subsequent study found that medical–surgical nurses at magnet hospitals were more satisfied with their jobs and reported feeling more empowered at their workplace (Upenieks, 2003a).

Higher salaries are not the sole criteria that retained nurses in these institutions. Characteristics common in magnet hospitals include

- Higher ratios of nurses to patients,
- Flexible schedules,
- Decentralized administration,
- Participatory management,
- Autonomy in decision making,
- Recognition, and
- Advancement opportunities.

To retain the current workforce and attract other nurses, health care organizations can take from the magnet program characteristics to improve work life conditions for nurses. Encouraging nurses to be full participants and to share a vested interest in the success of the organization can help alleviate the nursing shortage in those organizations and in the profession.

Floating

Another retention strategy suggested is the use of floating. **Floating** is the reassignment to a unit other than the one on which the nurse normally works. One hospital in

West Virginia implemented a successful floating system (Rudy & Sions, 2003). (See section in Chapter 18 about cross-training as a recruitment strategy.)

Several conditions enabled this program to succeed.

- Float assignments were rotated.
- A resource person was available on the unit receiving the float.
- Written information was available to the float.
- Ongoing feedback was solicited.
- A differential was offered for each float.

The hospital's floating program resulted in improving job satisfaction and reducing the vacancy rate (Rudy & Sions, 2003).

Mentoring

Mentoring is another strategy to improve retention. Mentors take a greater role than preceptors in developing staff. Precepting usually is associated with orientation of staff, whereas mentoring occurs over a much longer period and involves a bigger investment of personal energy.

A **mentor** is a wiser and more experienced person who guides, supports, and nurtures a less experienced person. Mentors tell you what you need to know and show you how to get it. Preceptors and preceptees are assigned to each other, whereas the mentor and mentee find one another, generally outside formal development programs. Mentors trust you with a job by giving assignments that are important; they test your limits and provide opportunities for learning. Mentors help by talking to you. They introduce you to people who may be helpful to your career development. Having a mentor instills a sense of greater personal satisfaction, increased self-confidence, and enhanced self-esteem. The relationship usually is intensely personal and rarely is hidden.

Mentors are usually the same sex as the protégé, 8 to 15 years older, highly placed in the organization, powerful, and willing to share their experiences. They are not threatened by the protégé's potential for equaling or exceeding them. Protégés are selected by mentors for several reasons: good performance, loyalty to people and the organization, a similar social background

---

KEY TERMS

Floating The reassignment to a unit other than the one on which the nurse normally works.

Mentor A more experienced person who guides, supports, and nurtures a less experienced person.

or a social acquaintance with each other, appropriate appearance, opportunity to demonstrate the extraordinary, and high visibility.

Mentor–protégé relationships seem to advance through several stages. The initiation stage usually lasts 6 months to a year, during which the relationship gets started. The protégé stage is that in which the protégé's work is not yet recognized for its own merit, but rather as a byproduct of the mentor's instruction, support, and encouragement. The mentor thus buffers the protégé from criticism.

A breakup stage may occur from 6 months to 2 years after a significant change in the relationship, usually resulting from the protégé's taking a job in another department or organization so that there is a physical separation of the two individuals. It also can occur if the mentor refuses to accept the protégé as a peer or when the relationship becomes dysfunctional for some reason. The lasting friendship stage is the final phase and will occur if the mentor accepts the protégé as a peer or if the relationship is reestablished after a significant separation. The complete mentor process usually includes the last stage.

Nurse managers can serve as mentors to their employees through some of the strategies already discussed in this chapter (e.g., coaching, giving positive feedback). Managers also can support their more senior staff to take on mentoring roles with newer staff.

Retaining productive staff is essential to be able to consistently provide quality nursing care. One nurse manager decreased voluntary turnover on her unit without incurring additional costs (see Case Study 22-1).

CASE STUDY 22-1: Retention

Mona Karnes is nurse manager of labor and delivery at a suburban hospital. Over the past 12 months, the voluntary turnover rate among full-time RNs has been 15 percent for her unit and 25 percent for the hospital as a whole. Despite increasing starting salary rates and offering signing bonuses, turnover rates have remained high. Administration is in the process of conducting an annual salary review as well as a benefits review.

Mona has collected information from exit interviews conducted by the human resources department. From this data, Mona has developed three strategies to aid in retention for her unit:

1. Rotating leadership responsibilities on the unit to offer all nurses the opportunity to develop leadership and management skills. These responsibilities currently include a weekly charge nurse role for each shift, education committee chair, physician relations liaison, women's health service line representative, and information technology representative. Other leadership roles will be added as appropriate.

2. Surveying staff to determine interests and strengths and connecting staff members with a mentor. For example, Debbie Edwards, RN, enjoys developing patient education modules. Debbie will work with Heather Adams, GN, to develop her patient education skills.

3. Scheduling monthly CEU offerings during staff meetings that are free of charge and presented by staff members, physicians, or pharmaceutical company representatives. By attending monthly staff meetings, most RNs will complete 90 percent of state-required CEUs for license renewal.

All three strategies are at no cost to the unit or hospital. After 6 months, the voluntary turnover rate on Mona's unit has decreased to 8 percent.

Manager's Checklist

The nurse manager is responsible for

- Understanding the financial impact of voluntary turnover on the unit and the organization,
- Gathering and analyzing data that provides insight into the reasons for voluntary turnover,
- Utilizing creative solutions to increase staff retention,
- Establishing open and effective communication with staff members,
- Evaluating retention strategies in a timely manner and adjusting processes as appropriate, and
- Communicating successful strategies to colleagues and administration.

What You Know Now

- Turnover may be functional or dysfunctional, but it is always costly to the organization.

- Turnover may lead to negative job attitudes, distorted workflow, and overtime.
- Positive outcomes of turnover include increased productivity, opportunities for promotion or transfer, and the avoidance of forced staff reductions.

- Turnover can be minimized by many factors, including hiring practices, job design, appropriate rewards, and the manager's interpersonal skills.

- Retaining staff involves financial considerations as well as the quality of work life of nurses.

- Pay-for-performance systems allow clinical nurses to be rewarded while staying at the bedside.

- Magnet hospital recognition programs have identified criteria that help retain nurses, including higher ratios of nurses to patients, flexible schedules, decentralized administration, participatory management, autonomy in decision making, recognition, and advancement opportunities.

- Floating and mentoring are additional strategies to help retain nurses.

Tools for Reducing Turnover, Retaining Staff

1. Recognize when turnover is voluntary or involuntary and when it is functional or dysfunctional.

2. Assess the reasons for voluntary, dysfunctional turnover.

3. Plan strategies individually and collectively to address voluntary, dysfunctional turnover, realizing the problem may be systemwide and beyond your control.

4. Consider the suggestions in the chapter for retaining staff. Try to implement those that are appropriate in your department or unit.

Questions to Challenge You

1. Is functional turnover a new concept to you? Can you recall instances where an employee's leaving has benefitted the organization? Describe what happened.

2. Have you voluntarily left a job?
   a. What was the reason? Was there more than one reason?
   b. What reason did you give your supervisor?
   c. Was it the same rationale that you answered in part a of this question?

3. In addition to ideas presented in the chapter, can you think of other ways to reduce voluntary dysfunctional turnover?

4. What suggestions to improve retention and reduce voluntary turnover would you recommend to administration of the organization where you work or have clinical experiences?

5. Have you seen managers be effective in retaining staff? What did they do that worked especially well?

6. If you were a manager, what specific actions would you take to retain staff?

Explore MediaLink

NCLEX review questions, essay activities, group activities, and other interactive resources for this chapter can be found on the Web site at http://www.prenhall.com/sullivan-decker. Click on "Chapter 22" to select activities for this chapter.

References

Aiken, L., Havens, D., & Sloane, D. (2000). The magnet nursing services recognition program: A comparison of two groups of magnet hospitals. *American Journal of Nursing, 100*(3), 26–35.

American Association of Colleges of Nursing. (2003). *Nursing shortage fact sheet*. Retrieved September 2003, from www. aacn.nche.edu/MediaBackgrounders/shortagefacts.htm

Benner, P. (2001). *From novice to expert: Excellence and power in clinical nursing practice*. Upper Saddle River, NJ: Prentice Hall.

Breaugh, J. A., & Dosset, D. L. (1989). Rethinking the use of personal history information. *Journal of Business and Psychology, 3*, 371–385.

Buchan, J. (1999). Still attractive after all these years? Magnet hospitals in a changing healthcare environment. *Journal of Advanced Nursing, 30*(1), 100–108.

Dalton, D., Krackhardt, D., & Porter, L. (1981). Functional turnover. *Journal of Applied Psychology, 66*, 716–721.

Greipp, M. E. (2003). Salary compression: Its effect on nurse recruitment and retention. *Journal of Nursing Administration, 33*(6), 321–323.

Hinrichs, J. (1975). Measurement of reasons for resignation of professionals: Questionnaire versus company and consultant interviews. *Journal of Applied Psychology, 60*, 530–532.

Joint Commission on the Accreditation of Healthcare Organizations. (2003). *Quick statistics on the nursing shortage*. Retrieved September 2003, from www.jcaho. org/news=roo/press=kits/quick=statistics=on=the= nursing=shortage.htm

Perry, G. (2003). A new performance-driven clinical ladder: Rewarding clinical excellence while keeping top nurses at the bedside. *Excellence in Nursing Administration, 4*(3). Retrieved September 2003, from www.nursingsociety. org/publication/EXCEL_NA3Q03.html

Rudy, S., & Sions, J. (2003). Floating: Managing a recruitment and retention issue. *Journal of Nursing Administration, 33*(4), 196–198.

Steers, R., & Stone, T. (1982). Organizational exit. In K. Rowland & G. Ferris (Eds.), *Personnel management.* Boston: Allyn and Bacon.

Triolo, P. K. (2003). Designing and launching a performance-driven clinical ladder. *Excellence in Nursing Admin-istration, 4*(3). Retrieved September 2003, from www.nursingsociety.org/publication/EXCEL_NA3Q03.html

Upenieks, V. (2003a). Recruitment and retention strategies: A magnet hospital prevention model. *Nursing Economics, 21*(1), 7–23.

Upenieks, V. (2003b). What's the attraction to magnet hospitals? *Nursing Management, 34*(2), 43–44.

Managing Absenteeism and Other Staff Problems

Absenteeism

A Model of Employee Attendance
Managing Employee Absenteeism
Absenteeism Policies
A Systems Perspective
Family and Medical Leave

Employees with Problems

Overachievers or Superachievers
Disgruntled Employees
Overstressed Employees
The Employee with a Substance
  Abuse Problem

Workplace Violence

Preventing Violence
Ensuring Safety

Looking Ahead

Chapter 23 addresses specific problems nurse managers face when interacting with a group of employees as a whole and with the individuals that make up that group. Difficulties ranging from absenteeism to overachievement to excessive stress to substance abuse begin with specific individuals and, in turn, affect group dynamics.

This chapter presents these issues and attempts to define strategies to help manage them.

Objectives

In this chapter, you will learn

- How to explain absenteeism.
- How to manage absenteeism.
- How to identify staff problems.
- How individual staff problems affect the work group.
- How to identify signs of a substance abuse problem.
- How to identify sources of potential violence.
- What steps are needed to ensure employee safety.

MediaLink www.prenhall.com/ sullivan-decker

Additional resources for this chapter can be found on the Companion Website at www.prenhall.com/ sullivan-decker. Click on "Chapter 23" to select the activities for this chapter.

- NCLEX Review
- Critical Thinking Activities
- Current Events
- MediaLinks
- *Nursing Leadership & Management in Action:* Understanding the Role of the State Board of Nursing; Developing Policies and Procedures

A major challenge confronting managers today is not only improving individual performance and productivity, but also enhancing the efforts of the entire work group. Some of the general techniques for enhancing performance described in Chapter 19 are ineffective because individual problems affect group functioning.

Problems with absenteeism, overachievers, disgruntled employees, overstressed employees, or employees abusing alcohol or drugs are addressed in this chapter. There are no proven methods for managing these problems; the strategies presented here are a starting point. Assistance from the human resources department often is needed.

Absenteeism

Although the extent or the cost of nurse absenteeism is difficult to determine, it is well established that absenteeism in health care organizations is both pervasive and expensive. The costs of absenteeism, however, go beyond its effects on patient care and dollar costs. Absenteeism can have a detrimental effect on the work lives of the other staff nurses. In some cases, they may have to work shorthanded; they are expected to cover the unit despite their missing colleagues. Working shorthanded, especially for an extended period of time, can create both physical and mental strain. These nurses may be forced to skip breaks, hurry through meals, work extended hours, abbreviate their interactions with patients, cancel scheduled nonwork activities, and so on. Even if temporary replacements are called in, the work flow of the unit will still be disrupted. For example, standard organizational procedure may need to be explained to replacement nurses.

Given the undesirable effects of absenteeism, it is not surprising that absenteeism has drawn a good deal of attention in the health care field. For the nurse manager, the question is what she or he can do to lessen the unit's recurrent absenteeism problem. But before considering ways to manage absenteeism, the manager must understand its causes. The following section presents a useful model for understanding nurse absenteeism or, conversely, nurse attendance.

A Model of Employee Attendance

To understand employee absenteeism, it is important to distinguish voluntary from involuntary absenteeism. For example, not coming to work in order to finish one's income taxes would be seen as **voluntary absenteeism** (i.e., absenteeism under the employee's control). In contrast, taking a sick day because of food poisoning would be considered **involuntary absenteeism** (i.e., largely outside of the employee's control). Although this distinction seems reasonable in theory, in practice it is often difficult to distinguish these two categories because of a lack of accurate information (few employees will admit to abusing sick leave).

Some organizations try to distinguish voluntary from involuntary absenteeism by the way they measure absenteeism. Traditionally, health care organizations have measured absenteeism in terms of **total time lost** (i.e., the number of scheduled days an employee misses). Given that one long illness can drastically affect this absenteeism index, total time lost is clearly not a perfect measure of voluntary absenteeism. In contrast, **absence frequency** (i.e., the total number of distinct absence periods, regardless of their duration) is somewhat insensitive to one long illness. Therefore, absence frequency has been used as an indirect estimate of voluntary absenteeism.

This distinction between absence frequency and total time lost should make sense to nurse managers. For example, an employee who missed nine Mondays in a row would have nine absence frequency periods as well as nine total days absent. In contrast, a person who missed nine consecutive days of work would have nine total days lost but only one absence frequency period. Intuitively, it seems likely that the first individual was much more prone to being absent voluntarily than the second.

Although there are many models of attendance/absenteeism behavior, a revised version of one developed by Rhodes and Steers (1990) is the basis of discussion in this chapter. According to this model (Figure 23-1), an employee's attendance at work is largely a function of two variables: the individual's ability to attend and motivation to attend.

MEDIALINK   Combating Absenteeism

KEY TERMS

Voluntary absenteeism   Absenteeism that is under the employee's control.

Involuntary absenteeism   Absenteeism that is not under the employee's control.

Total time lost   The number of scheduled days an employee misses.

Absence frequency   The total number of distinct absence periods, regardless of their duration.

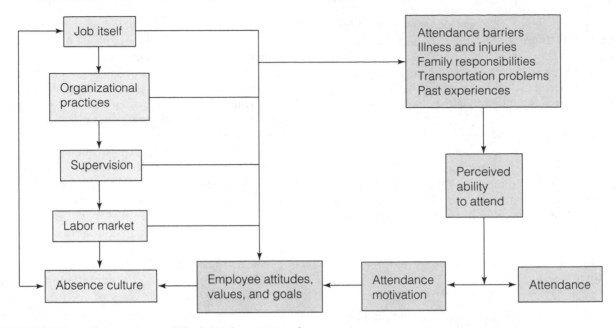

Figure 23-1 **A diagnostic model of employee attendance.**

As seen in Figure 23-1, an employee's ability to attend can be affected by such **attendance barriers** as

1. Personal illness or injury,
2. Family responsibilities (e.g., a sick child), or
3. Transportation problems (e.g., an unreliable automobile).

Although it is natural for a manager to view such barriers as resulting in involuntary absenteeism, sometimes this is too simplistic a judgment. For example, an employee whose car was not running may consciously have not made alternative arrangements to get to work the next day because he or she was not motivated to attend. This example illustrates that some of the distinctions portrayed in Figure 23-1 are not always clearcut. In trying to understand employee absenteeism, a manager will have to make assumptions about why the behavior is occurring (e.g., a manager cannot be certain that a person was actually ill).

According to the attendance model, an employee's motivation to attend is affected by several factors: the job itself, organizational practices, the absence culture, supervision, the labor market, and the employee's personal characteristics.

The Job Itself In assessing the job itself, employees holding more enriched jobs are less likely to be absent than those with more mundane jobs. Enriched jobs

may increase attendance motivation because employees believe that what they are doing is important and because they know that other employees are depending on the job holder (i.e., if the job holder doesn't do his or her job, other employees can't do theirs).

The nature of a job influences attendance through its effect on attendance motivation as well as on illness and injuries (i.e., attendance barriers). For example, a job that requires heavy lifting (e.g., moving patients from beds to stretchers) may increase the likelihood that a staff nurse will be injured. Similarly, a job that exposes a nurse to individuals with highly contagious conditions, such as in an outpatient clinic, may increase the likelihood of illness.

Organizational Practices As portrayed in Figure 23-1, organizational practices also can influence attendance motivation. Some health care organizations have absence control policies that reward employees for good attendance and/or punish them for excessive absenteeism. An organization also may be able to increase attendance motivation by carefully recruiting and selecting employees (see Chapter 18). In addition to affecting attendance motivation, organizational practices may influence an employee's ability to attend. Organizational activities, such as offering wellness programs, employee assistance programs, van pools, on-site child care, or coordinating car pools could influence an employee's ability to attend work.

Absence Culture The **absence culture** of a work unit (or an organization) can also influence employee attendance motivation. Some work units have an absence culture that reflects a tolerance for excessive absenteeism. Other units have a culture in which being absent is frowned upon. Although an organization's absence culture can be affected by organizational practices (e.g., attendance policies) and the nature of the jobs involved (e.g., people in higher-level jobs tend to be less accepting of co-workers calling in sick), it is also affected by informal norms that develop among work-group members. For example, people in a cohesive work group may develop an understanding that missing work, except for an emergency or a serious illness, is unacceptable. Such an attendance culture is likely to emerge if the employees work in jobs that they see as important (e.g., providing direct patient care) and if an employee being absent causes a hardship for co-workers (e.g., forced overtime, being called in on a day off).

Supervision Supervision also influences attendance motivation. A nurse manager can influence the nature of a staff nurse's job (e.g., the degree of responsibility given and participation in decision making), decisions about personnel, the consistency with which organizational practices are applied (e.g., whether sanctions are enforced for abuse of sick leave), and a work unit's absence culture by stressing the importance of good attendance.

Labor Market Another factor that influences attendance is the labor market. To the extent that the local employment market for nurses leads an employee to perceive it would be easy to find an equivalent job if she or he lost or disliked the current one, one would expect a lower level of attendance motivation than if market conditions were less favorable. This might happen during a nursing shortage.

Personal Characteristics Although features of the job itself, organizational practices, absence culture, supervision, and the labor market can all have a direct effect on employee attendance motivation, these factors also can interact with an employee's attitudes (e.g., job satisfaction), values (e.g., personal work ethic), or goals (e.g., desire to get promoted). If a person who seeks variety works in a job that does not provide it, the employee may become dissatisfied and thus more likely to abuse sick leave. Employee attitudes, values, and goals also can have a direct effect on attendance motivation. For example, a staff nurse with a high personal work ethic or who has a goal of getting promoted

should be more highly motivated to attend work than a nurse who lacks such a work ethic.

An employee's attendance behavior also is influenced by past experiences. For example, if an employee's perfect attendance in the previous year was not rewarded, we might expect the employee's attendance motivation to decrease in the coming year. Conversely, if a co-worker with an outstanding attendance record received a promotion, peers who value a promotion and who witnessed this linkage between performance and reward would be more motivated to attend work in the upcoming year.

Managing Employee Absenteeism

The attendance model in Figure 23-1 is useful not only for understanding why absenteeism occurs, but also for developing strategies to control it. Some causes of absenteeism, such as transportation difficulties or child care problems, may be beyond the direct control of nurse managers. The manager, however, should try to do what is possible, either in interactions with staff nurses or by attempting to get the organization to change policies that may be interfering with a nurse's ability or motivation to attend work. On the other hand, a manager must be careful that the steps taken do not go so far as to discourage the legitimate use of sick leave. Clearly, one does not want sick nurses coming to work and exposing patients and co-workers.

To diagnose the key factors leading to absenteeism, the manager needs information from several sources, including staff, the human resources department, other nurse managers, and administration. Absence patterns can answer such questions as

1. Is absenteeism equally distributed across staff nurses?
2. In comparison to other units, does your area of responsibility have a high absenteeism rate?
3. Are most absences of short or long duration?
4. Does the absenteeism have a consistent pattern (e.g., occur predominantly on weekends or shortly before a person quits)?

KEY TERMS

Attendance barriers The events that affect an employee's ability to attend (e.g., illness, family responsibilities).

Absence culture The informal norms within a work unit that determine how employees of that unit view absenteeism.

Although a manager may not be able to do much to affect the staff's ability to attend, the organization can take several actions. For example, to lessen child care problems, the organization could set up or sponsor a child care center. To reduce transportation problems, an organization could provide shuttle buses or coordinate car pools. Health fairs, exercise programs, and stress-reduction classes could be offered to promote health. Given that alcoholism and drug abuse are widely recognized as important causes of absenteeism, it may be prudent for an organization to offer access to an employee assistance plan. In addition to these organizational actions, a nurse manager, through coaching, may be able to influence a staff nurse's attendance. (See Chapter 21 for information on how to coach staff.)

Clearly, the best way for nurse managers to control absenteeism is by encouraging their staff's motivation to attend. Other absenteeism management strategies that a nurse manager might consider include

- Enriching the staff nurse's job by increasing its responsibility, variety, or challenge;
- Reducing job stress (e.g., by providing more timely and more concrete information);
- Creating a norm of excellent attendance (e.g., by emphasizing the negative impact of a nurse not coming to work);
- Enhancing advancement opportunities (e.g., by providing developmental experiences so that the best employees are promotable);
- Improving co-worker relations (e.g., by considering co-worker compatibility when scheduling work and/or creating work teams);
- Trying to select employees who will be satisfied with and committed to their jobs;
- Being a good role model by rarely taking sick days;
- Discussing the employee's attendance during the performance appraisal interview;
- Rewarding good attendance with salary increases and other rewards; and
- Enforcing absenteeism control policies (e.g., carrying through on employee discipline when there is an attendance problem).

Absenteeism Policies

Most organizational policies allow employees to accrue paid sick days—typically, 1 sick day for every month employed. Unused sick days accrue across time to some maximum number (e.g., 60 days). Typically, if an employee leaves the organization with accumulated sick leave or days above the maximum, the person simply loses it.

Although such a policy may seem reasonable, it may actually encourage unwanted behavior. For example, once a nurse has reached the maximum limit for accrued sick days, the person may see no reason for not using sick days that would otherwise be lost. Such a policy also encourages employees who know they will be leaving the organization (e.g., those about to retire or change jobs) to use accumulated sick leave.

An innovative approach for managing absenteeism is substituting personal days for unused sick days. Two problems arise if personal days are not given: Employees are forced to lie (i.e., say they are sick when they are not) to carry out what they see as legitimate activities (e.g., attending a conference with their child's teacher), and their manager has no warning and therefore may have difficulty covering for the absent employee.

By substituting personal days for sick days, the employee no longer has to lie, and the nurse manager may have time to plan for a replacement. In moving to a policy that incorporates the use of personal days, an organization typically allocates fewer paid sick days but adds personal days. For example, instead of 12 sick days, an employee may annually receive 9 sick days and 3 personal days. With the availability of personal days, a staff nurse can inform the nurse manager in advance of the need for a personal day off. In many cases, the two of them can arrive at a day off that is optimal for both of them.

Realizing that they have not been motivating good attendance, some progressive organizations have allowed sick days to accumulate without an upper limit. Then, when an employee leaves the organization, she or he is paid for unused sick days (e.g., one-half day's pay for each unused sick day). Other organizations allow retiring employees to add unused sick days to days worked. Still other organizations have paid employees for their sick days, allowed the conversion of sick days to vacation days or additional pay. Although uncommon, a few organizations have experimented with special financial incentives such as cash bonuses or other prizes as a reward for good attendance. Taunton and colleagues (1995) found low absence among staff nurses in a hospital with

1. Incentives for attendance (an extra earned holiday for perfect attendance for 6 months),
2. Deterrents for absence (no pay for first day of an absence episode), and
3. Clearly established policy with progressive discipline for infractions.

Obviously, changing an organization's paid sick leave policy is beyond the control of the nurse manager. However, a concerted effort by an organized group of nurse managers can be effective in getting the human resources department and the administration to initiate such changes. Considering the high costs of absenteeism, these changes can be quite cost effective.

Most health care organizations have formal policies concerning how much absenteeism is allowed. Once this limit is reached, disciplinary steps are prescribed. In disciplining an employee, the nurse manager must follow the discipline policy carefully. The effectiveness of discipline as a strategy for reducing absenteeism is limited. Most discipline policies only take effect after excessive absenteeism. Not surprisingly, most employees know what this is and are careful not to exceed it. In effect, the nurse manager is left with an absenteeism problem but not one that she or he is able to address through the use of discipline.

A Systems Perspective

Many of the managerial actions addressed in other chapters of this book are relevant to the control of absenteeism. For example, in recruiting employees, the use of a realistic job preview should increase the congruence between job characteristics and employee values and expectations. Similarly, basing merit pay and advancement opportunities on an employee's overall performance appraisal rating (which is partly based on attendance) will motivate better attendance. Also, leadership skills are important in getting the organization to change policy to lessen absenteeism (e.g., providing payment for unused sick days).

Two specific issues are relevant to employee selection: the use of personal characteristics and past behavior. Although personal characteristics (e.g., marital status, child care responsibility) have been linked to higher absenteeism rates, for legal reasons a nurse manager should not base a hiring decision on such personal characteristics. On the one hand, it is difficult to argue that every person within a category (e.g., married females with children) is likely to be prone to absenteeism.

On the other hand, the past behavior of a specific job candidate is potentially valuable information because absenteeism tendencies tend to be consistent from job to job (Breaugh, 1981). Although the reasons why some individuals have a higher level of absenteeism year after year are unclear (e.g., some people may be more susceptible to illness, others may have less of a work ethic), past behavior can be used as a predictor of future behavior. An applicant's previous absenteeism record may be acquired by written or telephone reference checks.

In a practical sense, nurse managers want strategies for dealing with employees with excessive absences. Several steps can be taken.

1. Set expectations with each new employee. Give her or him the attendance policy in writing, and clarify any questions.
2. Monitor each individual's attendance, and document it.
3. Intervene early and consistently, coaching and dealing with policy or procedure violations as appropriate.
4. If discipline is called for, use the key behaviors for disciplining in Chapter 21.
5. Be sure to reward staff who have good attendance. Ensure that any organizational rewards are delivered, and give your personal reward through feedback in performance appraisals.
6. Be a role model for good attendance yourself.

These steps will set a tone of intolerance for poor attendance.

Family and Medical Leave

The federal **Family and Medical Leave Act** (FMLA) took effect in 1993 and has a significant impact on employers. Under this act, all public employers (federal, state, and local) and all private employers employing 50 or more individuals must provide their eligible employees with leave of up to 12 weeks during any 12-month period for the employee's own serious illness, the birth or adoption of a child, the placement of a foster child into the household, or the care of a seriously ill child, spouse, or parent.

The FMLA also allows eligible employees to maintain health insurance coverage while on leave and allows them to return to the same or equivalent position at the

 MEDIALINK U.S. Bureau of Labor Statistics

KEY TERMS

Family and Medical Leave Act A federal law stating that employers must provide employees with leave when serious illness or family issues arise, while maintaining insurance and an equal position within the organization.

end of the leave period. The leave may be taken all at once, periodically (if the employer agrees) or by working part-time, such as after the birth of a child. The employee must be allowed to take leave for qualified purposes without pressure or discouragement by the employer or manager. More generous collective-bargaining agreements or state laws supersede the FMLA, but the FMLA supersedes any inconsistent or less generous provisions.

Employees are eligible to take leave if they

• Have worked for the employer for at least 12 months;
• Have worked at least 1,250 hours during the previous 12 months; and
• Are at a work site with 50 or more employees, or at a site where 50 workers are employed within 75 miles of the work site (50 employees/75 miles rule).

The FMLA is quite complex. Managers must be aware of multiple employee and employer responsibilities. State law and collective-bargaining agreements may make the organization's leave policy unique. Furthermore, the overlap and interaction between the Americans with Disabilities Act and the FMLA is complicated and largely unaddressed by federal regulation at this point. Only a fraction of the FMLA leave is disability related. It is important for the manager to work closely with the human resources department in executing the provisions of this law.

Employees with Problems

Overachievers or Superachievers

Even though superachievers are exceptionally productive, are technically proficient, and account for a large part of the organization's output, they can present management problems that equal or exceed their productivity.

Russell (1989) classified these superachiever nurses as the Bull or A-Bomb, the Killer Angel, or the Know-It-All. Bulls or A-Bombs, the most common type, are grouped together because the individual may show both characteristics. Bulls believe that their ideas, ways of doing things, and beliefs are the only way. Their main weapon is abusive, intimidating, and overwhelming behavior. The A-Bomb displays tantrum-like behaviors as a substitute for the direct attack. The tantrums can be physically dangerous. Strategies for managing Bulls and A-Bombs are as follows:

1. Let them run their course if no physical danger is involved. Give them time to cool off.

2. Present your position, which will require standing up to them. You may need to raise your voice to get their attention.
3. Do not argue, but continue to state your view firmly.
4. Outside of these confrontations, ask them for advice.
5. You will not change their behavior by yourself; professional help may be needed.

Killer Angels achieve their goals by digs and cutting remarks. Killer Angels feel the need to be right at the expense of others and take deliberate efforts to make other employees look less competent. They have a need to appear superior to all around them. Management strategies are as follows:

1. Confront the employee directly with the behavior. Confrontation lets the person know you know what she or he is doing.
2. Provide Killer Angels with a forum in which they can air their views, such as problem-solving meetings. Always set ground rules in these meetings, and do not let the Killer Angel dominate.
3. Seek the Killer Angel's advice.

The Know-It-All truly is an expert and wants everyone to know this. The Know-It-All is the least dangerous superachiever. He or she wants to be admired and thus gives advice on anything and everything. The best strategy is to mentally filter out the expert advice. However, if the Know-It-All causes problems with co-workers, confront the behavior in private. Coaching techniques often work with these employees.

In spite of the problems they pose to the manager and co-workers, superachievers are your best technical nurses. Carefully examine your strategy with each individual and seek appropriate help as needed.

Disgruntled Employees

Disgruntled employees are ones who are always complaining, behavior that affects morale on the unit. They complain about anything and everything, but they direct most complaints against the organization and may air them in public, which can affect how others view the organization. Although the temptation is to label this as an attitude problem, complaining is a behavior and as such can be addressed by the following:

1. Remember to set standards of performance and communicate them to the employee.

2. Keep notes about incidents of complaining in behavioral terms.
3. Take action early, and be consistent among employees.
4. Use key behaviors for coaching found in Chapter 21.
5. Follow up as scheduled.

Overstressed Employees

Stress, burnout, and lack of time management are major concerns in the nursing profession. Nurses daily confront pain, grief, dying, and death. In addition, they must often deal with the stress of having inadequate staff to care for high-acuity patients. Chapter 15 includes a model of stress and specific strategies for time management and stress reduction.

The Employee with a Substance Abuse Problem

As substance abuse has become increasingly prevalent in society, nursing has not remained immune. Substance abuse not only is detrimental to the impaired nurse, but also jeopardizes patients' care, thereby also exposing the employing agency to greater liability.

Early recognition of alcohol or drug dependency and prompt referral for treatment are generally recognized as responsibilities of the nurse manager, although the role of the nurse manager varies according to organizational policy.

Identifying the Employee with a Substance Abuse Problem   It is not easy to identify anyone who is abusing substances. The primary symptom is denial, which is present in the sufferer as well as in those around him or her. The person in denial really does not believe what seems obvious. Furthermore, alcohol or drug problems in women in general, as well as in nurses in particular, are stigmatized in today's society. This stigma, added to the profession's own negative attitudes regarding the disorder, encourages nurses—even those who break through their own denial—to continue to conceal their problem. The result is that nurses dependent on alcohol or drugs may continue practicing nursing, endangering both patients' and their own lives. Before obvious serious consequences take place, some general signs and symptoms may become evident as a nurse's dependency progresses (Boxes 23-1 and 23-2).

In addition to the signs and symptoms listed in Boxes 23-1 and 23-2, the nurse manager should be alert for frequently incorrect narcotics counts, alteration of narcotics vials, patient reports that their pain medications are ineffective, inaccurate recording of pain medication administration, discrepancies in narcotics records, large amounts of narcotic wastage, and marked shift variations in the quantity of drugs required on a unit.

If the manager discovers signs or symptoms in an employee or becomes aware of the unit changes described, further investigation is warranted, and administration should be informed. Often, with unit discrepancies, that simply means checking the schedule to see who was working when most of the errors occurred. Usually, one or two people emerge as those most likely to have been available during the time of the discrepancies. Further checking and observation may reveal individual behaviors suggesting a person has a substance abuse problem.

Box 23-1   Signs of Alcohol or Drug Dependency

- Family history of alcoholism or drug abuse
- Frequent change of work site (same or other institution)
- Prior medical history requiring pain control
- Conscientious worker with recent decrease in performance
- Decreased attention to personal appearance
- Frequent complaints of marital and family problems
- Reports of illness, minor accidents, and emergencies

- Complaints from co-workers
- Mood swings/depression/suicide attempts
- Strong interest in patients' pain control
- Frequent trips to the bathroom
- Increasing isolation (night shift request; eating alone)
- Elaborate excuses for tardiness
- Difficulty in meeting schedules/deadlines
- Inadequate explanation for missing work

From: Chemical Dependency in Nursing: The Deadly Diversion, by E. J. Sullivan, L. Bissell, and E. Williams, 1988, Menlo Park, CA: Addison-Wesley Nursing. Reprinted by permission of Pearson Education, Inc., Upper Saddle River, NJ.

> **Box 23-2   Physical Symptoms of Alcohol or Drug Dependency**
>
> - Shakiness, tremors of hands, jitteriness
> - Slurred speech
> - Watery eyes, dilated or constricted pupils
> - Diaphoresis
> - Unsteady gait
>
> - Runny nose
> - Nausea, vomiting, diarrhea
> - Weight loss or gain
> - Blackouts (memory losses while conscious)
> - Wears long-sleeved clothing continuously

From: Chemical Dependency in Nursing: The Deadly Diversion, by E. J. Sullivan, L. Bissell, and E. Williams, 1988, Menlo Park, CA: Addison-Wesley Nursing. Reprinted by permission of Pearson Education, Inc., Upper Saddle River, NJ.

Even if the manager is unsure of her or his perceptions or if the actions are so vague that the manager has many doubts about the identity of the person, the situation will be clarified in time. Untreated, addiction continues; as tolerance increases, use will increase, and the person will become increasingly careless about covering up actions. Thus, the manager will become more certain about a person's abuse problem. However, the longer it takes to identify the problem, the longer the nurse may continue to practice, jeopardizing both patients and self. Thus, the manager should carefully assess information about possible dependency problems but not wait too long. How long is a matter of judgment for the manager and administration.

Strategies for Intervention   Once the manager has identified a nurse with a substance abuse problem, intervention with that nurse must be planned. With the assistance of a superior, the manager should examine the organization's policies and procedures and licensure laws and prepare for the intervention. Reporting laws vary from state to state, as do consequences. Diversion programs offering referral, assistance, and monitoring may be offered in lieu of disciplinary action in some states.

Before intervening, the manager should collect all documentation or information about the nurse's behavior that would suggest an abuse problem. Documentation includes records of absenteeism and tardiness (especially recent changes), records of patient complaints about ineffective medications or poor care, staff complaints about job performance, records of controlled substances, and physical signs and symptoms noticed at different times. Dates, times, and behaviors should be carefully noted. Any one behavior means very little; it is the composite pattern that identifies the problem.

Next, the manager should identify appropriate resources to help the nurse. Internal resources include an employee assistance program (EAP) counselor, if the organization has one, or other nurses recovering from alcohol or drug dependency who have offered to help. External resources include the names and phone numbers of treatment center staff, other recovering nurses (if known), and Alcoholics Anonymous or Narcotics Anonymous. It is absolutely essential that several sources be provided so that the nurse knows that help from someone who knows how he or she feels is available and how to get it. This support cannot be emphasized enough. Failing to offer this assistance is like telling the diabetic he has diabetes and failing to tell him where he can get insulin.

In addition to assistance for the nurse, the manager should check on health insurance provisions for substance abuse treatment. Many insurance carriers have recognized that successful treatment reduces the use of other health care services and, thus, reduces the cost of health care. Accordingly, they offer coverage for treatment to encourage participants to enter recovery programs. Others, unfortunately, do not. Because many of an organization's employees may be covered under the same health care plan, the manager should be able to check these provisions. If the policy does not cover inpatient care, the nurse may be able to afford outpatient care, which is considerably less expensive. So, the nurse manager should not assume treatment is unavailable even when there is little or no insurance coverage. Alcoholics Anonymous and Narcotics Anonymous are effective alternatives, and both are free.

Before initiating the intervention, the manager must examine his or her own attitudes about the abuse problem. Probably, the drug or alcohol abuse has gone on for some time, and both the manager and the staff may have lost patience with the person whose performance and attendance may have forced others to do more than their fair share of the work. If substance abuse was suspected, others may have felt that the person should just "pull herself together," "stop doing it," and, as a last resort, should "know better." Once they understand that alcohol or drug dependency is an illness, however, they realize that none of these behaviors are possible; willpower and education have not prevented others from becoming addicted. The manager will need to deal with the staff's feelings later, but at this time it is enough to be certain that his or her own attitudes will not imperil the intervention. It is important that the message be clearly one of help and hope.

The goal of the intervention is to get the nurse to an appropriate place for an evaluation of the possible problem. Treatment centers or therapists who specialize in substance abuse are recommended to conduct the evaluation. They have the necessary experience for diagnosing and, if indicated, treating the disease.

The manager must also decide beforehand what action on the part of the nurse will be acceptable. If the nurse refuses to go for an evaluation, what will be the consequences? The organization's policies and the state board of nursing regulations must be met, and the manager must be clear about the consequences (e.g., discipline, termination) and willing to carry them out. Most experts in treating addictions in nurses recommend that the nurse be offered the option of substance abuse evaluation and, if needed, treatment. If she or he does not agree to that, then the manager should follow the usual disciplinary process and make a report to the state board of nursing, if indicated.

Once preparations have been made, the intervention should be scheduled as soon as possible. Others may be asked to join the manager, but the group should be small and restricted to only those involved in past problems, a substance abuse or human resource staff person, or the manager's supervisor. In some organizations, the top nursing administrator conducts all substance abuse interventions and, in that case, the nurse manager must fully inform the administrator of all circumstances leading to the intervention and provide all the documentation needed. Also, the manager should participate in the intervention so that all relevant information is presented and denial is kept to a minimum.

The intervention should be scheduled at a time and place when interruptions can be avoided. It is best to surprise the nurse with a request to come to the office. Denial can build, rationalizations can be developed, and defensiveness can increase if the nurse is given time to consider the problem.

The manager should present the nurse with the collected evidence showing a pattern of behaviors that suggests an abuse problem might be occurring and that an evaluation must be undertaken to know for sure. It is important to focus on the problem behaviors, not on the inadequacy of the person. The individual has already experienced shame and guilt about the use. The manager has an opportunity to help the nurse recognize that substance abuse is an illness that needs treatment; then the nurse will be better able to accept that a problem exists.

In the best-case scenario, the nurse admits the problem, is grateful to be getting help, and goes willingly to treatment. It is best to go directly to treatment from the work site if this can be arranged beforehand. It is important to move quickly before denial resurfaces.

Some nurses, of course, will continue to deny the obvious, in which case the manager must continue to confront the nurse with the reality of the circumstances. If the nurse refuses to go for an evaluation, the manager must follow the organization's disciplinary process. If the nurse is using alcohol or drugs at the time, immediate removal from patient care is necessary. The manager should arrange to have someone (either a family member or another staff member) drive the nurse home, whether the nurse is going to treatment or not. Not only do alcohol or drugs make the nurse an unsafe driver, but the stress of the intervention may distract the nurse even more.

If the nurse agrees to go for an evaluation and/or treatment, specific plans must be made. It should be clear to all parties when the nurse will contact the treatment center (the sooner the better, even if mood-altering chemicals are not being used at the time) and when the nurse will report back to the manager the recommended course of action. It is possible to arrange with a treatment facility for reports to be made directly to the manager, but federal regulations regarding confidentiality prohibit treatment staff from reporting a patient's status to anyone without that person's written consent. Because the goal of treatment is recovery, which includes returning to work, most facilities request that the nurse give this consent.

Treatment As with other forms of medical treatment, treatment for substance abuse has moved from the inpatient to the outpatient setting. Whereas a few years ago a patient could be expected to be admitted to a month-long hospitalization for substance abuse, today treatment is offered in several different formats along a continuum of care. These include

1. Inpatient treatment for detoxification (3 to 5 days),
2. Partial hospitalization (day treatment for 1 to 2 weeks),

3. Intensive outpatient treatment (e.g., 3 nights a week for 3 hours each night),
4. Traditional outpatient treatment (e.g., 4 hours a week, including some group therapy and one-to-one sessions), and
5. Weekly aftercare group sessions for 3 months.

The choices of treatments and their order ideally are based on the patient's status, environmental supports, and potential for relapse. Unfortunately, the decision is usually based on insurance coverage, which varies considerably among insurers.

The decision to allow an employee to return to work or even to require the employee to avoid returning for any period of time will be based on the recommended treatment. Withdrawal from narcotics very likely will require inpatient detoxification; partial hospitalization also may be recommended. If the employee needs time off for these treatments, sick leave can be used, or the employee may be given an unpaid leave of absence (see the section on the Americans with Disabilities Act and substance abuse).

Reentry Reentry to the workplace must be carefully planned, whether the employee has been absent for any length of time or not. It is especially important for the manager and administration to recognize the threat that access to the category of drugs the nurse was addicted to (e.g., narcotics) poses to recovery. Return to work is usually recommended, but not all treatment staff are familiar enough with nursing to be aware of the danger of putting the nurse in constant, daily contact with the drugs that may have been abused in the past. However, it is vitally important to the nurse's recovery that he or she return to work, preferably in the same setting.

This dilemma has often been dealt with in two ways. One method is to reassign the nurse for a period of time (possibly as long as 2 years) to a job or a unit where few mood-altering drugs are given, such as the nursery, department of education, rehabilitation, home care, or patient care audits. Although reassignment presents a problem for the organization and may be disappointing to the nurse, it is far better to make this accommodation than to jeopardize the nurse's recovery by providing access to drugs too soon. This is less a concern with nurses who abused only alcohol.

Another method is to retain the nurse on the unit but not allow administration of mood-altering medications. In fact, state law or organizational policy may require that recovering nurses in the early post-treatment period be restricted from handling controlled substances, carrying narcotic keys, being in charge, or working overtime. This method requires that other staff not only know about the nurse's problem but also be willing to give pain and sleep medications to that nurse's patients. Because this involves disclosing the nurse's addiction, management and staff must decide whether this is reasonable, and the nurse must agree.

Recovering nurses may be discouraged from working evening or night shifts. A reentry contract may be used to specify these restrictions. The contract also may require documentation of participation in recovery groups and random urine drug tests. Ideally, the reentering nurse should have an identified support person available at work.

These restrictions are usually necessary only for the nurse who was addicted to narcotics, but each case should be individually decided based on the amount of stress in the job, the need for rotating shifts, and other factors that may inhibit recovery.

Health care today requires that every employee function at peak efficiency and effectiveness. Health care organizations cannot afford to protect an employee whose professional functioning is impaired by substance abuse. Discharging the employee and allowing the person to go to another institution to continue practicing and endangering patients, as well as himself or herself, cannot be allowed. The nurse manager is the front-line contact with staff. He or she can be alert to the signs and symptoms of substance abuse problems, learn intervention techniques and skills, and help recovering nurses return to the workplace. Concern for patients' safety requires intervention, and humane concern for nurse colleagues mandates that such assistance be made available.

The Americans with Disabilities Act and Substance Abuse The Americans with Disabilities Act (ADA) went into effect in 1990 and applies to employers of 15 or more people. This law prohibits discrimination in personnel policies (such as hiring and firing) and other employment-related issues if an individual has a qualifying disability. Because alcohol or drug dependency limits one or more of the nurse's activities (see Chapters 5 and 18), it is considered a disability under the ADA. Only those who have been identified with substance abuse disorders, either diagnosed or self-reported, are protected under the law. A person using drugs or who is under the influence of alcohol in the workplace is not protected from the job-related consequences of that use.

The same consideration must be given to the nurse addict as to a nurse with a hearing impairment. This means providing sick leave and treatment opportunity, as well as making reasonable job accommodations. Several reasonable job accommodations have been mentioned previously: assignment to a unit where narcotics and sedatives are not given or are given infrequently, exemption from shift rotation, exemption from charge duties, and the like. Furthermore, the employee's drug abuse history must be kept private. The ADA confidentiality provisions require the employer to keep records on employee substance abuse (i.e., disability) in separate, locked files with access limited to a need-to-know basis.

As with other chronic diseases, alcohol and drug dependency is a disorder prone to relapse. How relapses will be treated under this law is not clear. As with many other personnel issues, it is wise for the nurse manager to consult with human resources and administration about ADA requirements.

Managers are faced with any number of other problems presented by employees. Case Study 23-1 describes one manager's experience with an employee.

CASE STUDY 23-1: Problem Staff

Gene Marshall is the nurse manager for a general medical–surgical unit in a veteran's hospital. His busy unit primarily serves elderly male patients. Felicia Ralston, RN, has worked on the medical–surgical unit for 3 years. Since her hiring, Felicia has obtained several body piercings, including her nose, eyebrow, and tongue. She usually wears large hoops or bars in her facial piercings. Felicia added a visible tattoo to the back of her neck and upper shoulder. Often her uniforms allow visualization of a tattoo on her lower back. Recently, she came to work after adding purple highlights to her hair.

As the number and prominence of Felicia's piercings and body art have increased, several patients and their family members expressed to Gene that they were "uncomfortable" having Felicia as their nurse. Some patients have felt intimidated by her unusual appearance. Gene spoke with Felicia about the patient and family member concerns and reviewed the hospital's dress code with her. Felicia became angry and told Gene that hair color, body piercings, and tattoos were a form of individual expression and had nothing to do with her performance as a nurse.

Later, Felicia told everyone on the unit about her discussion with Gene, speaking loudly and inappropriately in patient care areas. She asked the unit clerk if she knew which patients or family members had complained to Gene about her appearance. The following day, Felicia asked each of her assigned patients if they had a "problem with her." Felicia reported back to Gene that none of her patients expressed they had any problems with her or her appearance. After discussing the situation with the human resources department, Gene met with Felicia and provided her with a written warning regarding her body piercings, tattoos, and hair color, as well as her unprofessional behavior following their initial meeting. Gene told Felicia that she must remove jewelry from her nose and eyebrows prior to reporting for work and her hair color must be a natural color. He also told her that her tongue jewelry must be small and unnoticeable. Felicia's uniforms were to cover her tattoos completely.

Gene also provided Felicia with a copy of the federal court ruling in which the Court ruled that body piercings and tattoos were not considered protected as free speech and employers had the right to set standards of dress and appearance for their employees. Finally, Gene emphasized to Felicia that she should directly speak with him regarding any performance issues or problems and not involve staff or patients in the situation. If Felicia does not comply with these standards within 10 working days, she will be terminated from her position.

Manager's Checklist
The nurse manager is responsible for

- Understanding the human resource policies for their organization,
- Consistently applying policies to all employees,
- Providing timely and appropriate feedback when an employee is in violation of policies,
- Remaining professional at all times when dealing with an irate or angry employee,
- Maintaining accurate and thorough documentation of performance issues, and
- Following up with the human resources department as necessary.

Workplace Violence

Health care workers face a wide range of hazards on the job, including needlestick injuries, back injuries, latex allergy, stress, and violence. All are serious and efforts should be made to prevent accidents and injuries. Workplace violence is the focus of this discussion.

According to the U.S. Bureau of Labor Statistics, 44 percent of all workplace assaults and 8 percent of homicides occur in health care settings (Gray, Myers, & Myers, 1999). The U.S. Department of Labor (2003) reports, however, that workplace homicides were down about 5 percent in 2002 from the previous year and 44 percent from the highest recorded number of workplace homicides in 1994. Violence in health care is more likely to occur in psychiatric settings, emergency rooms, waiting rooms, and geriatric units (National Institute for Occupational Safety and Health [NIOSH], 2002).

By definition, **workplace violence** is any violent act, including physical assaults and threats of assault, directed toward persons at work or on duty. Most assaults are by patients, but assaults are also made by disgruntled family members, co-workers, employers, or employees. Some assaults are episodes of domestic violence that occur at work. Violence can range in intensity and cause physical injuries, temporary or permanent disability, psychological trauma, or death.

Violence in the workplace can affect worker morale, stress, absenteeism, turnover, mistrust of administration, and hostility (NIOSH, 2002). Although no workplace can be certain to be free from violence, some risk factors for potential violence in health care organizations are

- People under the influence of alcohol or drugs,
- Working understaffed, especially at meal times and visiting hours,
- Long waiting times,
- Overcrowded waiting rooms,
- Working alone,
- Unlimited public access, and
- Poorly lit corridors, rooms, and parking lots (NIOSH, 2002).

Preventing Violence

Signs of Potential Violence Everyone should learn how to watch for threatening behaviors to evaluate when a person is likely to become violent. Law enforcement personnel recommend watching for these behaviors:

- Clenched fists
- Blank stare

- Fighting stance (one foot back with arm pulled back ready to strike)
- Arms raised in a fighting position
- Standing too close or advancing toward you
- Holding anything that might be used as a weapon, such as a pen, letter opener, heavy object, or any actual weapon—a gun or knife
- Overt intent (say that they intend to "kick your—" or similar statements)
- Movement toward the exit to prevent you from leaving (Sullivan, 2004)

Policies to Prevent Violence The health care organization must set its violence prevention policies at zero tolerance. Appropriate personnel policies must state clearly what will happen if violence or the threat of using violence occurs. Policies regarding patients and visitors must do the same. Specifically, anyone who becomes violent or threatens to must be removed from the setting and authorities contacted.

Questions to ask when developing policies regarding violence prevention are shown in Box 23-3.

Ensuring Safety

A manager should make an effort to identify potential sources of violence and take whatever steps necessary to ensure employee safety. This includes

1. Assessing and reporting threats;
2. Supplying adequate staffing;
3. Providing training about recognizing potential assailants or agitators, conflict resolution, and deescalation tactics;
4. Instituting environmental controls (adequate lighting, security devices, bullet-resistant barriers in the emergency department, etc.);
5. Implementing safe work practices, such as
   a. Escort services;
   b. Judicious use of restraints or seclusion;
   c. Alerting staff about patients with histories of violent behavior, dementia, or intoxication; and

---

KEY TERMS

Workplace violence Any violent act, including physical assaults and threats of assault, directed toward persons at work or on duty.

Box 23-3   Preventing Violence: Questions to Ask

- Does your facility have a clear reporting procedure in the event that there's a workplace aggression incident?
- Whom does the staff inform of its concerns?
- What are the repercussions should individuals report an incident that makes them uneasy?

- Does your facility offer a mental health support program for staff? Is it effective in helping to reduce employee stress?
- When someone voices a concern to supervisory staff, is action taken to address the problem quickly?

From: "Escalating Workplace Aggression," by J. C. DelBel, 2003, *Nursing Management, 34*(9), pp. 30–34.

d. Not wearing health instruments (stethoscopes, hemostats, scissors) that could be used as weapons;

6. Teaching staff to watch for threatening behaviors.

What You Know Now

- Employee attendance is affected by the job, organizational practices, supervision, absence culture, labor market, and the employee's characteristics.

- An organization can improve employee attendance by addressing specific barriers, such as adding a child care center, coordinating car pools, or offering health promotion and employee assistance.

- Innovative solutions to absenteeism problems include substituting personal days for sick days, allowing sick days to accrue and unused days to be paid to the employee, or converting unused sick days to paid days at retirement.

- The behaviors of employees who are overachievers, are disgruntled, are overstressed, abuse substances, or are frequently absent affect work-group functioning.

- Nurse managers need to identify staff problems early and intervene if necessary.

- Identifying, intervening, and returning nurses with substance abuse problems to the workplace help the organization, the manager, and the affected nurse.

- Substance abuse not only is detrimental to the impaired nurse but also jeopardizes patient care and places the organization at increased liability.

- Risk factors for violence include drug and alcohol abuse, understaffing, long waiting times, overcrowded waiting rooms, and working alone.

- An effort should be made to identify potential sources of violence in the workplace and steps should be taken to ensure employee safety.

Tools for Managing Absenteeism and Other Staff Problems

1. Become familiar with signs and symptoms of potential problems.

2. Learn the steps of confrontation to intervene before problems escalate (see Chapter 21).

3. Identify risk factors for violence and alert staff and administration to these threats.

4. Initiate actions to prevent workplace violence.

5. Educate staff on maintaining safety in the workplace.

Questions to Challenge You

1. Have you ever worked or shared a class with a person who caused problems? (Most of us have.) How did the problem manifest itself? How was it handled? How do you wish the problem had been handled?

2. Are you familiar with the signs and symptoms of substance abuse? Have you seen someone exhibit these characteristics? What signs or symptoms did they exhibit? What happened?

3. For what reasons have you been absent from work or class?

4. As a nurse manager, what would you do to reduce absenteeism?

5. Evaluate your current workplace or clinical site. See if you can find potential opportunities that would allow violence to occur. Describe them.

6. What has your workplace or clinical site done to protect staff from violence? What more could you suggest?

Explore 🌐 MediaLink

NCLEX review questions, essay activities, group activities, and other interactive resources for this chapter can be found on the Web site at http://www.prenhall.com/

sullivan-decker. Click on "Chapter 23" to select activities for this chapter.

References

Breaugh, J. A. (1981). Predicting absenteeism from prior absenteeism and work attitudes. *Journal of Applied Psychology, 66,* 555–560.

Gray, G. R., Myers, D. W., & Myers, P. S. (1999). Workplace violence provision in private sector collective bargaining agreements. *Compensation and Working Conditions,* U.S. Bureau of Labor Statistics.

National Institute for Occupational Safety and Health. (2002). *Violence: Occupational hazards in hospitals.* Washington, DC: Author.

Rhodes, S., & Steers, R. (1990). *Managing employee absenteeism.* Reading, MA: Addison-Wesley.

Russell, L. N. (1989). Managing the "super-achiever" nurse. *Nursing Management, 20*(2), 38–39.

Sullivan, E. J. (2004). *Becoming influential: A guide for nurses.* Upper Saddle River, NJ: Prentice Hall.

Sullivan, E. J., Bissell, L., & Williams, E. (1988). *Chemical dependency in nursing: The deadly diversion.* Menlo Park, CA: Addison-Wesley.

Tawnton, R. L., Hope, K., Woods, C., & Bott, M. J. (1995). Predictors of absenteeism among hospital staff nurses. *Nursing Economic$, 13,* 217–219.

U. S. Bureau of Labor Statistics. (2003). *Most frequent types of work-related fatalities in 2002.* Washington, DC: Author.

Handling Collective-Bargaining Issues

Process of Unionization

Selecting a Bargaining Agent
Certifying the Contract
Administering the Contract
Decertifying the Contract
The Nurse Manager's Role
The Grievance Process

Collective Bargaining for Nurses

The Role of Professional
   Associations
Future of Collective Bargaining

Looking Ahead

What position do you take on the issue of collective bargaining? It is, after all, one of the most controversial issues facing nurses. The process of unionization, as well as issues in collective bargaining that are specific to nurses, are included in this chapter.

Objectives

In this chapter, you will learn

- What is involved in forming a union.
- How a contract is administered.
- What the nurse manager's role is.
- What is involved in the grievance process.
- How nurses are involved in collective bargaining.
- What roles professional associations play in collective bargaining.

MediaLink www.prenhall.com/ sullivan-decker

Additional resources for this chapter can be found on the Companion Website at www.prenhall.com/ sullivan-decker. Click on "Chapter 24" to select the activities for this chapter.

- NCLEX Review
- Critical Thinking Activities
- Current Events
- MediaLinks
- *Nursing Leadership & Management in Action:* The American Nurses Association and Collective Bargaining; Developing a Grievance Policy and Procedure

The purpose of this chapter is to clarify labor relations involving nurses in the health care setting. Collective bargaining is controlled primarily by the federal laws pertaining to it. The processes of achieving and losing union representation in a health care setting, the nurse manager's role in collective bargaining, and issues specific to nurses are explained. In addition the chapter includes the role of the American Nurses Association in collective bargaining.

Before federal laws governing labor relations in this country were enacted, disputes between the owners or managers of a company and the company's labor force were settled by the judiciary branch of government. During this period of American history, the courts often ruled that **collective bargaining,** collective action taken by workers to secure better wages or working conditions, was illegal. Today, however, labor laws enacted by Congress and decisions by the U. S. Supreme Court, guide labor relations between employers and employees.

Dissatisfaction with working conditions and administration has been cited as contributing to nurses' propensity to form unions, and first-line managers have the most impact on employee satisfaction (Friedrich, 2001). According to a study by Bilchik (2000), hospital administrators make their organizations more likely to unionize if they make three erroneous assumptions:

1. Believe that low wages cause the most job dissatisfaction
2. Believe that supervisors understand how front-line employees think about unionizing
3. Are ineffective in communicating with employees

Regardless of the reasons, health care organizations are susceptible to unionizing efforts, and nurses and nurse managers are often involved in negotiating contracts and dealing with grievances.

Process of Unionization

Selecting a Bargaining Agent

The process of establishing a union in any setting begins with the selection of a bargaining agent certified to conduct labor negotiations for a group of individuals. This process is known as a **representation election** and is presided over by the National Labor Relations Board (NLRB). For an election to occur, the union must demonstrate that interest is shown by at least 30 percent of the employees affected by this action. In this process, the union will ask eligible employees to sign a card authorizing an election. Once the 30 percent level is reached, the union can petition the NLRB to conduct an election. The NLRB then meets with both the union and the employer. At the conclusion of this meeting the NLRB will have determined three things:

1. Who is eligible to participate in the union. This is a problematic issue and not easily resolved, because registered nurses employed as staff nurses are eligible for collective bargaining, but registered nurses employed as management are not. Registered nurses who work for an organization, but in a capacity outside the traditional nursing department, such as a clinic, home health care, or in education, may or may not be eligible for membership. This issue alone can take many days or weeks to resolve.
2. Whether the signatories are employees of the organization.
3. A date for union election.

The election is conducted by the NLRB within 45 days, using a secret ballot. All individuals eligible for representation by the union are notified of the election time and date. On election day, eligible employees are asked to choose not only whether they wish to be represented by a union but also which union they want to represent them.

Many unions represent RNs in collective bargaining; therefore, the ballot may contain several choices for the **bargaining agent.** To place its name on the ballot, a union needs to show that at least one person eligible to vote in the election has signed an authorization card requesting that this union be a choice in the election.

The election outcome is determined by the group receiving a simple majority of the votes cast. Thus, if 500 people are eligible for coverage by the contract but only 100 people vote and union A receives 51 votes, union A wins. If no group receives a simple majority on the first ballot, a runoff election is held between the top two vote recipients. The union winning this election is certified to enter into contract negotiations with the employer.

The process of selecting a bargaining agent produces a tense, emotional climate that affects everyone in the organization. It is important for both nurse managers and staff nurses to remember that during this period, the rules of unfair labor practice apply. Nurse managers must refrain from any action that could be seen as interfering with the employees' right to determine their collective-bargaining representative. Such actions include individually questioning staff nurses about their knowledge of collective-bargaining activities and making promises or threats to individual staff members based on the outcome of the election. Promising raises or promotions if the union is defeated or promising pay cuts and demotions if the union succeeds are examples of unfair practices. Staff nurses also must be careful that their discussions regarding collective bargaining take place away from the work site and not on work time.

Certifying the Contract

Certification by the NLRB of a union to be the bargaining agent does not automatically mean employees have a contract. It does mean that a group of people have the right to enter into a contract with an employer, a concept known as **certification to contract.** The actual contract and its provisions must be written and voted on by the union membership, a process that may take some time.

Issues considered mandatory subjects of bargaining are

1. Rates of pay,
2. Wages,
3. Hours of employment,
4. Conditions of employment, and
5. Grievance procedures.

In addition, the contract may specify other areas provided that both parties agree they should be included. These can include

1. Union security clause,
2. Management rights clause,
3. Seniority,
4. Fringe benefits,
5. Layoffs and reductions in work,
6. Floating procedures,
7. Insurance provided,
8. Retirement policies, and
9. Professional issues.

The contract is considered to be in effect when both management of the organization and employees agree on its content. The final agreement is subject to a ratification vote by the affected employees. Passage of the contract, or **ratification,** is obtained by a simple majority of eligible members who vote.

Administering the Contract

The role of administering the contract then falls to an individual designated as the union representative. This individual may be an employee of the union or a member of the nursing staff. It is the duty of the union representative to provide fair and equal representation to all members of the unit. The role of the union representative is to explain the provisions of the contract to the union membership and be available to help in the grievance process.

Decertifying the Contract

Occasionally, members of a particular unit may decide that the union they have chosen to represent them may not be the union they want or that no union at all is needed. In such a case, the members of the bargaining unit have the right to either change their union affiliation or remove the union by using a process known as **decertification.** This process is essentially the same as that followed by the NLRB for a representation election. Once again, an employee who is a member of the bargaining unit must submit to the NLRB signed documents showing that at least 30 percent of the bargaining unit membership request an election to remove a union as their representative. Then the NLRB will review the signatures for authenticity, set a date and time, and conduct an election by secret ballot. The winner is determined by a majority of the cast ballots. Once an election has been conducted, the NLRB will

---

KEY TERMS

Collective bargaining   Collective action taken by workers to secure better wages or working conditions.

Representation election   The process of establishing a union through the selection of a bargaining agent certified to conduct labor negotiations for a group of individuals.

Bargaining agent   A union certified by the NLRB to conduct labor negotiations for a group of individuals.

Certification to contract   A process by which a union, certified by the NLRB as a bargaining agent, can enter into a contract with an employer that has been voted on by the union membership.

Ratification   Passage of the contract by a simple majority vote of the union membership.

Decertification   The process of changing union affiliation or removing the union altogether.

not return to the same work site for a vote by the same group for a period of 1 year (National Labor Relations Act [NLRA], Sec 9[e]2).

The Nurse Manager's Role

The nurse manager in a health care organization where nurses are organized into a collective-bargaining unit needs to be aware of the five categories of unfair labor practices described by the NLRA:

1. Interference with the right to organize
2. Domination
3. Encouraging or discouraging union membership
4. Discharging an employee for giving testimony or filing a charge with the NLRB
5. Refusal to bargain collectively

Another responsibility of the nurse manager is to participate in resolving **grievances,** using the agreed-upon grievance procedure. Grievances can usually be classified as:

a. Contract violations,
b. Violations of federal or state law,
c. Failure of management to meet its responsibilities, and
d. Violation of agency rules.

Grievances may be caused by misunderstandings that usually stem from circumstances surrounding the grievance, a lack of familiarity with the contract, or an inadequate labor agreement.

The grievance procedure used will be negotiated and clearly described in the labor agreement. Most likely, it will contain a series of progressive steps and time limits for submission/resolution of grievances.

The Grievance Process

The typical grievance process follows these steps.

Step 1. The employee talks informally with her or his direct supervisor, usually as soon as possible after the incident has occurred. A representative of the bargaining agent is allowed to be present. If the grievance is not adjusted in the informal discussion, a written request for the next step is given to the immediate supervisor within 10 work days. A written response must be received within 5 work days. The employee, supervisor, and agent will be present for any discussion.

Step 2. If the response to step 1 is not satisfactory, a written appeal may be submitted within 10 work days to the director of nursing or her or his designee. The employee, agent, grievance chairperson, and the top nursing administrator or designee can be present for discussion. Again, written response will be provided in 5 work days subsequent to these meetings. In most bargaining units, the positions of agent and grievance chairperson are separated. Generally, the grievance chairperson is an officer in the bargaining unit.

Step 3. The employee, agent, grievance chairperson, nursing administrator, and director of human resources meet for discussions. The 10- and 5-day time limits for appeal and answer are again observed.

Step 4. This final step is arbitration, which is invoked when no solution suggested is acceptable. An arbitrator who is a neutral third party is selected and is present at these meetings. The submission of a grievance may be required within 15 days after step 3 is completed.

Often, a statement included in each of the steps states that if the time limits are not observed by one party, the grievance may be considered resolved and further action barred. The contract also usually specifies how an arbitrator is selected.

Here are some suggestions that may be helpful in handling grievances (Beletz, 1977):

1. The objective of the grievance procedure is not to achieve conquest. You have to work with one another after resolution of the grievance, so treat each other with courtesy and respect. Don't threaten or bluff. Don't withhold facts or information relating to the grievance.
2. Do not, whatever your position, allow disagreements or disputes among members of your team (e.g., management) to be public. Both the bargaining unit and the management team must present a solid front when faced with one another.
3. Expedience is a must; delaying tactics serve only to heighten emotions. However, allow time to consider all of the facts.
4. Stay objective. Emotionalism usually leads to further problems. If discussions escalate into angry exchanges, adjourn and reschedule later.
5. Implementing decisions or filing grievances requires planning. Get all the facts and information, witnesses, and documentation. Evaluate and anticipate the other party's position and possible response. Know the strengths and weaknesses of the issue for both sides. Find out whether any similar situations occurred and what decision was reached. Use all the resources available. Seek guidance from those higher in administrative positions.

6. Never refuse to meet with the grievant's representatives. The right to representation is one of the advantages of being under the auspices of a collective-bargaining unit.

7. The bargaining unit representative, though in a unique position, is not immune from reprimand or discipline. When not involved in bargaining unit activities, the agent is an employee who must observe the rules and regulations of the organization, and the employer has the right to a full day's work and an acceptable level of performance. However, while handling grievances, the employee/agent is not really considered an employee. She or he is considered the representative and advocate of the employee who filed the grievance.

8. Integral to bargaining are solutions that may also accommodate future changes and needs. Therefore, think ahead. Once a grievance is filed, a chain reaction may occur, and almost any imaginable outcome may end up as the solution. However, a carefully written grievance procedure should obviate this possibility.

9. Be prepared to give or take acceptable compromises and alternative solutions within the framework of the contract, no matter which party suggests them. Know your bottom line for compromise. Do not submit to emotional appeals as to what is fair. The contract is the sole determinant of what is fair; if necessary, a neutral third party will be called on to interpret the contract. What one person considers fair may not necessarily be seen in the same light by the other.

10. Pat formulas do not settle grievances or solve problems. A formula would negate the needed judgment and flexibility that are so necessary to grievance handling.

11. Observe the time limits. If you do not, the bargaining unit may lose the right to continue the grievance to the next level, or both the bargaining unit and management may lose in an eventual arbitration.

12. In adjusting a grievance, knowledge is very important. As with any interaction between people, your statement is colored by your temperament and is interpreted by the other party in accordance with his or her own temperament.

13. Gloating over a win is human, but remember that you may lose the next one; don't become overconfident. Similarly, don't blame the other side for taking advantage of your mistakes. Learn from them, and don't repeat them the next time.

The Grievance Hearing   In the grievance hearing, remember these key behaviors (Trotta, 1976):

1. Put the grievant at ease. Do not interrupt or disagree. Let the grievant have her or his say.

2. Listen openly and carefully. Search for what the employee is trying to say. Take notes.

3. Discuss the problem calmly and with an open mind. Avoid arguments, avoid antagonizing others, and avoid the urge to win. Negotiate.

4. Get the story straight. Get all the facts. Ask logical questions to clarify doubtful points. Distinguish fact from opinion.

5. Consider the grievant's viewpoint. Do not assume she or he is automatically wrong.

6. Avoid snap judgments. Do not jump to conclusions. But be willing to admit mistakes.

7. Make an equitable decision, then give it to the grievant promptly. Do not pass the buck.

Strikes   When an agreement cannot be reached through collective bargaining, employees usually **strike.** A strike is an organized stoppage of work by employees within the union. Striking is not commonly used by nurses. By law, a 10-day notice must be given to allow hospitals the opportunity to prepare for striking nurses' absences. Also, employers have the right to permanently replace striking employees.

Collective Bargaining for Nurses

To ensure the balance between the rights of employees and the rights of the public to health care, Congress passed a special set of dispute-settling procedures to be applied in the health care industry:

1. Before changing or terminating a contract, one party must notify the other of its intent to do so 90 days prior to the contract expiration date. This is 30 days more than specified for other industries.

2. If after 30 days of this notification both sides cannot agree, then the Federal Mediation and Conciliation Service (FMCS) must be notified.

KEY TERMS

Grievances   Formal expressions of complaints, generally classified as misunderstandings, contract violations, or an inadequate labor agreement.

Strike   The organized stoppage of work by employees within the union.

3. The FMCS will appoint either a mediator or an inquiry board within 30 days.
4. The mediator or board must make recommendations within 15 days.
5. If after 15 more days both sides cannot agree, then a strike vote can be conducted and a strike scheduled.

If a strike vote is affirmed, then a 10-day written notice must be given to management indicating the date, time, and place of the strike. This is to ensure that a hospital has adequate time to provide for continuity of patient care in the event of a strike.

To enforce these amendments, the NLRB established separate provisions for the health care industry. These provisions include

1. Recognition of appropriate bargaining units for health care employees so that the hospital would not have to conduct separate contract negotiations with many different unions. Registered nurses are a separate bargaining unit in health care.
2. Determination of locations where unions could solicit members and distribute literature in the hospital without disrupting patient care or interfering with work time. Currently, solicitation of members can occur in hospital cafeterias, gift shops, and main lobbies.

The Role of Professional Associations

Since its inception, the American Nurses Association (ANA) has had an active interest in the economic security of nurses. One of the purposes of ANA was "to promote the usefulness and honor, the financial and other interests of the nursing profession" (Flannigan, 1976, p. 169). Although this statement was useful in helping to shape the role of the profession in supporting collective bargaining for nurses, the ANA did not officially adopt an economic security program that included collective bargaining until 1946 (Flannigan, 1976). Since that time, the ANA has actively promoted collective bargaining for nurses through the Economic and General Welfare Program, which now is called the Department of Labor Relations and Work Place Advocacy.

The American Nurses Association is a registered labor organization, but it does not engage in direct collective bargaining. The actual certification of units, negotiation of contracts, and administration of contracts is conducted by the state nurses associations (SNAs). Although the ANA supports collective bargaining and takes an active role in promoting collective

bargaining, the SNAs have the freedom to independently decide their own level of participation regarding collective bargaining. All of the SNAs have a labor relations program as a part of their purpose and conduct programs to address the needs of the nurses in their state regarding financial and job security.

In 1999 the ANA House of Delegates changed its bylaws to create the United American Nurses (UAN) as the labor arm of the ANA. UAN held its first National Labor Assembly (NLA) in June 2000. Under the UAN bylaws, state nurses associations or their collective-bargaining units are members of the UAN, which is designed to provide national support to nurses' collective-bargaining efforts.

Complicating the collective-bargaining issue today are numerous other efforts to organize nurses. Established unions in a variety of fields (e.g., steelworkers, textile workers, food workers, UAW Teamsters, AFL/CIO) are attempting to recruit nurses. Employees of individual health care organizations are forming their own collective-bargaining organization and include nurses. So collective bargaining in nursing runs the gamut from national collaboration of state organizations to coordination with other employees in health care to individual units of nurses.

Future of Collective Bargaining

The use of collective bargaining as a way for nurses to influence the practice environment and to ensure their economic security holds both concerns and promises, especially with the radical changes occurring in health care today. The concerns are that the very processes of collective bargaining separate rather than unite nurses, notably between staff nurses and those in management. What the future holds for collective bargaining in nursing is uncertain and unknown.

What You Know Now

- Nurse dissatisfaction is often the impetus for establishing a union.
- The process of achieving unionization involves selecting a bargaining agent, developing a contract between the employer and the employees, and ratifying the contract.
- The contract specifies workplace policies and employee benefits, among other conditions.
- Disagreements between employees and employers are handled by a structured, formal arrangement known as the grievance process.

- A collective-bargaining unit can be decertified in much the same way it was originally certified.
- Certain conditions of labor law apply in health care to protect patients and the public.
- The American Nurses Association (through its state nurses associations and its recently established labor arm, the United American Nurses) provides collective-bargaining services to nurses, but the ANA is not the only union that represents nurses.
- The future of collective bargaining for nurses is uncertain and unknown.

Tools for Handling Collective-Bargaining Issues

1. Determine if your organization has a collective-bargaining arrangement with its registered nurse employees.
2. If so, become familiar with provisions of the policy and grievance procedures.
3. Contact administration for any questions you may have with contract policies.
4. If your organization does not have a union contract, be aware of the possibility that efforts to establish a collective-bargaining unit may be initiated.
5. If attempts are made to unionize your workplace, obtain information on the legal obligations you have as an employee and/or manager.
6. Remember, collective bargaining is an agreement between an employer and its employees; it does not need to be adversarial.

Questions to Challenge You

1. Are you a member of a collective-bargaining unit? Do you know anyone who is?
2. Have you been involved in union organizing? What happened during and after the process?

3. If you have not been involved in union organizing, find someone who has been and ask them what happened.
4. What is your opinion of unions for nurses? Name the pros and cons.
5. You are negotiating a union contract on behalf of the nurses. List your demands in priority order.
6. You are negotiating a union contract on behalf of administration. Respond to the demands on your list generated in question 5.

Explore 🌐 MediaLink

NCLEX review questions, essay activities, group activities, and other interactive resources for this chapter can be found on the Web site at http://www.prenhall.com/sullivan-decker. Click on "Chapter 24" to select activities for this chapter.

References

Beletz, E. (1977, August). Some pointers for grievance handlers. *Supervisory Nurse, 8,* 56.

Bilchik, G. S. (2000). Norma Rae, RN. *Hospitals and Health Networks, 74*(11), 40–44.

Flannigan, L. (1976). *One strong voice: The history of the American Nurses Association.* Kansas City, MO: American Nurses Association.

Friedrich, B. (2001). Staying power: Unions. *Nursing Management, 32*(7), 26–28.

Trotta, M. S. (1976). *Handling grievances: A guide for management and labor.* Washington, DC: Bureau of National Affairs.

Index

Page numbers in *italics* denote figures; those followed by *t* denote tables.